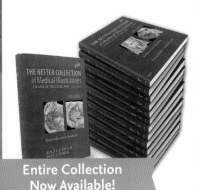
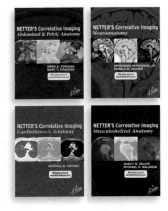

Netter's Concise Neurology – UPDATED EDITION

Karl E. Misulis, MD, PhD
Thomas C. Head, MD

Illustrations by Frank H. Netter, MD

Contributing Illustrators
John A. Craig, MD
Carlos A. G. Machado, MD

ELSEVIER

ELSEVIER

1600 John F. Kennedy Blvd.
Ste 1800
Philadelphia, PA 19103-2899

NETTER'S CONCISE NEUROLOGY – UPDATED EDITION ISBN: 978-0-323-48254-7

Notice

Knowledge and best practice in this field are constantly changing. As new research and experience broaden our knowledge, changes in practice, treatment and drug therapy may become necessary or appropriate. Readers are advised to check the most current information provided (i) on procedures featured or (ii) by the manufacturer of each product to be administered, to verify the recommended dose or formula, the method and duration of administration, and contraindications. It is the responsibility of the practitioner, relying on their own experience and knowledge of the patient, to make diagnoses, to determine dosages and the best treatment for each individual patient, and to take all appropriate safety precautions. To the fullest extent of the law, neither the Publisher nor the Authors assume any liability for any injury and/or damage to persons or property arising out of or related to any use of the material contained in this book.

The Publisher

Library of Congress Cataloging-in-Publication Data
Names: Misulis, Karl E., author. | Head, Thomas C. (Thomas Channing), 1963-
    author. | Netter, Frank H. (Frank Henry), 1906-1991, illustrator.
Title: Netter's concise neurology/Karl E. Misulis, Thomas C. Head ;
    illustrations by Frank H. Netter ; contributing illustrators, John A.
    Craig, Carlos A. G. Machado.
Other titles: Concise neurology
Description: Updated edition. | Philadelphia, PA : Elsevier, [2017] |
    Includes index.
Identifiers: LCCN 2016017028 | ISBN 9780323482547 (pbk. : alk. paper)
Subjects: | MESH: Nervous System Diseases—diagnosis | Neurologic
    Examination—methods | Nervous System Diseases—therapy | Handbooks
Classification: LCC RC355 | NLM WL 39 | DDC 616.8—dc23 LC record available at https://lccn.loc.gov/2016017028

Acquisitions Editor: Elyse O'Grady
Developmental Editor: Marybeth Thiel
Publishing Services Manager: Linda Van Pelt
Project Manager: Melanie Peirson Johnstone
Design Direction: Lou Forgione

Working together to grow
libraries in developing countries

www.elsevier.com | www.bookaid.org | www.sabre.org

ELSEVIER   BOOK AID
             International   Sabre Foundation

Printed in China
Last digit is the print number: 9 8 7 6 5 4 3 2 1

To our mentors:

Vivian Abrahams, Russell Durkovic, Gerald Fenichel, Wolf Dettbarn, Shin Oh, and to the memory of John Whitaker

Netter's Concise Neurology is the product of more than two years of composition. We wrote this book to provide a helpful aid to the evaluation and management of patients with neurologic conditions.

Neurologic diseases are often complex and there is often a broad differential diagnosis. Therefore, diagnosis must begin with a systematic evaluation. First, localize the lesion, then narrow the differential diagnosis. Likewise, management of neurologic disorders can be complex with multiple options and alternative approaches. Strict protocols will never be employed in neurology, as the field is too complex and fluid, but guidance on approaches to management are appropriate.

Netter's Concise Neurology is divided into sections which are in order of clinical encounter. The first section reviews the neurologic and medical examination with a discussion of clinical implications of findings. The second section describes an approach to specific complaints. The third section describes important neurologic disorders with information on diagnosis, management, and clinical course.

The information is organized as tabular text enhanced by the accompanying anatomical and clinical artwork of Frank H. Netter, MD. Dr. John Craig has contributed excellent new art to this work as well as adapting some existing art, along with Dr. Carlos Machado.

We hope this book will be a help to physicians in all stages of training and practice.

Karl E. Misulis and Thomas C. Head

Acknowledgments

The authors would like to express their appreciation to everyone who has been involved in this book. Special thanks are offered to Dr. John Craig for wonderful artwork and to the folks at Elsevier who have done so much for the editing, production, and promotion of the text.

The authors would also like to acknowledge those who have shaped our knowledge, practice style, and teaching style: teachers, colleagues, students, and friends.

Karl E. Misulis, MD, PhD is Clinical Professor of Neurology at Vanderbilt University and Neurologist at the Semmes-Murphey Clinic in Jackson, Tennessee. He received his BSc from Queen's University (Canada), MD from Vanderbilt University, and PhD from State University of New York Health Sciences Center at Syracuse. He is the author of 16 books and has contributed chapters to many others. Dr. Misulis lectures extensively to practicing physicians, medical students, residents, fellows, and patient groups. His lecture style derives, in part, from his experience as a stand-up comedian. He is the keyboardist for the charity rock band, *Hearts & Minds*.

Thomas C. Head, MD is Neurologist at the Semmes-Murphey Clinic in Jackson, Tennessee. A former student and faculty member at University of Alabama, Birmingham, he has extensive experience in general neurology and neuromuscular disease. Having taught at all levels of medicine, from medical students to practicing physicians, Dr. Head is a sought after speaker for his authoritative information and dynamic style. This is his second collaboration with Karl Misulis, having co-authored *Essentials of Clinical Neurophysiology* 3rd edition (Elsevier). He performs percussion and vocals for the charity rock band, *Hearts & Minds*.

Frank H. Netter was born in 1906, in New York City. He studied art at the Art Student's League and the National Academy of Design before entering medical school at New York University, where he received his MD degree in 1931. During his student years, Dr. Netter's notebook sketches attracted the attention of the medical faculty and other physicians, allowing him to augment his income by illustrating articles and textbooks. He continued illustrating as a sideline after establishing a surgical practice in 1933, but he ultimately opted to give up his practice in favor of a full-time commitment to art. After service in the United States Army during World War II, Dr. Netter began his long collaboration with the CIBA Pharmaceutical Company (now Novartis Pharmaceuticals). This 45-year partnership resulted in the production of the extraordinary collection of medical art so familiar to physicians and other medical professionals worldwide.

Icon Learning Systems acquired the Netter Collection in July 2000 and continued to update Dr. Netter's original paintings and to add newly commissioned paintings by artists trained in the style of Dr. Netter. In 2005, Elsevier, Inc. purchased the Netter Collection and all publications from Icon Learning Systems. There are now over 50 publications featuring the art of Dr. Netter available through Elsevier, Inc.

Dr. Netter's works are among the finest examples of the use of illustration in the teaching of medical concepts. The 13-book *Netter Collection of Medical Illustrations*, which includes the greater part of the more than 20,000 paintings created by Dr. Netter, became and remains one of the most famous medical works ever published. *The Netter Atlas of Human Anatomy*, first published in 1989, presents the anatomical paintings from the Netter Collection. Now translated into 16 languages, it is the anatomy atlas of choice among medical and health professions students the world over.

The Netter illustrations are appreciated not only for their aesthetic qualities, but, more importantly, for their intellectual content. As Dr. Netter wrote in 1949,". . . clarification of a subject is the aim and goal of illustration. No matter how beautifully painted, how delicately and subtly rendered a subject may be, it is of little value as a *medical illustration* if it does not serve to make clear some medical point." Dr. Netter's planning, conception, point of view, and approach are what inform his paintings and what make them so intellectually valuable.

Frank H. Netter, MD, physician and artist, died in 1991.

Table of Contents

Table of Contents

Table of Contents

7 DISORDERS—PAIN

8 DISORDERS—IMMUNE

9 DISORDERS—NEUROMUSCULAR

Table of Contents

⑩ DISORDERS—INFECTIONS

⑪ DISORDERS—TUMORS

⑫ DISORDERS—TOXIC/METABOLIC

Table of Contents

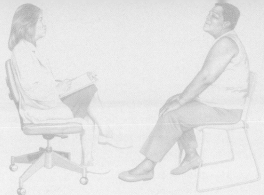

1 History

HISTORY	

Goals of the history	• Determine why the patient has come to the physician.
	• Characterize the presentation, including:
	  • Symptoms
	  • Duration
	  • Frequency
	  • Precipitating factors
	  • Alleviating factors
	  • Previous related problems
	  • Family history of similar or related problems
	• Determine the predisposing factors to the presentation.
	• Determine which parts of the exam require particular focus.

Components of the History	
COMPONENT	**IMPORTANT ELEMENTS**
Chief complaint	• It is the problem that causes presentation. • Usually stated in the patient's own words. • Other complaints may be described, which may or may not be related to the chief complaint.
Patient characteristics	• Age • Gender • Handedness

History of present illness	Regarding patient's symptoms, ask:
	  • How have they developed?
	  • How long have they have been present?
	  • How often do they occur, and how long do they last (if episodic)?
	  • What is the character of the symptoms?
	  • Where are they located?
	  • What factors worsen or improve them?

Past medical history	Ask about:
	  • Previous medical problems, regardless of whether they seem to be related to the chief complaint
	  • Specific problems that might be related to the patient's complaints

Past surgical history	Ask about:
	  • All past surgeries, even in childhood
	  • Any complications of past procedures

COMPONENT	IMPORTANT ELEMENTS
Medications and allergies	Ask about: · All current and previous medications · Allergic reactions and hypersensitivities to medications and/or certain foods. Allergies to contrast dye, which might be used in diagnostic testing
Review of systems	Detailed review should cover all systems, concentrating on those relevant to the complaints. One or more elements in each component of patient's history should be asked about: · General symptoms, well-being, and pain · Neurologic and psychological · Eyes, ears, nose, and mouth, including sight · Cardiac and vascular · Respiratory · Gastrointestinal · Genitourinary and breast · Musculoskeletal · Skin · Allergy and immunologic · Hematologic · Endocrine, including hormonal
Social history	· Marital status and/or sexual history · Occupation and occupational history · Habits, including tobacco, alcohol, and illicit drugs

Name:_____ **Age:**_____ **Sex:**_____ **Handedness:**_____
Date:_____
Referring clinician:_____
Chief complaint:_____
History of present illness:

_____
_____
_____
_____

Past medical history:

o Hypertension	o Stroke	o Immune disorders
o Diabetes	o Cancer/tumors	o Trauma
o Hyperlipidemia	o Arthritis/DJD	o Other:_____
o MI/CAD	o Infections	

Past surgical history:

o Cranial	o PPM	o Pulmonary
o Neurovascular	o Spine	o Other:_____
o Cardiovascular	o Orthopedic	
o Peripheral vascular	o Gastrointestinal	

Family history:

o Diabetes	o Cancer	o Arthritis
o Hypertension	o Stroke	o Other: _____
o Dementia	o Movement disorder	

Review of systems:

Constitutional
   o Fever/chills
   o Weight loss/gain
Visual
   o Vision loss
   o Double vision
Ear, nose, throat
   o Hearing loss/ringing
   o Allergies
Heart
   o Chest pain
   o Palpitations
   o Irregular heartbeat
   o Pacemaker
Lungs/Chest
   o Shortness of breath
   o Cough
   o Breast lumps/mass

Gastrointestinal
   o Abdominal pain
   o Constipation/diarrhea
   o Ulcers
Genital and urinary
   o Sexual dysfunction
   o Incontinence
Muscle and skeletal
   o Muscle pain
   o Cramps
   o Weakness
   o Arthritis
Blood
   o Anemia
   o Bleeding
Skin
   o Growths/moles
   o Bruising

Psychiatric
   o Depression
   o Anxiety
Neurologic
   o Memory loss/dementia
   o Ataxia – Gait/Limb
   o Headache
   o Limb pain
   o Weakness – Prox/Distal
   o Sensation – Loss/Pain
   o Sleep disturbance
Endocrine/hormonal
   o Diabetes
   o Adrenal
   o Thyroid
Other
   o _____
   o _____

Current and recent medicines, vitamins, supplements:

o _____	o _____	o _____
o _____	o _____	o _____
o _____	o _____	o _____
o _____	o _____	o _____
o _____	o _____	o _____

Medication allergies:

o _____	o _____	o _____

Habits:

o Tobacco	o Drugs	o Hobbies
o Alcohol	o Exercise	o Diet

| COMPONENTS OF MENTAL STATUS EXAMINATION ||
Exam Component	Method
Orientation	Ask patient to name: • Person (his own name) • Place • Time and date
Short-term memory	• Give patient three objects to remember and recall. • After 5 minutes, ask patient to recall the three objects again.
Remote memory	• Ask patient to recall events from his/her past. • Must be verifiable by the examiner • Patient's family can be of great help in this task
Constructions	• Ask patient to copy a figure. • Examples are intersecting pentagons or a three-dimensional wireframe cube. • The angles and intersecting points should all be correct.
Calculations	Simple calculations, such as making change, should be tested.
Naming	Ask patient to identify: • Others in the room • Common objects, such as a watch and comb
Conversation	• Routine office conversation reveals mental status, including intellectual function, organization, and mood. • Pay attention not only to what is said, but how the story is told.
Concentration	Ask patient to perform tasks: • Serial 7s: count backward from 100 by 7s for 5 iterations, to 65. • Backward spelling: spell the word "world," first forward, then backward. A second chance is given if needed.

| MENTAL STATUS EXAM INTERPRETATION ||
Finding	Possible Causes
Poor short-term memory	• Dementia from any cause • Encephalopathy, which produces an acute or subacute deficit • Frontal or temporal structural lesions
Aphasia	• Left hemisphere lesion with frontocentral location, producing expressive aphasia and/or temporal-parietal lesions, producing receptive difficulty • Degenerative dementia can present with aphasia.
Poor naming	• Dementia from any cause • Left central/posterior frontal lesion
Poor calculations	• Dementia from any cause • Encephalopathy of any cause • Left parietal lesion

Mental Status Examination *continued*

Finding	Possible Causes
Poor constructions	• Dementia, especially Alzheimer's disease • Right hemisphere lesion, especially in the central and parietal regions • Encephalopathy, which produces an acute or subacute deficit

Testing for Defects of Higher Cortical Function

A. Appearance and interpersonal behavior

Pleasant, neatly dressed, good spirits

Depressed, sloppily dressed, careless

Belligerent

B. Language

Good   Defective

Doctor : "Write me a brief paragraph about your work."

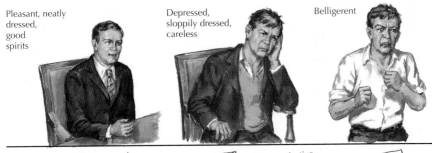

I have been an executive secretary to the vice president of the Zilch corporation for many years. My working conditions are satisfactory and I look forward to each day's business activity. I tend to many details for and supervise other ...

I don't mush much do it yestiday way busy day five aclock when no to go to a job when

C. Memory

Doctor: "Here are 3 objects: a pipe, a pen, and a picture of Abraham Lincoln. I want you to remember them, and in 5 minutes I will ask you what they were."

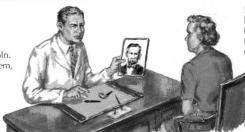

5 minutes later: Patient: "I'm sorry, I can't remember. Did you show me something?"

D. Constructional praxis and visual-spatial function

Doctor: "Draw me a simple picture of a house."

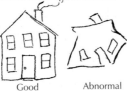

Good   Abnormal

"Draw a clock face for me."

Good   Abnormal

| COMPONENTS OF LANGUAGE EXAMINATION ||
Components	Methods
Spontaneous speech	Listen to the patient tell a story. This gives information on: • Reception/understanding questions • Expression while speaking • Searching for words/composing language • Mental status This is not a substitute for formal language and mental status testing.
Naming	Ask the patient to name common objects, such as a watch or comb.
Repetition	Ask the patient to repeat a short phrase, such as "No ifs, ands, or buts."
Reading	Ask the patient to read a short passage aloud. The accuracy of the reading and subsequent comprehension is assessed.
Writing	Ask the patient to write a brief passage, preferably spontaneous rather than from dictation.

| LANGUAGE ABNORMALITIES |||
Abnormality	Features	Implications
Anomia	Impaired naming of objects	Left hemisphere lesion, but generally of imprecise localizing implications. Can be seen in aging and dementia.
Expressive aphasia	Speech difficulty with preserved comprehension	Structural lesion in Broca's area, posterior aspect of left inferior frontal lobe
Receptive aphasia	Comprehension difficulty with preserved speech, although speech is devoid of complex content	Structural lesion in Wernicke's area, left superior temporal gyrus
Global aphasia	Inability to comprehend or express language in any form	Lesions of the left hemisphere, which affect both Broca's and Wernicke's areas
Conduction aphasia	Inability to repeat well	Left superior temporal or inferior parietal regions affecting the arcuate fasciculus, usually a structural lesion
Aphemia	Impaired speech without writing deficit	Structural lesion of Broca's area or subcortical white matter, usually a small lesion
Alexia without agraphia	Inability to read with preserved writing	Lesion of the projections from the occipital lobes to the left temporal-parietal region
Transcortical motor aphasia	Expressive difficulty with preserved repetition	Inferior frontal lobe, adjacent to Broca's area
Transcortical sensory aphasia	Comprehension difficulty with preserved repetition	Posterior temporal region, behind Wernicke's area

Dominant-Hemisphere Language Dysfunction

Clinical syndromes related to site of region

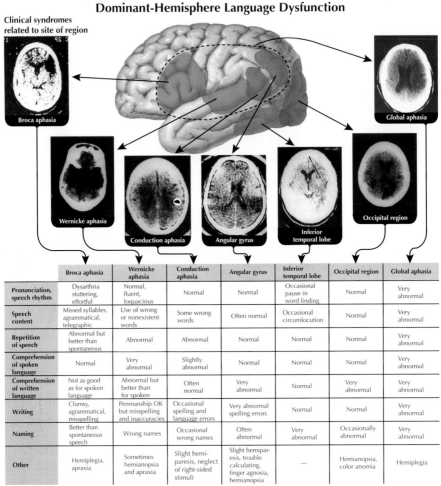

	Broca aphasia	Wernicke aphasia	Conduction aphasia	Angular gyrus	Inferior temporal lobe	Occipital region	Global aphasia
Pronunciation, speech rhythm	Dysarthria stuttering, effortful	Normal, fluent, loquacious	Normal	Normal	Occasional pause in word finding	Normal	Very abnormal
Speech content	Missed syllables, agrammatical, telegraphic	Use of wrong or nonexistent words	Some wrong words	Often normal	Occasional circumlocution	Normal	Very abnormal
Repetition of speech	Abnormal but better than spontaneous	Abnormal	Abnormal	Normal	Normal	Normal	Very abnormal
Comprehension of spoken language	Normal	Very abnormal	Slightly abnormal	Normal	Normal	Normal	Very abnormal
Comprehension of written language	Not as good as for spoken language	Abnormal but better than for spoken	Often normal	Very abnormal	Normal	Very abnormal	Very abnormal
Writing	Clumsy, agrammatical, misspelling	Penmanship OK but misspelling and inaccuracies	Occasional spelling and language errors	Very abnormal spelling errors	Normal	Normal	Very abnormal
Naming	Better than spontaneous speech	Wrong names	Occasional wrong names	Often abnormal	Very abnormal	Occasionally abnormal	Very abnormal
Other	Hemiplegia, apraxia	Sometimes hemianopsia and apraxia	Slight hemiparesis, neglect of right-sided stimuli	Very abnormal spelling errors	Slight hemiparesis, trouble calculating, finger agnosia, hemianopsia	—	Hemianopsia, color anomia	Hemiplegia

CRANIAL NERVE EXAMINATION	
Cranial nerve examination	• Eye movement examination studies multiple important cranial nerves. • Visual field testing more commonly detects an optic radiation abnormality than an optic nerve abnormality.

How much to test?	Minimal testing includes:
	   • Eye movement exam
	   • Pupil exam
	   • Facial movement assessment
	   • Visual fields
	   • Listening to speech during the history allows evaluation of oropharyngeal function.
	• Abnormalities on screening exam indicate a need for more detailed exam.
	• Olfaction is rarely tested, and is seldom a useful test.

What can be determined?	• Visual field defect, eye movement abnormality, or weakness of facial or oropharyngeal muscles can raise awareness and concern about local cranial nerve and brainstem pathology. • Differential diagnosis can be narrowed by clearly defining the deficit. • Comparing the cranial nerve defect with axial and appendicular deficits is crucial to anatomic localization.
What can be missed?	• Visual field defect is the most commonly missed finding on examination. • Hemianopia to extinction (simultaneous stimulation of both visual fields) is often missed, yet has important structural implications.

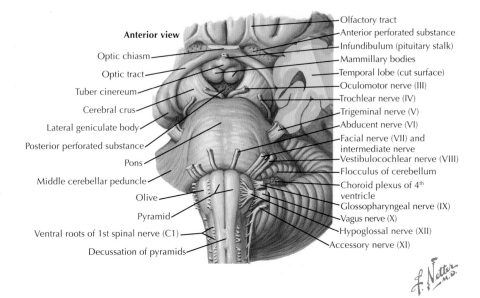

Anterior view

Optic chiasm

Optic tract

Tuber cinereum

Cerebral crus

Lateral geniculate body

Posterior perforated substance

Pons

Middle cerebellar peduncle

Olive

Pyramid

Ventral roots of 1st spinal nerve (C1)

Decussation of pyramids

Olfactory tract

Anterior perforated substance

Infundibulum (pituitary stalk)

Mammillary bodies

Temporal lobe (cut surface)

Oculomotor nerve (III)

Trochlear nerve (IV)

Trigeminal nerve (V)

Abducent nerve (VI)

Facial nerve (VII) and intermediate nerve

Vestibulocochlear nerve (VIII)

Flocculus of cerebellum

Choroid plexus of 4th ventricle

Glossopharyngeal nerve (IX)

Vagus nerve (X)

Hypoglossal nerve (XII)

Accessory nerve (XI)

CRANIAL NERVE I-XII FUNCTIONS		
Nerve	**Motor**	**Sensory**
Olfactory (CN-I)		Smell
Optic (CN-II)		Vision
Oculomotor (CN-III)	Eye movement—superior, inferior, and medial recti; inferior oblique; pupil and ciliary muscles	
Trochlear (CN-IV)	Eye movement—superior oblique muscle	
Trigeminal (CN-V)	Muscles of mastication	• Sensation of face in ophthalmic (V1), maxillary (V2), and mandibular (V3) distributions • Sinuses, external ear, and cornea are also supplied.
Abducens (CN-VI)	Eye movement—lateral gaze	
Facial (CN-VII)	Facial movement—grimace and forced eye closure	• Soft palate • Taste—anterior 2/3 of tongue
Vestibulocochlear (CN-VIII)		• Hearing • Position sense of the head in space • Rotation and acceleration
Glossopharyngeal (CN-IX)	• Pharyngeal muscles • Stylopharyngeus muscle	• Pharynx • Taste—posterior third of tongue
Vagus (CN-X)	• Pharynx • Larynx • Thoracic and abdominal viscera	• Pharynx • Larynx • External auditory canal • Thoracic and abdominal viscera
Accessory (CN-XI)	• Sternocleidomastoid and trapezius muscles • Some laryngeal muscles	
Hypoglossal (CN-XII)	• Tongue movement • Indirect innervation of the geniohyoid and infrahyoid muscles	

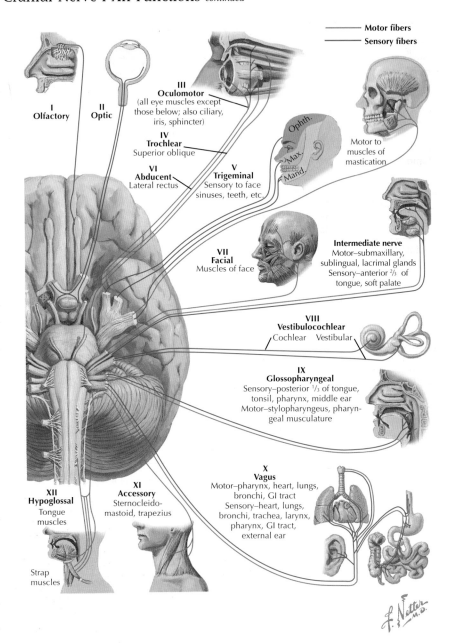

Motor fibers
Sensory fibers

I Olfactory

II Optic

III Oculomotor
(all eye muscles except those below; also ciliary, iris, sphincter)

IV Trochlear
Superior oblique

VI Abducent
Lateral rectus

V Trigeminal
Sensory to face sinuses, teeth, etc.

Ophth.

Max.

Mand.

Motor to muscles of mastication

VII Facial
Muscles of face

Intermediate nerve
Motor–submaxillary, sublingual, lacrimal glands
Sensory–anterior ⅔ of tongue, soft palate

VIII Vestibulocochlear
Cochlear   Vestibular

IX Glossopharyngeal
Sensory–posterior ⅓ of tongue, tonsil, pharynx, middle ear
Motor–stylopharyngeus, pharyngeal musculature

X Vagus
Motor–pharynx, heart, lungs, bronchi, GI tract
Sensory–heart, lungs, bronchi, trachea, larynx, pharynx, GI tract, external ear

XII Hypoglossal
Tongue muscles

Strap muscles

XI Accessory
Sternocleidomastoid, trapezius

CRANIAL NERVES I-XII FUNCTION TESTING		
Nerve	Motor Function Testing	Sensory Function Testing
Olfactory (CN-I)		• Smell of coffee grounds • Do not use mint (trigeminal irritant)
Optic (CN-II)		• Vision in each eye • Combine this with visual fields.
Oculomotor (CN-III)	• Eye movements of both eyes, vertically, horizontally, and both directions diagonally	
Trochlear (CN-IV)	• Tested as part of eye movement examination, looking down while eye is turned in	
Trigeminal (CN-V)	• Observation of chewing, although muscles of mastication are hard to examine	• Sensation in ophthalmic (V1), maxillary (V2) and mandibular (V3) distributions. • Corneal reflex: Lightly touch the outer edge of the cornea with a wisp of cotton. Watch for closure of both eyes.
Abducens (CN-VI)	• With testing of eye movements, abduction of the eye	
Facial (CN-VII)	• Smile • Eye closure, including corneal reflex • Observation of facial symmetry • Examine upper and lower facial movement	• Taste on each side of the tongue, usually using a sugar solution.
Vestibulocochlear (CN-VIII)		• Hearing in both ears • Weber's test: place tuning fork on the forehead, and ask where the patient hears the sound—midline or lateralized. • Rinne's test: place tuning fork on the mastoid, and when the sound abates, move the end of the fork to immediately outside of the pinna, comparing air versus bone conduction. • Baranay maneuvers (head position)
Glossopharyngeal (CN-IX)	*Cannot test these muscles*	• Gag reflex depends on glossopharyngeal nerve for afferent limb, although efferent is vagal.

Nerve	Motor Function Testing	Sensory Function Testing
Vagus (CN-X)	• Gag reflex, efferent limb	*Not routinely tested*
Accessory (CN-XI)	• Head turning with observation specifically of the sternocleidomastoid muscles	
Hypoglossal (CN-XII)	• Tongue protrusion	

Cranial Nerve Nuclei in Brainstem: Schema

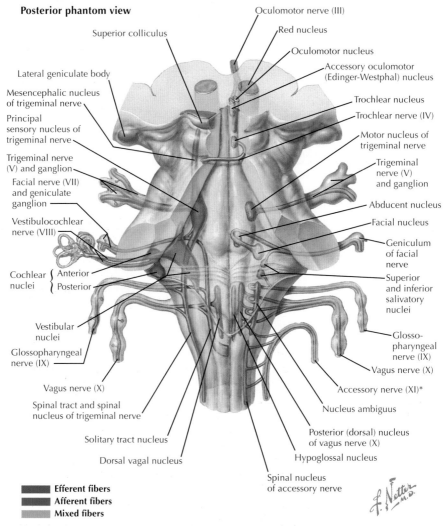

Posterior phantom view

Oculomotor nerve (III)
Superior colliculus
Red nucleus
Oculomotor nucleus
Accessory oculomotor (Edinger-Westphal) nucleus
Lateral geniculate body
Mesencephalic nucleus of trigeminal nerve
Trochlear nucleus
Principal sensory nucleus of trigeminal nerve
Trochlear nerve (IV)
Motor nucleus of trigeminal nerve
Trigeminal nerve (V) and ganglion
Trigeminal nerve (V) and ganglion
Facial nerve (VII) and geniculate ganglion
Abducent nucleus
Vestibulocochlear nerve (VIII)
Facial nucleus
Geniculum of facial nerve
Cochlear { Anterior / Posterior } nuclei
Superior and inferior salivatory nuclei
Vestibular nuclei
Glossopharyngeal nerve (IX)
Glosso-pharyngeal nerve (IX)
Vagus nerve (X)
Vagus nerve (X)
Accessory nerve (XI)*
Spinal tract and spinal nucleus of trigeminal nerve
Nucleus ambiguus
Solitary tract nucleus
Posterior (dorsal) nucleus of vagus nerve (X)
Dorsal vagal nucleus
Hypoglossal nucleus
Spinal nucleus of accessory nerve

■ Efferent fibers
■ Afferent fibers
■ Mixed fibers

*Recent evidence suggests that the accessory nerve lacks a cranial root and has no connection to the vagus nerve. Verification of this finding awaits further investigation.

| FINDINGS WITH LESIONS OF THE CRANIAL NERVES ||
Cranial Nerve	Clinical Findings and Diagnostic Implications
Olfactory (CN-I)	• Loss of smell • Smell disorders must be differentiated from loss of taste. • Most common after head injury, but also consider olfactory groove meningioma or sinus disease
Optic (CN-II)	• Loss of vision • Monocular loss suggests optic nerve lesion. • Hemianopia suggests optic radiation lesion behind the chiasm. • Incongruous deficits, from both eyes, suggest a lesion near the chiasm. • Common causes include nerve compression, optic neuritis, and multiple sclerosis.
Oculomotor (CN-III)	• Diplopia and often ptosis • Diplopia cannot be corrected by head tilt or looking to just one side. • There is a vertical component to the diplopia. • Common causes include compression in the midbrain and surrounding areas, cavernous sinus, or orbit. Nerve infarction can develop especially in diabetics.
Trochlear (CN-IV)	• Diplopia • External rotation of the affected eye, resulting in head tilt to the side opposite the lesion • Nerve may be damaged in the CSF or in the orbit.
Trigeminal (CN-V)	• Loss of sensation on one side of the face • May be lancinating pain with trigeminal neuralgia • Causes may be idiopathic, mass lesion in the cerebellopontine angle or cavernous sinus, or idiopathic.
Abducens (CN-VI)	• Diplopia, which is enhanced with gaze, toward the side of the lesion • Inability to abduct the eye, with compensatory nystagmus of the other eye • Affected by compression or infarction most likely in the CSF. Also, pontine infarction can produce CN-VI palsy, although with other signs.
Facial (CN-VII)	• Facial weakness on one side. Rarely, bilateral facial palsy can occur. • Loss of taste is often found, if the lesion is in the facial canal. • Facial nerve lesion affects upper and lower face, whereas cerebral lesions produce predominantly lower facial weakness. • Common causes include Bell's palsy or nerve compression at the cerebellopontine angle.

Cranial Nerve	Clinical Findings and Diagnostic Implications
Vestibulocochlear (CN-VIII)	• Hearing loss from damage to the acoustic branch • Vertigo, imbalance from damage to the vestibular branch • Tinnitus is common. • Common causes are acoustic neuroma, other cerebellopontine angle mass, trauma, toxins (e.g., some chemotherapies and antibiotics).
Glossopharyngeal (CN-IX)	• Glossopharyngeal neuralgia is the most common condition, which affects solely this nerve. This is neuropathic pain in the tonsillar area and ear. • Usually idiopathic. Can be due to tumor or vascular abnormality.
Vagus (CN-X)	• Unilateral paralysis of the soft palate, which is apparent with direct visualization • Unilateral paralysis of the vocal cord, which produces hoarse voice, but cannot be seen on routine exam
Accessory (CN-XI)	• Weakness of the ipsilateral sternocleidomastoid muscle, affecting head turning to the side opposite the lesion • Atrophy may be present and evident on exam. Usually seen with other cranial nerve deficits. • Extracranial compressive lesions can be the cause.
Hypoglossal (CN-XII)	• Ipsilateral weakness of the tongue • With protrusion, tongue deviates to the side of the lesion. • Oropharyngeal mass and destructive lesions can affect CN-XII.

COMPONENTS OF EYE MOVEMENT EXAMINATION	
Components of the exam	• Funduscopic exam • Eye movement exam • Visual field testing
Components	**Methods**
Funduscopic exam	• Examine the fundus of each eye. • Look for papilledema, hemorrhages, exudates, or signs of plaque.
Eye-movement exam	• Ask patient to look in all of the cardinal directions: lateral, medial, up, down, and diagonally up and down; left and right. • Defect in movement of either eye should be documented. • Look for nystagmus of either eye with movement.
Visual-field testing	• Measure visual acuity in each eye. • Test visual field of both eyes, medial and lateral hemifields, and superior and inferior quadrants of each hemifield. • Double simultaneous stimulation is more sensitive for optic tract and occipital lesions than pure visual perception.

COMMON EYE MOVEMENT ABNORMALITIES		
Exam Finding	**Anatomic Localization**	**Clinical Implications**
Impaired abduction of one eye	Abducens (CN-VI) palsy	Microvascular disease affecting the VITH nerve. Can be produced by increased intracranial pressure.
Defects in muscles supplied by more than one cranial nerve in both eyes	Defective neuromuscular transmission of the ocular muscles	Myasthenia. May be ocular myasthenia or ocular manifestation of systemic myasthenia.
Skew deviation—one eye is higher than the other	Brainstem or cerebellum	Indicates brainstem dysfunction rather than single ocular motor dysfunction
Reflexive eye movements are relatively preserved compared to command movements	Supranuclear palsy. Descending influences from the cerebrum to the brainstem are damaged.	Can be due to degenerative condition (e.g., progressive supranuclear palsy [PSP]) or extensive cerebral dysfunction
Gaze preference to one side	Hemisphere lesion on the side of the gaze or pontine lesion on the opposite side	Usually due to stroke
Oculomotor (CN-III) palsy, pupil sparing	Lesions of the oculomotor nerve, sparing pupillary axons on the periphery of the nerve bundle	Microvascular disease. Commonly seen in patients with diabetes and hypertension.

Exam Finding	Anatomic Localization	Clinical Implications
Oculomotor (CN-III) palsy, with pupillary dilation	Lesions of the oculomotor nerve affecting the pupillary axons, often compressive	Compressive lesions of the oculomotor nerve, including aneurysm and other mass lesions. Can be vascular.
Inability to adduct one eye	Internuclear ophthalmoplegia, lesion of the medial longitudinal fasciculus	Parenchymal brainstem lesions, especially multiple sclerosis and vascular disease.
Inability to look upward, dilated and nonreactive pupils	Parinaud's syndrome. Lesion of the midbrain.	Usually compressive lesions, such as a pineal tumor
Small pupil on one side with ptosis and anhydrosis	Horner's syndrome from damage to the sympathetic nerves	Ipsilateral brainstem, spinal cord, lower brachial plexus, or cervical sympathetic chain can be seen with carotid occlusive disease.
Horizontal nystagmus, unilateral	Brainstem or cerebellar lesions	Stroke or tumor is most common.
Vertical nystagmus, fast phase downward	Downbeat nystagmus indicates lesion at the craniocervical junction.	Tumors, Chiari malformation, and other craniocervical lesions

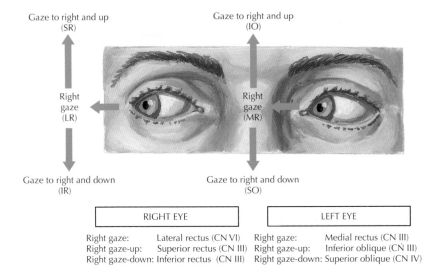

Gaze to right and up
(SR)

Gaze to right and up
(IO)

Right
gaze
(LR)

Right
gaze
(MR)

Gaze to right and down
(IR)

Gaze to right and down
(SO)

RIGHT EYE	LEFT EYE

Right gaze:	Lateral rectus (CN VI)	Right gaze:	Medial rectus (CN III)
Right gaze-up:	Superior rectus (CN III)	Right gaze-up:	Inferior oblique (CN III)
Right gaze-down:	Inferior rectus (CN III)	Right gaze-down:	Superior oblique (CN IV)

Gaze to left and up
(IO)

Gaze to left and up
(SR)

Left
gaze
(MR)

Left
gaze
(LR)

Gaze to left and down
(S.O.)

Gaze to left and down
(IR)

RIGHT EYE	LEFT EYE

Left gaze:	Medial rectus (CN III)	Left gaze:	Lateral rectus (CN VI)
Left gaze-up:	Inferior oblique (CN III)	Left gaze-up:	Superior rectus (CN III)
Left gaze-down:	Superior oblique (CN IV)	Left gaze-down:	Inferior rectus (CN IV)

Six cardinal positions of gaze place each eye in the field of action
of a single extraocular muscle, and allows testing of the action
of each muscle and its innervation.

JOHN A.CRAIG—AD

VISUAL FIELD DEFECTS	
Defect	**Localization**
Monocular visual loss	Optic nerve or retina lesion. Consider optic neuritis, optic nerve compression.
Hemifield defect affecting both eyes similarly	Contralateral optic radiations or occipital cortex. Can be stroke, tumor, or other structural lesion.
Hemifield defect affecting each eye differently	Optic chiasm lesion, usually compressive from tumor
Hemianopia affecting both eyes sparing the macula	Occipital lobe lesion sparing the pole, usually posterior cerebral artery infarction, because the macular region of the occipital pole is supplied by the middle cerebral artery
Superior quadrant defect in both eyes	Contralateral temporal lobe lesion, usually stroke or tumor, affecting Meyer's loop, the portion of the optic radiations that loops into the temporal lobe
Binasal hemianopia	Optic chiasm or perichiasmal lesion, usually from pituitary or other parasellar tumor
Bitemporal hemianopia	Optic chiasm lesion, especially pituitary tumor

Anatomy and Relations of Optic Chiasm

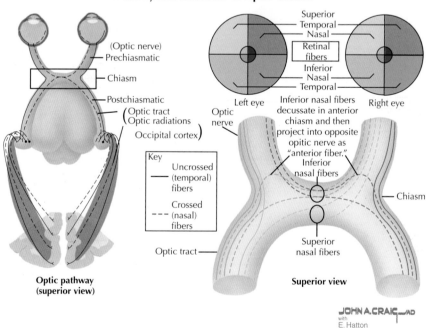

(Optic nerve) Prechiasmatic

Chiasm

Postchiasmatic
(Optic tract
Optic radiations
Occipital cortex)

Key
Uncrossed —— (temporal) fibers

Crossed --- (nasal) fibers

Optic tract

Optic pathway (superior view)

Superior
Temporal
Nasal
Retinal fibers
Inferior
Nasal
Temporal

Left eye   Right eye

Optic nerve

Inferior nasal fibers decussate in anterior chiasm and then project into opposite optic nerve as "anterior fiber."

Inferior nasal fibers

Chiasm

Superior nasal fibers

Superior view

JOHN A.CRAIG_AD
with
E. Hatton

COMPONENTS OF MOTOR EXAMINATION	

- Muscle tone
- Muscle strength
- Muscle consistency

Component	Method
Muscle tone	• Tested by moving the elbow joint, wrist, or knee and feeling for stiffness and resistance • Increased in patients with spasticity and in those with parkinsonism • Decreased in patients with acute causes of paralysis
Muscle strength	• Strength of representative muscles is tested, including muscles from each limb. • Both sides are tested for symmetry. • Typical testing protocol for the arm includes deltoid, biceps, and hand grip (long finger flexors). • Typical testing protocol for the leg includes tibialis anterior and quadriceps.
Muscle consistency	• Muscle consistency can be difficult to evaluate • Muscular dystrophies may produce fibrosis of the muscle.

INTERPRETATION OF THE MOTOR EXAMINATION	
Clinical Finding	Interpretation
Weakness with decreased tone	• Peripheral lesion that is producing weakness • Acute central lesions can also do this, with differentiation on the basis of acuteness and distribution of the lesion.
Weakness with increased tone	• Central lesion with corticospinal tract involvement. Pathological reflexes, such as extensor plantar response and accentuated tendon reflexes, are common.
Normal strength with increased muscle tone	• Fibrosing lesion of the muscle, such as with muscular dystrophy or repetitive intramuscular injections • Parkinsonism can produce increased tone with normal strength, although mobility and coordination are impaired. • Spasticity from corticospinal tract defect can occasionally produce increased tone with preserved strength.
Normal strength with decreased tone	• No clinical significance if there is no other deficit • Cerebellar lesions can produce impaired coordination, decreased tone, and normal strength.

Primary Sites of Motor Disorders

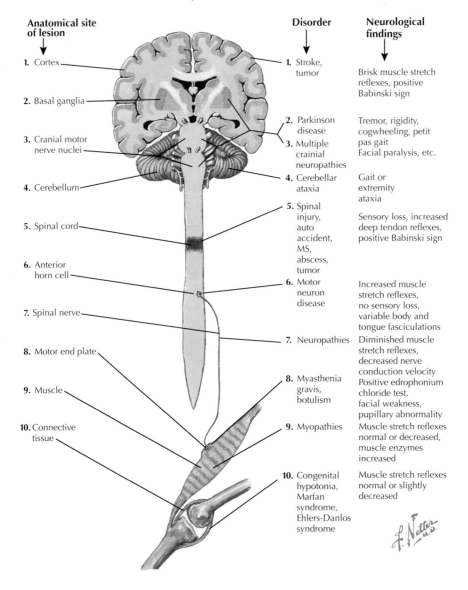

Anatomical site of lesion	Disorder	Neurological findings
1. Cortex	1. Stroke, tumor	Brisk muscle stretch reflexes, positive Babinski sign
2. Basal ganglia	2. Parkinson disease	Tremor, rigidity, cogwheeling, petit pas gait
3. Cranial motor nerve nuclei	3. Multiple crainial neuropathies	Facial paralysis, etc.
4. Cerebellum	4. Cerebellar ataxia	Gait or extremity ataxia
5. Spinal cord	5. Spinal injury, auto accident, MS, abscess, tumor	Sensory loss, increased deep tendon reflexes, positive Babinski sign
6. Anterior horn cell	6. Motor neuron disease	Increased muscle stretch reflexes, no sensory loss, variable body and tongue fasciculations
7. Spinal nerve	7. Neuropathies	Diminished muscle stretch reflexes, decreased nerve conduction velocity
8. Motor end plate	8. Myasthenia gravis, botulism	Positive edrophonium chloride test, facial weakness, pupillary abnormality
9. Muscle	9. Myopathies	Muscle stretch reflexes normal or decreased, muscle enzymes increased
10. Connective tissue	10. Congenital hypotonia, Marfan syndrome, Ehlers-Danlos syndrome	Muscle stretch reflexes normal or slightly decreased

MUSCLES TO TEST IN ROUTINE NEUROLOGIC EXAMINATION*			
Muscle	Action	Nerve	Root
Infraspinatus	External rotation of arm	Suprascapular	C5
Biceps	Flexion of forearm	Musculocutaneous	C5–6
Deltoid	Abduction of arm	Axillary	C5
Triceps	Extension of forearm	Radial	C7
Extensor digitorum	Extension of fingers	Posterior interosseous of radial	C7–8
Flexor digitorum	Grip	Median	C7–8
APB/opponens pollicis	Abducting thumb and touching tip to fifth finger	Median	C8–T1
Dorsal interossei	Spread fingers apart	Ulnar	C8
Iliopsoas	Flexion of thigh	Femoral	L2–3
Quadriceps	Extension of leg	Femoral	L3–4
Hamstring	Flexion of knee	Sciatic	S1
Gluteus medius	Abduction of thigh	Superior gluteal	L5
Gluteus maximus	Extension of thigh	Inferior gluteal	S1
Tibialis anterior	Dorsiflexion of foot	Deep peroneal	L5
Tibialis posterior	Inversion of foot	Tibial	L5
Peroneus longus	Eversion of foot	Superficial peroneal	L5, S1
Gastrocnemius	Plantar flexion of foot	Tibial	S1–2

*APB indicates abductor pollicis brevis.
From Jones, H: *Netter's Neurology,* Carlstadt, NJ: Icon Learning Systems, 2005.

Sensory Examination

SENSORY EXAMINATION	
Modality	Method
Touch	• Touch lightly with the unraveled end of a cotton swab or specialized von Frey hair.
Sharp sensation	• Touch with Neurotip or other single-use sharp device. • Differentiation of sharp from light touch is also assessed.
Position sense	• Move a joint while stabilizing the proximal bone. • Do not put pressure on the pad of the digit, which could otherwise suggest the direction of movement.
Vibration	• Touch vibrating tuning fork to the skin. • Testing of proximal and distal parts can be helpful.

INTERPRETATION OF SENSORY ABNORMALITIES	
Feature	Interpretation
SENSORY LOSS	
Cutaneous loss in a neural distribution	Peripheral nerve lesion, appropriate to the neurotome affected.
Cutaneous loss in a dermatomal distribution	Nerve root dysfunction, usually due to osteophyte, disc, or inflammation
Loss on one side of the body	Thalamic disorder or spinothalamic tract disorder
Loss at and below a spinal level	Spinothalamic tract at or above the respective level in the spinal cord
Facial sensory loss	Trigeminal nerve lesion
ALTERED SENSORY PERCEPTION	
Hyperpathia	Pain due to damage to the peripheral nerve. If on one side of the body, can be thalamic pain.
Sensory hallucinations	Cortical sensory disorder, occasionally seen after amputation
Paresthesias	Abnormal spontaneous sensation due to nerve damage, usually peripheral
Dysesthesias	Abnormal perception of evoked sensation, due to nerve damage, usually peripheral
Unilateral facial pain	Trigeminal neuralgia, occasionally due to vascular compression of the trigeminal nerve

Dermatomes

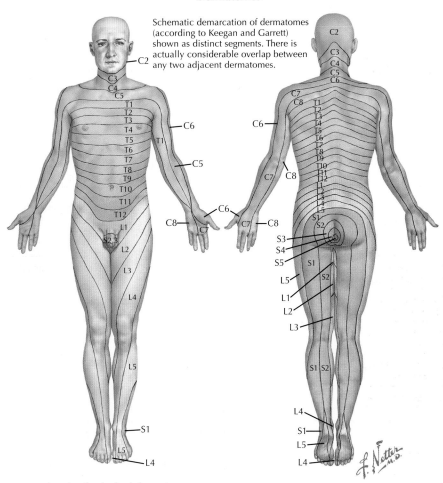

Schematic demarcation of dermatomes (according to Keegan and Garrett) shown as distinct segments. There is actually considerable overlap between any two adjacent dermatomes.

Levels of principal dermatomes

C5	Clavicles
C5, 6, 7	Lateral parts of upper limbs
C8, T1	Medial sides of upper limbs
C6	Thumb
C6, 7, 8	Hand
C8	Ring and little fingers
T4	Level of nipples
T10	Level of umbilicus
T12	Inguinal or groin regions
L1, 2, 3, 4	Anterior and inner surfaces of lower limbs
L4, 5, S1	Foot
L4	Medial side of great toe
S1, 2, L5	Posterior and outer surfaces of lower limbs
S1	Lateral margin of foot and little toe
S2, 3, 4	Perineum

Coordination Examination

COORDINATION EXAMINATION	
Modality	**Method**
Finger-nose-finger (FNF)	Finger moves between examiner's finger and patient's nose quickly, but carefully. Emphasis is on accuracy, not speed, although overly deliberate movements should not be made.
Heel-knee-shin (HKS)	Leg moves so that the heel runs carefully up and down the tibia.
Rapid alternating movements	Patient alternately slaps the front and back of the hand on the thigh.
Finger tapping	Patient taps index finger and thumb repeatedly. Remind patient to make good finger excursions.
Arm drift and movement	Arms are extended with palms up then the eyes closed. After stability is assessed, the patient is asked to touch the nose with each index finger.

IMPORTANT ABNORMALITIES ON COORDINATION EXAMINATION	
Abnormality	**Implications**
Wavering of the finger near the target on FNF testing	Cerebellar appendicular ataxia, usually due to a lesion of the cerebellar hemisphere on the side of the deficit.
Wavering of the heel on the shin on HKS testing	Cerebellar appendicular ataxia, with deficit affecting the cerebellar hemisphere on the side of the deficit.
Reduced excursion of the fingers on finger tapping	Extrapyramidal lesion. Most often seen in parkinsonism. In this case, the tapping is of reduced excursion yet rapid and slightly irregular.
Inaccurate and arrhythmic rapid alternating movements	Cerebellar dysfunction causes inability to easily make the alternating movements. Extrapyramidal and pyramidal can also affect this through stiffness and weakness, although the appearance differs from the arrhythmic action of cerebellar dysfunction.
Downward arm drift	Corticospinal tract dysfunction. Often has cupping of the palm and fingers and mild pronation of the hand.

IMPORTANT CAUSES OF COORDINATION DEFICITS	
Exam Finding	**Interpretation**
Essential tremor	• Tremor of the hands with movement and posture • No coordination deficit other than for the superimposed tremor
Parkinsonism	• Impaired finger tapping, with reduced excursions • Slowness and stiffness on coordination testing
Cerebellar ataxia	• Wavering on finger-nose-finger and heel-knee-shin testing • Normal or reduced tone
Chorea, athetosis	• Poorly-directed movements • Superimposed spontaneous writhing or jerky movements
Hemiballismus	• Involuntary flinging of an arm and/or leg on one side • Patient is able to move the limb and remains conscious during the episode.

Appendicular Ataxia

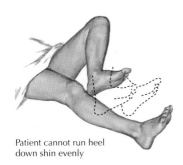

Patient cannot run heel down shin evenly

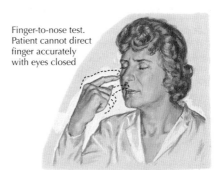

Finger-to-nose test. Patient cannot direct finger accurately with eyes closed

Gait Examination

GAIT EXAMINATION	
Modality	**Methods**
Stance	• Patient stands with narrow base, eyes open, and looking ahead. • Watch for wavering of stance.
Normal gait	• Patient walks linear distance and turns. • More than one lap is usually required for evaluation • Watch for wavering and side-step.
Tandem gait	• Patient walks heel-toe, as if on a tightrope. • Watch for side-step and inability to walk tandem.
Romberg testing	• Patient stands with eyes open, then closes eyes. Examiner pulls patient backward, off balance. • Watch for fall or side-step. • If the patient cannot stand with eyes open, this is not a positive response. Test is only positive if there is loss of posture after the eyes close.

INTERPRETATION OF GAIT EXAMINATION	
Clinical Finding	**Interpretation**
Positive Romberg, unable to stand when closes eyes	• Dorsal column abnormality, may be spinal cord.
Wide-based stance and broad-based, ataxic gait	• Cerebellar disorder • Occasionally seen with hydrocephalus
Stiff gait, narrow base, short steps	• Spasticity, suggesting corticospinal tract abnormality. • Unilateral suggests brain; bilateral suggests spinal lesion.
Narrow base, short steps, stooped posture	• Basal ganglia or frontal lobe lesion • Consider parkinsonism, frontal lobe ataxia

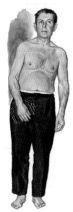

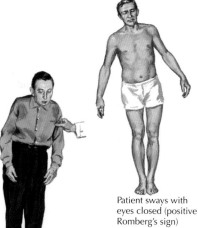

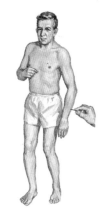

Unilateral involvement; blank facies; affected arm in semiflexed position with tremor; patient leans to unaffected side

Pronounced gait disturbances and moderate generalized disability; postural instability with tendency to fall

Patient sways with eyes closed (positive Romberg's sign)

Left hemiparesis with decreased arm swing sometimes associated with limited sensation secondary to a corticospinal tract lesion

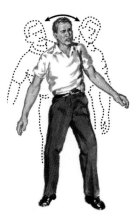

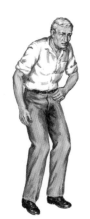

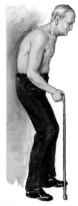

Wide-based gait of midline cerebellar tumor or other lesion

Apraxic gait of normal-pressure hydrocephalus

Patient with lumbar spinal stenosis with forward flexion gait

Reflex Examination

REFLEX EXAMINATION	
Modality	Methods
Tendon reflexes	• Stretch reflexes, elicited by tapping, to lengthen a muscle • Depressed reflex suggests a peripheral lesion. • Exaggerated reflex suggests a spinal or cerebral lesion.
Plantar reflex	• Prototypic sign of corticospinal tract function • Down-going plantar response is normal. • Up-going plantar response indicates a corticospinal tract lesion.
Release signs	• Normally absent in adults, but may be present in children • Sign of cerebral damage, although not of precise localizing value • Lesions of frontal lobes and basal ganglia are most likely cause of abnormal signs. • Components include: glabellar, palmomental, snout, and grasp.

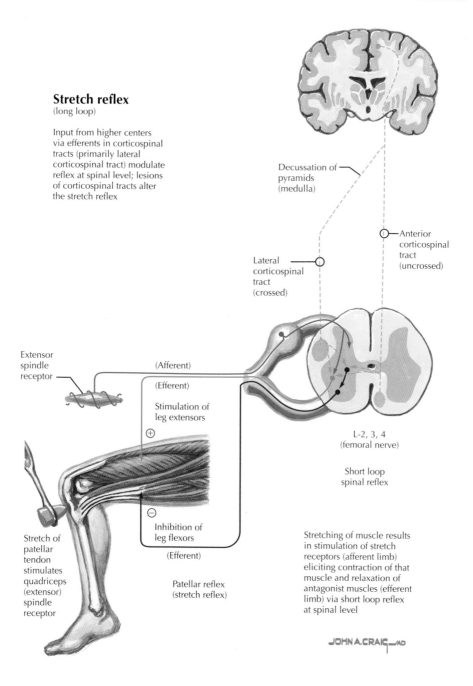

Stretch reflex
(long loop)

Input from higher centers via efferents in corticospinal tracts (primarily lateral corticospinal tract) modulate reflex at spinal level; lesions of corticospinal tracts alter the stretch reflex

Decussation of pyramids (medulla)

Anterior corticospinal tract (uncrossed)

Lateral corticospinal tract (crossed)

Extensor spindle receptor

(Afferent)

(Efferent)

Stimulation of leg extensors

⊕

L-2, 3, 4 (femoral nerve)

Short loop spinal reflex

⊖

Inhibition of leg flexors

(Efferent)

Stretch of patellar tendon stimulates quadriceps (extensor) spindle receptor

Patellar reflex (stretch reflex)

Stretching of muscle results in stimulation of stretch receptors (afferent limb) eliciting contraction of that muscle and relaxation of antagonist muscles (efferent limb) via short loop reflex at spinal level

JOHN A.CRAIG—MD

PHYSIOLOGY AND METHODS OF REFLEXES		
Reflex	**Anatomy**	**Method**
Biceps	Musculocutaneous nerve, C6 root	Tap your finger, which is on the biceps tendon, medial and superior to the antecubital fossa.
Triceps	Radial nerve, C7 root	Tap the triceps tendon just superior to the elbow, posteriorly, with the elbow bent, either on the lap or with the arm abducted and held by the examiner.
Brachioradialis	Radial nerve, C6 root	Tap on the radius and observe for pronation of the arm.
Patellar (knee)	Femoral nerve, lumbar plexus, L2–4 roots	Tap tendon below patella while patient is sitting with leg hanging without foot on floor.
Achilles	Sciatic, sacral plexus, S1 root	• Tap on the ankle tendon while the patient is sitting with the foot off of the floor. • Watch for contraction of the gastrocnemius with plantar flexion.

CLINICAL INTERPRETATION OF TENDON REFLEXES		
Reflex Abnormality	**Pathology**	**Disorders**
Individual reflex absence	Defect in the respective nerve root conduction	• Radiculopathy is the most common cause. • Mononeuropathy should also be considered.
Increased tendon reflex	Corticospinal tract lesion	• Stroke, tumors, head injuries, and other causes of focal cerebral and brainstem dysfunction
Achilles is absent.	Defect in the S1 nerve root loop to the spinal cord	• Bilateral loss common in peripheral neuropathy • Unilateral loss S1 radiculopathy
Decrease or absence of all reflexes	Defect in peripheral nerve roots or nerves	• Peripheral neuropathy • When subacute, suggests Guillain-Barré syndrome.

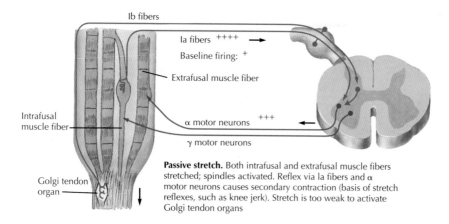

Ib fibers

Ia fibers ++++ →

Baseline firing: +

Extrafusal muscle fiber

Intrafusal muscle fiber

α motor neurons +++ ←

γ motor neurons

Golgi tendon organ

Passive stretch. Both intrafusal and extrafusal muscle fibers stretched; spindles activated. Reflex via Ia fibers and α motor neurons causes secondary contraction (basis of stretch reflexes, such as knee jerk). Stretch is too weak to activate Golgi tendon organs

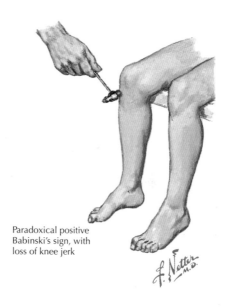

Paradoxical positive Babinski's sign, with loss of knee jerk

PHYSIOLOGY AND METHODS OF PATHOLOGIC REFLEXES		
Reflex	**Anatomy**	**Method**
Grasp	• Afferent: Palmar nerves to spinal cord and frontal lobes • Efferent: Descending corticospinal tract fibers to the arm, median, and ulnar nerves	• Stroke the palmar aspect of the hand with your fingers. • Watch for closure of the hand around your fingers. • A positive response may be merely curling of the fingers or forced closure of the hand.
Palmomental	• As above for grasp, but the efferent limb is the face through facial nerve (CN-VII).	• Stroke the palm of the hand, and watch for contraction of perioral muscles on the same side.
Snout	• Trigeminal nerve (CN-V) afferent to the brainstem	• Tap the skin between the upper lip and nose. • Watch for pursing of the lips.
Glabellar	• As above for snout, with efferent muscles differing by eye blink and afferent being V1	• Tap between the eyebrows, keeping the hand away from the line of sight. • Watch for eye blink that the patient cannot suppress.
Babinski	• Sole of the foot to spinal cord • Efferent is motoneurons of the leg, especially the extensor hallucis.	• Stroke the bottom of the foot from the midsole to the base of the toes. • Watch for upward movement of the great toe.

CLINICAL INTERPRETATION OF PATHOLOGIC REFLEXES		
Reflex Abnormality	**Pathology**	**Disorders**
Grasp, snout, and palmomental are present.	• Disorder of frontal lobe function	• Dementia • Frontal lobe structural lesions, e.g., tumors, hydrocephalus, and subdural hematoma
Glabellar is present.	• Abnormal cerebral subcortical reflex	• Parkinson's disease. When positive, glabellar is isolated. • Dementia or frontal lobe dysfunction, in combination with other pathologic reflexes
Babinski testing shows up-going plantar response.	• Corticospinal tract defect • Bilateral defect suggests spinal cord lesion • Unilateral defect suggests brain lesion	• Stroke, mass lesion, abscess, or any other lesion of brain corticospinal tracts • Spinal cord compression or infarction • Degenerative disease of the corticospinal tract, including amyotrophic lateral sclerosis (ALS) and primary lateral sclerosis (PLS)

Snout Reflex

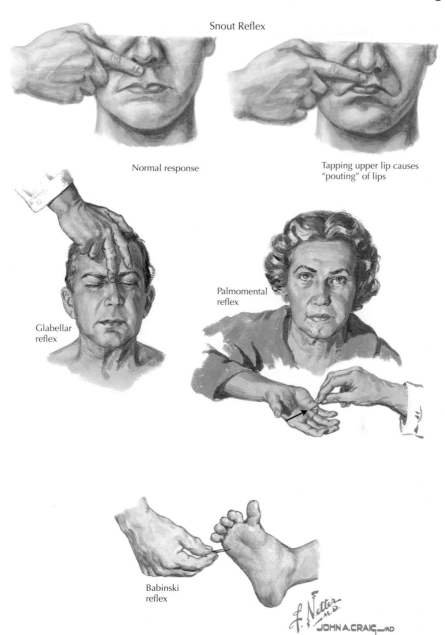

Normal response

Tapping upper lip causes "pouting" of lips

Glabellar reflex

Palmomental reflex

Babinski reflex

IMPORTANT ELEMENTS OF THE MEDICAL EXAM	
Element	Focus Points of Exam
Vascular	• Listen for carotid bruits. • Feel for peripheral pulses. • Observe for cyanosis and edema. • Examine temporal arteries.
Cardiac	• Listen for murmurs. • Listen for irregular rhythm.
Respiratory	• Listen for congestion and wheezes; assess ventilatory function.
Skin	• Look for rashes, ulcers, and dystrophic changes.
Skeletal	• Observe for scoliosis, kyphosis, and skeletal deformity, which may suggest a developmental or traumatic abnormality.

ABNORMALITIES OF THE MEDICAL EXAM	
Finding	Implications
Carotid bruit	• May indicate flow-limiting stenosis of the internal carotid artery • Bruits need further vascular evaluation, but may be benign, due to either insignificant stenosis or stenosis of the external carotid. • Absence of carotid bruit is not reassuring, so this finding is of interest only if present. High-grade stenosis may have insufficient flow to generate a bruit.
Absent or reduced peripheral pulse(s)	• Vascular insufficiency, which can suggest peripheral ischemic disease
Heart murmur	• Valvular disease, which may place patient at risk for stroke • Murmurs are often benign flow murmurs
Irregular rhythm	• May be atrial fibrillation which increases stroke risk
Tender, swollen temporal artery	• Temporal arteritis, which is especially examined in senior patients with headache and temporal pain
Tachypnea, and other signs of ventilatory insufficiency	• Wide differential diagnosis, which can include primary cardiac and respiratory causes • Can indicate neuromuscular failure, such as Guillain-Barre syndrome, myasthenia gravis, amyotrophic lateral sclerosis (ALS), or another paralyzing condition
Rash	• In a patient with weakness, it can suggest dermatomyositis. • In a patient with stroke, it can suggest vasculitis.
Scoliosis or kyphosis	• Can predispose to myelopathy, radiculopathy, or lesions of the cauda equina

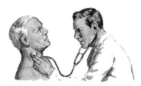

Auscultation

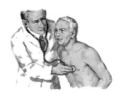

Cardiac

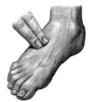

Pulses, color, temperature,
and skin status assessed

JOHN A.CRAIG—MD

D. Mascaro

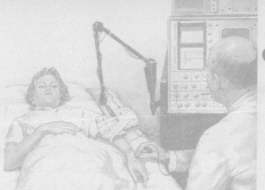

② Diagnosis

2 Approach to Diagnosis

APPROACH TO DIAGNOSIS	
Overview of diagnosis	• Obtain history to isolate the medical problems. • Use historical information to focus the examination. • Use the examination to localize the lesion. • Evaluate the mechanisms of disease. • Develop a list of possible diagnoses—the differential diagnosis. • Reach a provisional diagnosis. • Critically examine the diagnosis, test the possibilities. • Establish the diagnosis and begin subsequent management based on this conclusion, considering the possibility of other diagnoses possibilities.
Steps to Diagnosis	**Methods**
Localize the lesion	• With knowledge of anatomy, determine the location of the lesion. This greatly narrows the differential diagnosis. • A localization may be focal, multifocal, or diffuse.

Evaluate mechanisms of disease.	Consider the cardinal mechanisms of disease to arrive at a differential diagnosis:
	  • Degenerative
	  • Genetic
	  • Immune-mediated
	  • Infectious
	  • Metabolic/toxic
	  • Neoplasmic
	  • Trauma
	  • Vascular

Reach a differential diagnosis.	• Determine which diseases best fit the data. • List the differential diagnoses.
Critically examine the diagnosis.	• Perform tests to determine which diagnosis is the most likely on the basis of the data.
Post-diagnosis consideration	• Continue to reevaluate the diagnosis, considering other diagnostic possibilities throughout the patient's course.

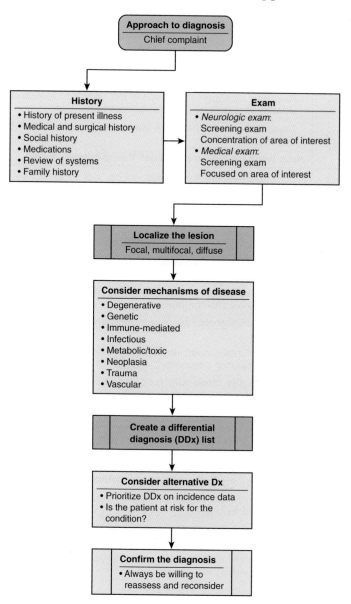

NEURODIAGNOSTIC TESTS FOR EVALUATION	
Description	• Neurodiagnostic tests are used for aids to diagnosis. Some are structural and some are functional. • *Structural tests* show interior anatomy. • *Functional tests* are an extension of the neurologic examination, showing metabolic or electrical function of the body. • Tissue and body fluid analyses are needed for diagnosis of some disorders. Note: Individual tests are discussed throughout this chapter.
Structural tests	• *Computed tomography (CT)* for patients with stroke, transient ischemic attack (TIA), head injury, possible subarachnoid hemorrhage, hydrocephalus, and other conditions • *Magnetic resonance imaging (MRI)* for numerous neurologic conditions with structural findings: stroke, tumor, infections, degenerative conditions, and immune abnormalities • *Magnetic resonance angiography (MRA)* for patients with stroke and TIA, or suspected aneurysm • *Magnetic resonance venography (MRV)* for patients with suspected intracranial venous thrombosis • *Catheter angiography* for patients with stroke and TIA, or suspected aneurysm • *Computed tomographic angiography (CTA)* for patients with stroke and TIA, or suspected aneurysm • *Carotid duplex sonography (CDS)* for patients with stroke and TIA • *Echocardiography (Echo)* for patients with stroke and TIA • *Myelography* for spinal cord lesions
Functional tests	• *Electroencephalography (EEG)* for seizures, encephalopathy, and brain death • *Nerve conduction study* (NCS) and *electromyography* (EMG) for neuropathy, myopathy, and neuromuscular transmission disorders • *Evoked potentials (EP)* for multiple sclerosis, acoustic neuroma, and spinal cord lesions • *Positron emission tomography (PET)* for degenerative diseases and brain tumors. PET of the body is performed for systemic neoplasms • *Single photon emission computed tomography (SPECT)* for degenerative diseases such as Alzheimer's disease
Tissue and body fluid analysis	• *Blood and urine* for a variety of tests • *Muscle biopsy* for possible myopathy, especially muscular dystrophies, metabolic myopathies, and inflammatory myopathies • *Nerve biopsy* for possible neuropathy, especially inflammatory neuropathies • *Lumbar puncture (LP)* for CSF analysis for infection, tumor, and demyelinating disease

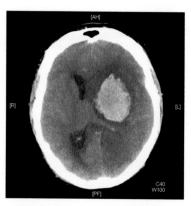

Computerized tomography (CT) of the brain showing a large intraparenchymal hematoma

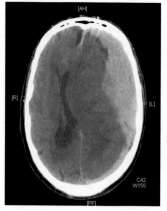

CT of the brain showing large subdural hematoma

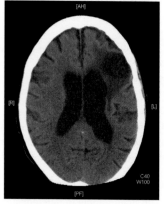

CT of the brain showing remote infarction in the left frontal region

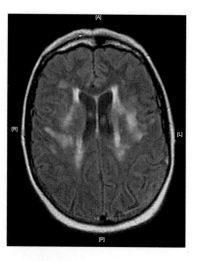

Magnetic resonance imaging (MRI) showing extensive white matter ischemic disease

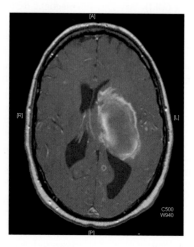

MRI with gadolinium enhancement showing large neoplasm

BRAIN AND SPINE IMAGING: CT, MRI, SPECT, PET

Imaging is a prominent part of the diagnostic armamentarium. Many recent advances have concentrated on brain and spine imaging.

Diagnostic modalities include:

- CT
- MRI
- SPECT
- PET

Individual Modalities	Features
Computed tomography (CT)	• X-rays are transmitted through the body and picked up by a detector array. The data are reformatted to produce a series of stacked, two dimensional (2-D) images. 3-D reconstruction can be performed with limited resolution.
	• Performed in the emergency department for evaluation of a number of conditions that present with acute neurologic deficit
	• Can be performed on patients with implanted electronic devices.
	• It is more sensitive than MRI for detection of subarachnoid hemorrhage, but less sensitive for detection of acute infarction.
	• High-speed, high-resolution contrasted CT can be used to visualize vessels (CT angiography).
Magnetic resonance imaging (MRI)	• Radiofrequency pulses are delivered in the setting of a powerful magnetic field. Signals detected from this are reconstructed into images of the body in almost any plane.
	• It is the most sensitive imaging modality for acute stroke, demyelinating disease, tumor, and infection.
	• Cannot be done well on uncooperative patients, because motion degrades the images more than with CT
	• Cannot be performed on patients with most implanted devices, including deep brain stimulators, permanent pacemakers, and implanted defibrillators. Some prosthetic heart valves preclude MRI, but not all.
	• Can be used to visualize vessels
Single photon emission computed tomography (SPECT)	• Uses metabolism of radioactive elements to show regions of hypo- and hypermetabolism
	• Patients with vascular and degenerative process may have no specific abnormalities on CT and MRI, yet show regional hypometabolism on SPECT.
Positron emission tomography (PET)	• Uses radioisotopes to evaluate cellular metabolism
	• *Brain PET* can show a typical pattern for Alzheimer's disease, although the PET is not always abnormal, especially early in the course.
	• *Body PET* is performed to look for systemic neoplasm.
	• Can be used for patients with brain tumors to differentiate recurrent tumor from radiation necrosis

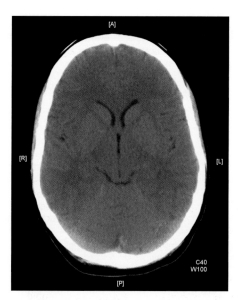

CT of the brain, normal

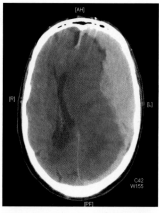

CT scan showing large subdural hematoma

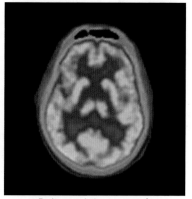

Positron emission tomography (PET) of the brain, normal

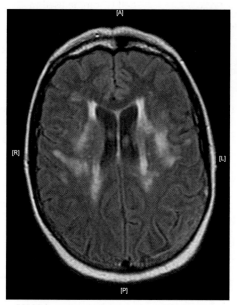

MRI of the brain, FLAIR imaging, showing extensive white matter lesions

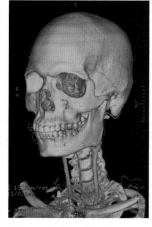

3-D reconstruction from CT, normal

VASCULAR IMAGING: CATHETER ANGIOGRAPHY, CDS, TTE, TEE, MRA, MRV, CTA
Vascular imaging is performed in a variety of ways for identification of arterial and venous anatomy of patients. The indications differ slightly between techniques. Imaging modalities include: · Catheter angiography · CDS · TTE · TEE · MRA · MRV · CTA

Catheter Angiography	
Description	An invasive technique that involves intra-arterial injection of iodinated contrast while rapidly imaging the vessels
Indications	Includes patients with infarction or hemorrhage who are considered for surgical or endovascular intervention. CTA can give much of the same information, but conventional catheter angiography is still considered the gold-standard for evaluation of the cerebral vasculature.
Contraindications	Includes anticoagulation, renal failure, and hypersensitivity to iodinated contrast, although these problems can usually be circumvented.
Interpretation	May reveal any of numerous abnormalities, including arterial occlusion, vascular malformation, aneurysm, dissection. Venous abnormalities can also show on the angiography.

Carotid Duplex Sonography (CDS)	
Description	The use of ultrasound to visualize much of the extracranial carotid vascular system. Parts of the vertebral system may also be seen on CDS, although this is not the main purpose of this technique.
Indications	Includes stroke, TIA, and suspected carotid artery dissection. The CDS should be considered to be a screening test, with significant findings re-evaluated by MRA, CTA, or catheter angiography.
Contraindications	None; catheter in neck may make performance difficult.
Interpretation	Can show occlusion, stenosis, ulcerated plaque, or dissection of the carotid artery. Thickness of the neck, patient movement, or even heavy calcification of the walls of the arteries can easily degrade images. Therefore, nondiagnostic study reports are occasionally generated, and restudy with one of the other modalities should be considered.

Transthoracic Echocardiogram (TTE)	
Description	Echo comes in two forms, transthoracic and transesophageal. TTE is performed by use of an ultrasonic emitter and transducer running over the surface of the chest.
Indications	Includes stroke, which might be due to cardiac emboli, suspected heart failure, or suspected valvular abnormality. TTE can assess right-to-left shunt with a bubble study, though this is better assessed by TEE.
Contraindications	None

VASCULAR IMAGING: CATHETER ANGIOGRAPHY, CDS, TTE, TEE, MRA, MRV, CTA–cont'd	
Interpretations	Can show regions of the heart that would predispose to stroke, including valvular disease, akinetic myocardium often with associated mural thrombus, increased left atrial size, reduced ejection fraction, cardiac aneurysm, or right-to-left shunt.

Transesophageal Echocardiogram (TEE)

Description	Performed for selected patients for identification of sources of cardiac emboli. An ultrasound emitter and a transducer module are part of a tube inserted down the esophagus. This method allows better visualization, especially of posterior aspects of the heart and in patients in whom the chest wall has interfered with adequate visualization on TTE.
Indications	Includes suspected cardiac emboli with the absence of source identified on routine testing
Contraindications	Few, but would include instability of the patient for sedation and insertion of the esophageal probe or inability to swallow
Interpretation	Can reveal akinetic myocardium, dilated atrium, ventricular aneurysm, valvular abnormality, or septal defect predisposing to right-to-left shunt

Magnetic Resonance Angiography (MRA)

Description	A noninvasive technique to visualize the arterial structure. MRI uses a magnetic field to image the brain and vessels. The arteries can be visualized without injection of contrast material, although intravenous magnetic contrast results in improved visualization.
	Used mainly as a screening test for vascular pathology. If there are lesions that might need surgery or which are not adequately seen on MRA, then CTA or catheter angiography is performed.
Indications	Stroke, TIA, hemorrhage, or suspicion of aneurysm
Contraindications	Pacemaker or other implanted electronic device, metallic valve, or other object that could place the patient at risk if there should be movement in response to the magnetic field.
Interpretation	Computer viewing of the images. Serial 3-D reconstructs of the arteries can be manipulated on display to give an excellent 3-D visualization of the vessels.

Magnetic Resonance Venography (MRV)

Description	Use of the MRI to show the venous structures of the brain. This is not routinely performed during MRA, so this study has to be specifically requested.
Indications	Suspected venous thrombosis or other venous outflow obstruction
Contraindications	The same as for MRI, including pacemaker or other implanted electronic device or metallic heart valve.
Interpretation	Best viewed on a computer monitor, which allows for 3-D reconstructions of the venous system to be visualized

VASCULAR IMAGING: CATHETER ANGIOGRAPHY, CDS, TTE, TEE, MRA, MRV, CTA–cont'd	
Computed Tomographic Angiography (CTA)	
Description	A noninvasive technique that involves injection of iodinated contract intravenously and performance of a high-resolution, high-speed CT. The vessels are imaged, and computerized reconstruction generates a 3-D view of the vessels. Both arteries and veins can be visualized.
Indications	Infarction and hemorrhage. Patients who are considered for surgery can often use CTA as the definitive imaging modality for the vessels. Patients with subarachnoid hemorrhage may have all but the smallest aneurysms visualized by CTA.
Contraindications	Allergy to contrast media and renal failure, although allergy can be circumvented in most patients if the study absolutely needs to be done
Interpretation	Facilitated by direct viewing on the computer; viewing on film degrades the 3-D view and impairs interpretation. Areas of narrowing, plaque formation, aneurysmal dilatation, and occlusion are visualized on CTA.

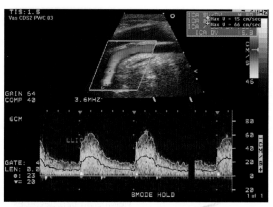

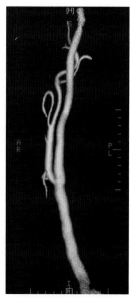

Carotid duplex sonography (CDS) showing normal flow in the internal carotid artery

CT angiography (CTA) of the carotid artery with bifurcation, mild disease

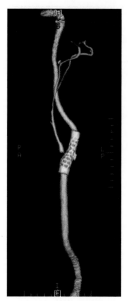

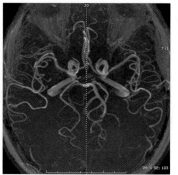

Magnetic resonance angiography (MRA) of the brain, projection from above, normal

CTA of the carotid artery with a stent in place

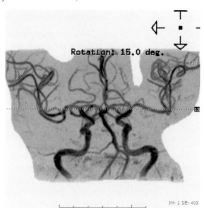

MRA of the brain, projection from the rear, normal (inversed values on image)

CLINICAL NEUROPHYSIOLOGY: EEG, NCS AND EMG, EP	
Neurophysiologic tests are a useful adjunct to examination for identification, localization, and characterization of neurologic lesions of the central and peripheral nervous system.	
Electroencephalography (EEG)	
Description	A recording of the electrical activity from the cerebral cortex. A routine EEG is performed using scalp leads, making this a noninvasive test. Epileptologists use invasive electrodes for presurgical monitoring and mapping of an epileptogenic focus.
Indications	• Includes suspected seizures, encephalopathy due to infection, hypoxia, and in some cases of dementia • With suspected infection, EEG can help to distinguish herpes simplex encephalitis from other causes. • With dementia, EEG can show patterns suggestive of metabolic derangement, prion disease, or other encephalopathy. • With hypoxic encephalopathy, the EEG can look for seizure activity and give some prognostic information.
Contraindications	Only skin lesions affecting the scalp, which would increase the risk for infection with electrode placement.
Interpretation	Can reveal ictal or interictal seizure activity, slowing suggestive of encephalopathy, focal abnormalities suggestive of a structural lesion, or one of a number of specific abnormalities that suggest specific diagnoses
Nerve Conduction Studies (NCS) and Electromyography (EMG)	
Description	• The recording of the velocity and amplitude of the compound action potentials of the sensory and motor nerves. Multiple nerves can be tested; while most nerves are mixed sensory and motor nerves, recording from a muscle means that the entire response is motor, and recording from a digit means that the entire response is sensory. • EMG is the recording of electrical activity from the muscles. A needle contains a small electrode that records the extracellular potentials from the muscle. Therefore, the EMG makes a statement about the motor axons, but does not assess sensory axons. • NCS and EMG are partnered for evaluation of the patient, and the specific subtest routines are determined by the examiner, usually a physician specializing in neurology.
Indications	Suspected peripheral neuropathy, myopathy, or neuromuscular transmission defect
Contraindications	Contraindications for NCS are few, although care has to be exercised if the patient has some stimulators that might be affected by the electrical nerve stimulation. Patients with burns or other extensive skin lesions may not be candidates to have skin electrodes placed.
Interpretation	May reveal mononeuropathy, polyneuropathy, mononeuropathy multiplex, myopathy, or neuromuscular transmission abnormality. Among the transmission defects, special studies are often able to suggest myasthenia versus botulism versus Lambert-Eaton myasthenic syndrome.

CLINICAL NEUROPHYSIOLOGY: EEG, NCS AND EMG, EP–cont'd	
Evoked Potentials (EP)	
Description	The responses from the body, usually to sensory stimuli. Motor evoked potentials can also be studied, but are not in routine use. Sensory modalities include visual, auditory, and somatosensory. The products are the visual evoked potential (VEP), brainstem auditory evoked potential (BAEP), and somatosensory evoked potential (SSEP).
Indications	Includes: • Suspected multiple sclerosis, where all modalities can be used to look for clinically silent lesions. • BAEP is used for premature infants as a measure of brainstem maturity. • SSEPs are used for evaluation of spinal cord function in patients before or during spine surgery.
Contraindications	Essentially none. Skin lesions that would prohibit placement of the electrodes are uncommon, but would interfere with the test.
Interpretation	May indicate conduction deficits, which would indicate a functional correlate to structural imaging showing a lesion

Electrodiagnostic Studies in Compression Neuropathy

Electromyography (EMG)

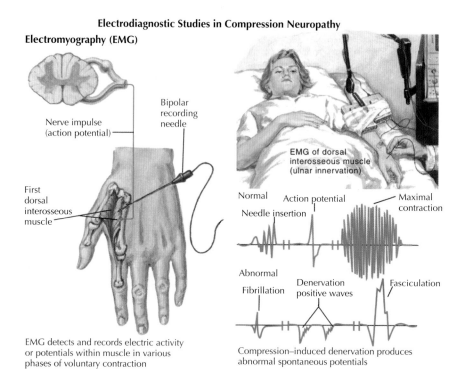

Nerve impulse
(action potential)

Bipolar
recording
needle

First
dorsal
interosseous
muscle

EMG of dorsal
interosseous muscle
(ulnar innervation)

Normal   Action potential   Maximal contraction

Needle insertion

Abnormal

Fibrillation   Denervation positive waves   Fasciculation

EMG detects and records electric activity
or potentials within muscle in various
phases of voluntary contraction

Compression–induced denervation produces
abnormal spontaneous potentials

Nerve conduction studies

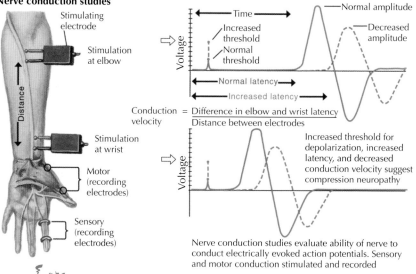

Stimulating
electrode

Stimulation
at elbow

Distance

Normal amplitude

Time

Increased
threshold

Decreased
amplitude

Normal
threshold

Voltage

Normal latency

Increased latency

$$\text{Conduction velocity} = \frac{\text{Difference in elbow and wrist latency}}{\text{Distance between electrodes}}$$

Stimulation
at wrist

Motor
(recording
electrodes)

Voltage

Increased threshold for
depolarization, increased
latency, and decreased
conduction velocity suggest
compression neuropathy

Sensory
(recording
electrodes)

Nerve conduction studies evaluate ability of nerve to
conduct electrically evoked action potentials. Sensory
and motor conduction stimulated and recorded

JOHN A. CRAIG—AD

Mechanisms of Electroencephalography (EEG)

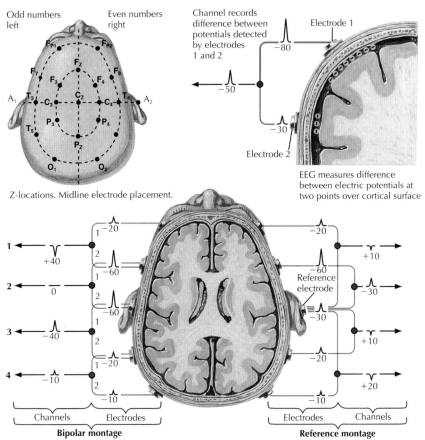

Odd numbers left   Even numbers right

Channel records difference between potentials detected by electrodes 1 and 2

Electrode 1

−80

−50

−30

Electrode 2

Z-locations. Midline electrode placement.

EEG measures difference between electric potentials at two points over cortical surface

Bipolar montage

Channels | Electrodes

Arranged as overlapping chain with adjacent channels (derivations) sharing common electrode. Recording reflects relative gradient between adjacent electrodes. Note phase reversal between channels 1 and 3

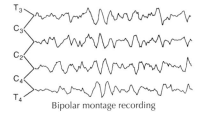

Bipolar montage recording

Reference montage

Electrodes | Channels

All channels share common reference electrode. Channel recordings reflect relative gradient between active electrode and reference. Reference electrode involved in electrical field

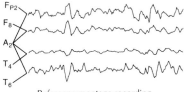

Reference montage recording

JOHN A.CRAIG—AD

LUMBAR PUNCTURE (LP)	
Description	A sampling of the CSF by placing a needle into the spinal sac
Indications	• Indicated for evaluation of suspected meningitis and encephalitis • Used to measure and reduce CSF pressure in patients with pseudotumor cerebri • Performed for injection of isotope or dye for performance of cisternography and myelography, respectively
Contraindications	• Cerebral mass lesion places the patient at increased risk for downward herniation. • Spinal mass lesion places the patient at increased risk for spinal cord damage from LP, although myelography can be helpful for identification and characterization of spinal mass lesions. • Hydrocephalus places the patient at increased risk for herniation. • Anticoagulation places the patient at increase risk for spinal epidural hematoma.
Methods	• Should only be performed by someone trained and experienced in this technique • The lower lumbar spine is cleaned and prepared in sterile fashion. Local anesthetic is often injected under the skin. Then, a spinal needle is inserted between the spinous processes, into the spinal sac. • CSF pressure is often measured, and this is especially important if pseudotumor cerebri is considered. CSF is collected, with usually 10–20 mL withdrawn. If the purpose of the LP is to reduce CSF pressure, more CSF may be removed.
Interpretation	• CSF analysis is routinely performed for cell count and differential, glucose, and protein. • When infection is considered, bacterial, mycobacterial, and fungal smears and cultures are performed. Cryptococcal antigen is performed for identification of cryptococcal meningitis. CSF-VDRL is performed for identification of syphilis. Herpes Simplex Virus assay and West Nile Virus assay are often performed if encephalitis is suspected. • Cytology is performed when neoplastic cells are suspected in the CSF. • Additional special testing is available, depending on the condition.

Cerebrospinal fluid

Patient with subarachnoid hemmorhage

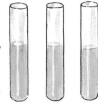

Three successive
fluid samples
collected. Shortly
after or during
bleeding, all 3
samples frankly
bloody or orange

Later, on repeat tap,
all 3 samples
are xanthochromic
(yellow) as a result
of hemoglobin
release or bilirubin
formation

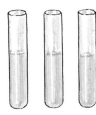

If blood is due to
traumatic tap, fluid
clears progressively
in successive samples

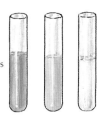

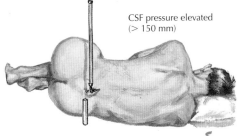

CSF pressure elevated
(> 150 mm)

CLASSIFICATION OF MENTAL STATUS CHANGE		
Types of Changes	**Features**	**Important Diagnoses**
Acute mental status change	• Confusion, usually with alteration of consciousness • Disturbance of the sleep-wake cycle	• Delirium from intercurrent medical illness • Side effect from medications • Stroke • Intoxications • Hypoxia, hypercarbia
Subacute mental status change	• Encephalopathy, confusion, and/or memory loss • May be alteration of consciousness	• Side effect from medications • Stroke • Metabolic encephalopathies • Decompensation of incipient dementia by medical illness
Chronic mental status change	• Confusion without disturbance of consciousness • Changes in judgment, behavior, and other aspects of cognitive function	• Alzheimer's disease • Other degenerative dementias • Vascular dementia • Dementia with Lewy bodies

SOME IMPORTANT CAUSES OF ACUTE MENTAL STATUS CHANGE		
Diagnosis	**Features**	**Causes**
Delirium	• Confusion and often agitation associated with an intercurrent illness • Most often seen in hospitalized patients	• Hospitalization of elderly patients especially with multiple medical problems predisposes to delirium.
Side effects of medications	• Confusion without focal signs • Usually develops about the time of a medication change or when liver or kidney insufficiency has altered metabolism of medication(s)	• Wide range of medications, including sedatives, antidepressants, neuroleptics, anticonvulsants, selected antihypertensives, and others
Global cerebral hypoperfusion	• Episodic confusion or loss of consciousness without focal symptoms or signs • May have tachycardia and hypertension after the episode as a hyperadrenergic reaction to the hypotension	• Cardiac arrhythmia • Vasovagal syncope • Orthostatic hypotension • May be exacerbated by fixed cerebrovascular disease
Seizure	• Episodic disturbance of consciousness, usually with automatisms or other motor activity suggesting seizure	• Complex partial epilepsy • Absence epilepsy

Diagnosis	Features	Causes
TIA or CVA	• Episodic loss of focal neurologic function • Confusion is unusual in the absence of other deficits: motor, sensory, language, or coordination.	• Vascular disease from atherothrombosis or vasculitis • Cardiogenic emboli • Hypertension • Diabetes • Hyperlipidemia
Transient global amnesia	• Confusion, with preservation of much elementary function • Duration of several hours • No neurologic deficits during or after the episode other than the cognitive changes	• Felt to be related to migraine, but only occurs in older people at risk for vascular disease.
Metabolic encephalopathy	• Confusion, often with a depression of the level of consciousness • No focal findings on examination	• Electrolyte abnormalities and hypocortisolism can be subacute to acute. • Thyroid and nutritional deficiencies are more insidious.

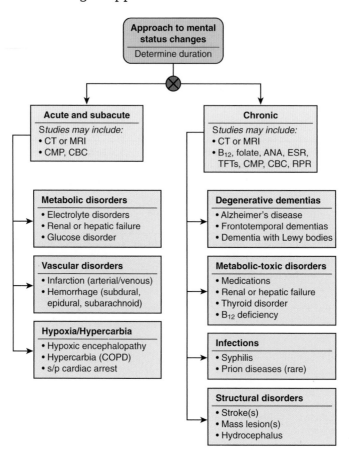

Lumbar Puncture

DIFFERENTIAL DIAGNOSIS OF SUBACUTE MENTAL STATUS CHANGE		
Diagnosis	**Features**	**Causes**
Medications	• Confusion • Alteration of consciousness • Ataxia is often present.	• Anticholinergics • Sedative/hypnotics • Antidepressants
Stroke	• Confusion with other neurologic deficits • Other deficits can include hemiparesis, hemianopia, language defects, or neglect.	• Anterior cerebral artery with ataxia, leg weakness • Middle cerebral artery with language disturbance (left hemisphere) or neglect (right hemisphere) • Posterior cerebral artery with hemianopia
Intercurrent illness	• Confusion • Disturbance of sleep-wake cycle • May be alteration of consciousness • Agitation is common.	• Urinary tract or sinopulmonary infection in a patient with mild cognitive impairment or incipient dementia • This is typically a loss of compensatory mechanisms for mild organic brain syndrome.

DIFFERENTIAL DIAGNOSIS OF CHRONIC MENTAL STATUS CHANGE		
Diagnosis	**Features**	**Causes**
Alzheimer's disease	• Confusion • Memory loss • Impaired judgment and other cognitive spheres • Language disturbance is common.	• Degenerative process • Genetic predisposition is likely for many patients. • Environmental trigger is possible.

Vascular dementia	• Stepwise or progressive dementia, with confusion and memory loss, but without disturbance of consciousness
	• Vascular risk factors are present.
		• Multiple strokes from:
		  • Diabetes
		  • Hypertension
		  • Cardiac emboli
		  • Vasculitis

Frontotemporal dementia	• Dementia with memory loss, confusion, and behavioral disturbance • Frontal lobe disinhibition symptoms	• Degenerative disease • No known precipitating features
Dementia with Lewy bodies (DLB)	• Dementia with parkinsonism • Dementia features include memory loss, confusion, and loss of awareness. • Parkinsonian features are indistinguishable from idiopathic Parkinson's disease—resting tremor, rigidity, bradykinesia, loss of postural reflexes.	• Degenerative disease • No known precipitating features

DIAGNOSIS OF DELIRIUM	
Definition	Acute change in mental status with confusion and impaired attention
Clinical features	• Confusion and memory loss • Speech changes are common, with language disturbance both receptive and expressive. • Hallucinations are common.
Important causes	• Medications • Toxins • Metabolic derangements, including renal and hepatic disease, electrolyte abnormalities, and thyroid abnormalities, including both hyper- and hypothyroidism • Nutritional causes, including thiamine, B_{12}, and possibly folate deficiency • Alcohol intoxication or withdrawal • Sleep deprivation • Hypoxia • Hypercarbia • Infections—primary central nervous system (CNS) infections, such as meningitis or encephalitis, or indirectly with systemic infection, producing mental status changes
Diagnostic tests	• Blood and urine tests are performed on most patients. • Imaging with CT or MRI is performed when no cause is evident from initial evaluation. • EEG is performed when patient could have seizure activity. • LP is performed when meningitis or encephalitis is a possible cause.

Diagnostic Tests	Implications
Blood and urine	• Comprehensive metabolic panel (CMP) and magnesium (Mg)—screen for electrolyte, renal, and hepatic causes. • *Thyroid function tests*—screen for hyper- and hypothyroidism. • *Complete blood count (CBC)*—screen for anemia (hemoglobin [Hgb] and red blood count [RBC]) and signs of infection (white blood count [WBC]). • *Drug screen*—urine drug screen and focused blood as indicated • *Arterial blood gas*—screen for hypoxia and hypercarbia, especially in patients with chronic obstructive pulmonary disease (COPD), asthma, and other disorders. • *B_{12} and folate levels*—screen for patients with possible nutritional deficiencies, especially seniors, the poor, cancer patient, and other serious medical illnesses. • Thiamine is not routinely assessed by laboratory studies, so replacement is usually given empirically.

Diagnostic Tests	Implications
Brain imaging—CT or MRI	• CT is performed as a rapid screen for hemorrhage, mass lesion, and infarction. May miss early infarction. • MRI is more sensitive than CT for infarction, especially in early stages. May miss subarachnoid hemorrhage, as it is better seen on CT. May be impossible to perform on uncooperative patients.
LP	• Required for identification of meningitis and usually for encephalitis • Indicated especially if the patient has fever, meningeal signs on examination, or seizures • Usually not performed prior to imaging because of the possibility of a cerebral or brainstem mass lesion, which could be made worse by LP
EEG	• Usually shows slowing of the brain waves in patients with encephalopathy or delirium • Patients with absence status epilepticus and complex partial status epilepticus can present with mental status changes without overt motor signs of seizures, and this is diagnosed by EEG. • Periodic discharges from one side suggest acute focal brain destruction from stroke or encephalitis.

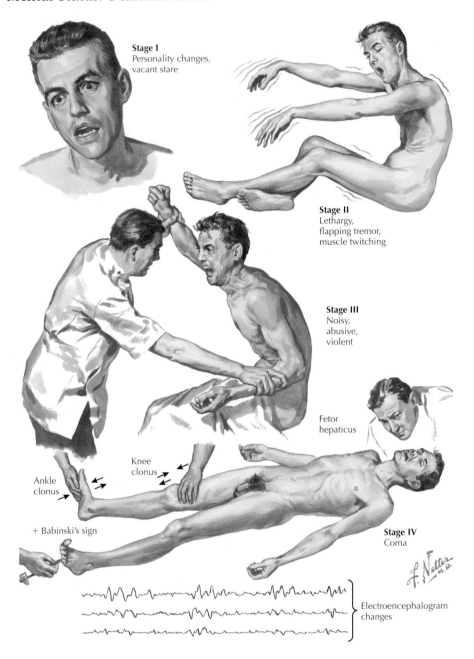

Stage I
Personality changes, vacant stare

Stage II
Lethargy, flapping tremor, muscle twitching

Stage III
Noisy, abusive, violent

Fetor hepaticus

Knee clonus

Ankle clonus

+ Babinski's sign

Stage IV
Coma

Electroencephalogram changes

DIFFERENTIAL DIAGNOSIS OF DELIRIUM		
Disorder	**Distinguishing Clinical Features**	**Making the Diagnosis**
Electrolyte abnormalities	• Delirium without focal signs • May have diffuse weakness • Seizures can occur, especially with hyponatremia.	• Abnormalities on CMP, especially sodium, potassium, or calcium.
Hyperglycemia	• Stroke-like focal deficits may occur. • Patient usually has history of DM.	• Elevated blood glucose • Increased osmolarity
Hypoglycemia	• Most patients have a history of DM. • Tremulous and sweaty	• Low blood glucose
Alcohol intoxication	• Dysarthric speech • Ataxia • Apathetic or agitated • Smells of alcohol	• Elevated blood alcohol • Often associated with electrolyte abnormalities
Alcohol withdrawal	• Confusion with agitation, often with hallucinations • Seizures may occur.	• History of alcohol use. Consider unreliability of self-reporting. • Rule out subdural hematoma, electrolyte abnormality, and other important causes.
Hyperthyroidism	• Confusion with agitation • Occasionally lethargic, especially in seniors	• Thyroid function tests
Hypothyroidism	• Memory loss and slowness of thought processes, often with motor slowing • Reflexes are hung-up, a classic though uncommon sign.	• Thyroid function tests
Stroke	• Confusion, usually with other signs including hemiparesis, aphasia, or hemianopia • Mild-to-moderate aphasia from a middle-cerebral artery infarct may look like mental status change.	• CT or MRI evidence of stroke • Subsequent evaluation for cause, including vascular imaging and risk-factor management is performed.
Medications	• Confusion often with alteration of responsiveness • Related to change in medication	• Drug screen • Ask about changes in medications prior to the delirium, even over-the-counter (OTCs) and nutritional supplements.
Toxins	• Industrial and farm chemicals • Intoxication with illicit drugs is common.	• Urine toxin screen • Blood levels of certain measurable agents, such as cholinesterase inhibitors (insecticides, nerve agents)

Disorder	Distinguishing Clinical Features	Making the Diagnosis
Meningitis	• Headache • Neck pain • Meningeal signs on examination • Imaging of the brain is normal. • Fever is common with bacterial meningitis, but uncommon with other causes.	• LP shows elevated WBC. • Specific CSF analysis is performed to look for individual agents. Bacterial, viral, and fungal infections are considered.
Encephalitis	• Confusion, with alteration in mental status • Seizures may develop. • Patients can develop marked encephalopathy and coma with cerebral edema or CNS destruction. • Fever is common but not invariable.	• MRI may show temporal lobe abnormalities with herpes simplex encephalitis. • CT is usually normal, or may show edema in severe cases. • Blood can be tested for multiple causes of encephalitis. • CSF shows increased WBC and often protein, may show increased RBC (with HSV).
Hypoxia and hypercarbia	• Confusion, usually with respiratory difficulty • COPD, neuromuscular disorder, or sleep apnea can be causes of ventilatory insufficiency • Pulmonary emboli are considered, especially if patient has chest pain and/or has been at bed rest.	• ABGs • CXR for infiltrate, pneumothorax • Chest CT with pulmonary embolism protocol or ventilation-perfusion lung scan for pulmonary emboli • Sleep study may be needed for possible sleep disorder

DIAGNOSIS OF DEMENTIA	
Definition	• Progressive decline in intellectual function • Deficits in memory and other aspects of cognition
Clinical features	• Memory loss that affects short-term, more than long-term, memory • Language deficits are common, including partial aphasia.
Important causes	• Alzheimer's disease (AD) • Frontotemporal dementia (FTD) • Dementia with Lewy bodies (DLB) • Vascular dementia (VaD) • Normal pressure hydrocephalus (NPH) • Pseudodementia
Diagnostic tests	• Neuropsychological testing • Blood and urine • Brain imaging with CT, MRI, and PET • EEG • LP

Diagnostic Tests	Implications
Neuropsychological testing	• First goal of testing is differentiation between pseudodementia, dementia, and mild cognitive impairment. • Can suggest differentiation between cortical dementias (e.g., AD) and subcortical dementias (e.g., VaD) • Neuropsychological testing is not always needed
Blood and urine	• CMP for metabolic derangement, especially renal and hepatic failure, although these produce delirium or subacute encephalopathy rather than dementia. • B_{12} and folate levels for nutritional deficiency, which can cause dementia. • Thyroid function tests and RPR
Brain imaging	• CT is adequate for most patients to rule out strokes, mass lesions, and hydrocephalus. • MRI for younger patients in whom multiple sclerosis, infiltrating lesions, or other more subtle abnormalities are considered. • PET is rarely performed, but can differentiate AD from other degenerative dementias and vascular dementia.
Electroencephalography (EEG)	• EEG is rarely performed for dementia, but can show periodic discharges in some patients with prion diseases.
Lumbar puncture (LP)	• LP can show chronic meningitis, which can present with dementia, such as cryptococcal meningitis. • LP can show abnormalities supportive of prion diseases and paraneoplastic degenerations in some patients. • Rarely done for uncomplicated dementia

DIFFERENTIATING CORTICAL VERSUS SUBCORTICAL DEMENTIAS

Dementias are differentiated into *cortical* and *subcortical*. This is a helpful differentiation that can aid diagnosis and management. The prototypic cortical dementia is Alzheimer's disease. Subcortical dementias include vascular dementia (VaD), multiple sclerosis (MS), and progressive supranuclear palsy (PSP).

Feature	Cortical Dementia	Subcortical Dementia
Pathophysiology	• Damage to cortical neurons, usually degenerative	• Damage to white matter and subcortical gray matter • Can be vascular, inflammatory, or degenerative
Clinical features	• Confusion and memory loss • Apraxia and language difficulties are common.	• Confusion and memory loss • Gait and coordination deficits are common. • Apraxia and language disturbance are uncommon.
Important causes	• Alzheimer's disease • Frontotemporal dementia • Creutzfeldt-Jakob disease	• Vascular dementia • Multiple sclerosis • Progressive supranuclear palsy • Huntington's disease

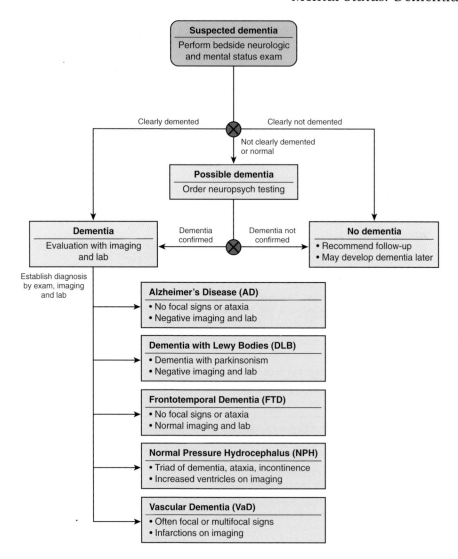

DIFFERENTIAL DIAGNOSIS OF DEMENTIA		
Disorder	**Distinguishing Clinical Features**	**Making the Diagnosis**
Alzheimer's disease (AD)	• Dementia, with the remainder of the neurologic exam relatively normal • Language dysfunction typical. • Absence of motor, coordination, and gait deficits is a major distinguishing feature. Most other causes of dementia have abnormalities in these areas.	• Clinical features • No laboratory abnormalities • No structural abnormalities on imaging • PET may show specific abnormalities, but is rarely needed.
Frontotemporal dementia (FTD)	• Early behavioral abnormalities, which suggest a frontal lobe dysfunction • Obsessive-compulsive features are typical.	• Clinical features • PET can help distinguish this from AD. • Neuropsych testing can help distinguish.
Dementia with Lewy bodies (DLB)	• Dementia with parkinsonism • Psychotic features, including hallucinations, are common.	• Clinical features of parkinsonism and progressive dementia • Absence of hydrocephalus or multiple infarctions on imaging
Vascular dementia (VaD)	• Dementia with a stepwise or progressive course • Vascular risk factors or previous vascular events	• Imaging showing multifocal infarctions • Neuropsych testing can help to distinguish a coexistent degenerative dementia with vascular disease.
Normal pressure hydrocephalus (NPH)	• Triad is dementia, ataxia, and urinary incontinence. Not all are present in all patients.	• Imaging shows ventricular enlargement out of proportion to brain atrophy.
Creutzfeldt-Jakob disease (CJD)	• Dementia with myoclonus, more rapidly progressive than AD • May have corticospinal tract signs	• MRI may show suggestive abnormalities in the basal ganglia. • EEG shows periodic discharges in most patients at some point in their disease. • LP may show supportive, but not diagnostic, abnormalities.
Pseudodementia	• Complaints of memory loss without objective deficit on mental status examination	• Neuropsych testing shows normal mental status or depression without dementia. • Further evaluation is usually not needed, but clinical follow-up is recommended for most patients.
Mild cognitive impairment (MCI)	• Mild memory deficit, but not enough to meet the criteria for a diagnosis of dementia	• Clinical diagnosis, usually supported by neuropsych testing. • Imaging and blood studies are often done to screen for causes, but are usually normal.

Alzheimer's Disease

In neocortex, major involvement of association areas (especially temporoparietal and frontal) with relative sparing of primary sensory cortices (except olfactory) and motor cortices. Stippling shows relative distribution of plaques

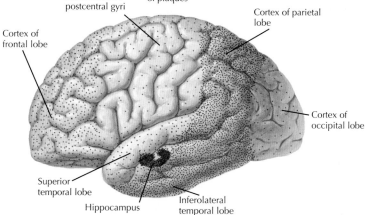

Precentral and postcentral gyri

Cortex of frontal lobe

Cortex of parietal lobe

Cortex of occipital lobe

Superior temporal lobe

Hippocampus

Inferolateral temporal lobe

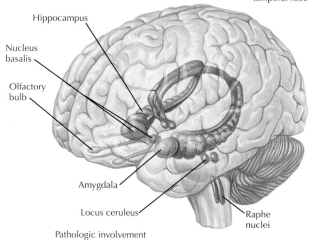

Hippocampus

Nucleus basalis

Olfactory bulb

Amygdala

Locus ceruleus

Raphe nuclei

Pathologic involvement of limbic system and subcortical nuclei projecting to cortex

Frontotemporal dementias (FTDs)

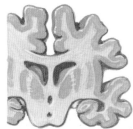

Atrophy of frontal and/or temporal areas

JOHN A. CRAIG—AD

C. Machado
—M.D.

DIAGNOSIS OF COMA	
Definition	• A state of profound unresponsiveness
Clinical features	• No spontaneous movement • Unresponsive to stimulation by various means
Important causes	• Stroke • Anoxia • Intoxication—medications and drugs • Head injury • Metabolic derangements—hyponatremia, hypo- and hyperglycemia • Locked-in syndrome • Pseudocoma (psychological unresponsiveness)
Diagnostic tests	• Lab—drug screen, blood levels of certain prescribed medications, electrolytes • Imaging—CT or MRI

Glasgow Coma Scale

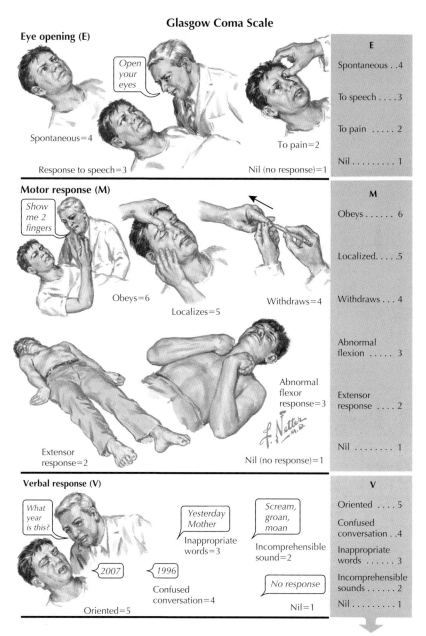

Eye opening (E)

Open your eyes

Spontaneous=4

Response to speech=3

To pain=2

Nil (no response)=1

E	
Spontaneous	..4
To speech	3
To pain	2
Nil	1

Motor response (M)

Show me 2 fingers

Obeys=6

Localizes=5

Withdraws=4

Abnormal flexor response=3

Extensor response=2

Nil (no response)=1

F. Netter M.D.

M	
Obeys	6
Localized	5
Withdraws	...4
Abnormal flexion	3
Extensor response	2
Nil	1

Verbal response (V)

What year is this?

2007

Oriented=5

1996

Confused conversation=4

Yesterday Mother

Inappropriate words=3

Scream, groan, moan

Incomprehensible sound=2

No response

Nil=1

V	
Oriented	5
Confused conversation	..4
Inappropriate words	3
Incomprehensible sounds	2
Nil	1

Coma score (E+M+V)=3 to 15

DIFFERENTIAL DIAGNOSIS OF COMA		
Disorder	**Distinguishing Clinical Features**	**Making the Diagnosis**
Stroke	• Acute onset of deficit • Neurologic deficits, including corticospinal tract signs, eye movement deficit, and/or reflex asymmetries	• Clinical diagnosis of coma plus signs of severe brain damage in a focal distribution appropriate to the coma • Imaging showing infarcts or hemorrhage
Anoxia	• Coma following an episode of anoxia • Myoclonus and/or seizures are often seen. • There may be multifocal signs with unequal regions of anoxic damage.	• History of cardiac arrest or other causes of anoxia • Clinical features of coma with or without myoclonus
Intoxication	• Coma, often with loss of brainstem reflexes, but without other focal signs • History of substance ingestion	• Clinical features are nonspecific. Suspicion is key. • Drug screen is critical.
Head injury	• Coma, following head injury, with or without focal signs • Mental status may fluctuate with cerebral edema and other factors. • Overt signs of injury are present.	• Clinical features • History of recent head injury • Imaging, which may be normal or show contusions, edema, and/or hemorrhage
Metabolic derangements	• Metabolic derangements are an uncommon cause of coma, more often encephalopathy. • Coma with preserved brainstem function can be seen. Seizures can occur.	• Lab results that show the abnormalities, including electrolyte problems, etc. • Imaging and lab results do not show other causes— consider alternative causes.
Locked-in syndrome, from brainstem infarction	• Patient is immobile, and may, on casual observation, appear to be comatose. However, the patient retains vertical eye movements and communication is possible with this condition.	• Able to communicate with eye movements • Brainstem infarction may show on MRI or CT.

Pseudocoma	• Clinical appearance of coma with preservation of brain function
	• Patient may be unaware of the pseudocoma (conversion reaction) or be intentionally unresponsive (malingering).
		Evidence from exam of preserved response:
		  • Hold arm over head and let it fall—with pseudocoma the arm falls so that the face is not hit.
		  • May suggest that an intravenous injection will give 15 seconds of responsiveness. Injection is either sham or saline.
		  • Evidence from studies of normal response, e.g., EEG

Disorder	Distinguishing Clinical Features	Making the Diagnosis
Persistent vegetative state (PVS)	• State of unconsciousness with preserved reflex responsiveness • Differentiated from coma by the ability to make elementary responses to stimuli • Patients may appear awake or asleep, but exam shows that they are unable to appreciate their environment, commands, and situations.	• Clinical exam • Findings of maintained brainstem response to stimuli • Imaging and lab results show causes for the unresponsiveness.

Differential Diagnosis of Coma

Clinical features	Pathology (examples)	Etiologies

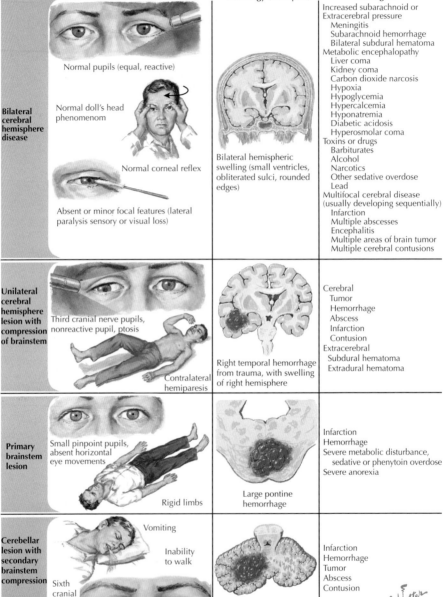

Bilateral cerebral hemisphere disease

Normal pupils (equal, reactive)

Normal doll's head phenomenom

Normal corneal reflex

Absent or minor focal features (lateral paralysis sensory or visual loss)

Bilateral hemispheric swelling (small ventricles, obliterated sulci, rounded edges)

Increased subarachnoid or
Extracerebral pressure
  Meningitis
  Subarachnoid hemorrhage
  Bilateral subdural hematoma
Metabolic encephalopathy
  Liver coma
  Kidney coma
  Carbon dioxide narcosis
  Hypoxia
  Hypoglycemia
  Hypercalcemia
  Hyponatremia
  Diabetic acidosis
  Hyperosmolar coma
Toxins or drugs
  Barbiturates
  Alcohol
  Narcotics
  Other sedative overdose
  Lead
Multifocal cerebral disease
(usually developing sequentially)
  Infarction
  Multiple abscesses
  Encephalitis
  Multiple areas of brain tumor
  Multiple cerebral contusions

Unilateral cerebral hemisphere lesion with compression of brainstem

Third cranial nerve pupils, nonreactive pupil, ptosis

Contralateral hemiparesis

Right temporal hemorrhage from trauma, with swelling of right hemisphere

Cerebral
  Tumor
  Hemorrhage
  Abscess
  Infarction
  Contusion
Extracerebral
  Subdural hematoma
  Extradural hematoma

Primary brainstem lesion

Small pinpoint pupils, absent horizontal eye movements

Rigid limbs

Large pontine hemorrhage

Infarction
Hemorrhage
Severe metabolic disturbance, sedative or phenytoin overdose
Severe anorexia

Cerebellar lesion with secondary brainstem compression

Vomiting

Inability to walk

Sixth cranial nerve palsy

Large cerebellar hemorrhage

Infarction
Hemorrhage
Tumor
Abscess
Contusion

f. Netter M.D.

DIAGNOSIS OF BRAIN DEATH	
Definition and criteria	• Cessation of all brain function • Cessation is irreversible • Cause is known
Clinical features	• Most common presentation is of a patient with anoxic encephalopathy or stroke who suffers neurologic deterioration and loses all clinical signs of brain function. • Evaluation for brain death occurs to determine whether additional life supports should be given to the patient and whether the patient is a candidate for organ donation.
Important causes	• Cardiac arrest with anoxic encephalopathy • Stroke with subsequent severe brain damage and cerebral edema • Head injury with edema, contusion, hemorrhage

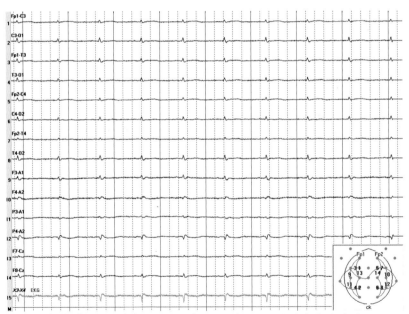

Brain death: Electroencephalogram (EEG) of patients who meets criteria for brain death. There is no significant electrical activity from the brain. The small blips at approximately 1-second intervals are from cardiac activity.

DETERMINATION OF BRAIN DEATH	
Cessation of all brain function	• No response to auditory or visual stimuli • No pupillary response • No corneal reflex • No response to "doll's head maneuver" • No response to ice water caloric testing • No respiratory effort with apnea testing

Cessation is not reversible	Causes of brain dysfunction that are reversible should be ruled-out by ensuring:
	  • No toxic levels of CNS depressants
	  • Temperature of at least 90°F
	  • Systolic blood pressure of at least 80 mm Hg
	  • No neuromuscular blockade
	  • Examination is repeated after a period of observation with all of the above parameters as noted. This ensures that the patient is not recovering form some intoxication or injury.

Cause is known	• Most patients have a cause that is obvious at the time of evaluation. • If the cause is unknown, most clinicians adopt a very conservative view about brain death, because one cannot be sure of toxic or metabolic causes.
Period of observation	• Period of observation between exams depends on the cause of the coma and whether or not there is a confirmatory test performed. • If the cause is anoxia and there is no confirmatory test = 24 hours. • If the cause is anoxia and there is a confirmatory test = 12 hours. • If the cause is not anoxia and there is no confirmatory test = 12 hours. • If the cause is not anoxia and there is a confirmatory test = 6 hours.

Confirmatory tests	Confirmatory tests routinely used include:
	  • EEG
	  • Radionucleotide flow study
	  • Angiogram

Method of apnea testing	Performed in a variety of ways. One common approach is:
	  • Place catheter with oxygen jet near the level of the carina.
	  • Monitor oximetry and can measure CO_2 while watching for signs of respiratory effort.
	  • Test ends if the patient makes any respiratory effort, has significant reduction in oxygen, elevated pCO_2 to at least 60 mm Hg, or has a complication of the test (e.g., cardiac arrest is a rare occurrence).

DETERMINATION OF BRAIN DEATH–cont'd	
What to do after determination of brain death	• Next-of-kin and other medical personnel are informed that the patient has expired. Determination of brain death is not a subject of philosophical debate when rigorously determined.
	• Patient is usually taken off the life supports when the family has had adequate time to visit the deceased. Organ donor issues come into play here, and most hospitals have protocols for evaluation of potential donors.
	• Sensitivity on the part of the medical staff indicates a "hard-line approach" should usually not be taken with the family.

DIAGNOSIS OF CRANIAL NERVE DEFICITS		
Symptom	**Cranial Nerve(s)**	**Possible Causes**
Anosmia	Olfactory (CN-I)	• Meningioma • Sinusitis • Head injury • Increased ICP
Diplopia	Oculomotor (CN-III) Trochlear (CN-IV) Abducens (CN-VI)	• Vascular disease affecting the oculomotor or abducens nerve • Oculomotor nerve compression • Abducens nerve dysfunction from increased ICP • Cavernous sinus thrombosis • Myasthenia gravis, affecting muscles from any of these nerves • Multiple sclerosis • Stroke
Facial and/or ear pain	Trigeminal (CN-V) or Glossopharyngeal (CN-IX)	• Trigeminal neuralgia • Glossopharyngeal neuralgia • Cavernous sinus thrombosis
Face weakness	Facial (CN-VII)	• Bell's palsy • Stroke (affecting the upper motor neurons)
Hearing loss and tinnitus	Vestibulocochlear (CN-VIII)	• Acoustic neuroma • Cerebellopontine angle lesion (often with other brainstem and cranial nerve deficits)
Loss of taste	Facial (CN-VII), and Glossopharyngeal (CN-IX), though CN-IX lesions rarely result in clinical taste loss and the nerve is difficult to test.	• Bell's palsy, when the area of involvement is from the middle ear through the facial canal, affecting the chorda tympani—the bundle of nerves serving taste

IMPORTANT DISORDERS WITH CRANIAL NERVE DEFICITS		
Disorder	**Cranial Nerve(s) Affected**	**Clinical Findings**
Olfactory groove meningioma	Olfactory (CN-I)	• Anosmia • May have disinhibition, cognitive dysfunction, and/or seizures from frontal lobe involvement
Optic neuritis	Optic (CN-II)	• Loss of vision in one or both eyes (if bilateral involvement) • Pain behind the eyes worsened by movement may occur. • No ocular motor deficit
Oculomotor palsy from compression	Oculomotor (CN-III)	• Diplopia, which usually has both horizontal and vertical components • Pupil is typically dilated and of less reactivity, a helpful differentiating feature from vascular lesion.
Oculomotor palsy from ischemia	Oculomotor (CN-III)	• Diplopia, often with both horizontal and vertical components • Pupil is typically spared, a helpful differentiating feature from compressive lesion.
Myasthenia gravis	Muscles of oculomotor (CN-III), trochlear (CN-IV), and abducens (CN-VI) nerves	• Diplopia, which localizes to muscles supplied by more than one nerve, and both eyes are typically affected. • No sensory symptoms or signs
Cavernous sinus thrombosis	Oculomotor (CN-III) Trochlear (CN-IV) Trigeminal (CN-V) Abducens (CN-VI)	• Painful ophthalmoplegia, around one eye • Diplopia, with any of the ocular motor nerves affected • Facial pain and sensory loss may occur.
Abducens palsy from increased intracranial pressure	Abducens (CN-VI)	• Horizontal diplopia, which is worsened by looking to the side of the lesion, and lessened by looking to the opposite side • Headache and papilledema are common.
Trigeminal neuralgia	Trigeminal (CN-V)	• Lancinating pain on the face • Symptoms worsened by speaking and chewing • No motor or sensory deficit
Bell's palsy	Facial (CN-VII)	• Unilateral (rarely bilateral) face weakness affecting the upper and lower face • Taste may be affected on the anterior tongue. • No sensory deficit on the face
Acoustic neuroma	Vestibulocochlear (CN-VIII)	• Tinnitus and hearing loss, unilateral or bilateral • Vertigo can occur, but is uncommon.

Disorder	Cranial Nerve(s) Affected	Clinical Findings
Cerebellopontine angle mass	Trigeminal (CN-V), Facial (CN-VII), vestibulocochlear (CN-VIII)	• Face pain and weakness • Hearing loss, tinnitus, and/or vertigo • May be signs of brainstem compression with diplopia, ataxia, and other sites of weakness
Glossopharyngeal neuralgia	Glossopharyngeal (CN-IX)	• Lancinating pain in the tonsillar region • No motor or sensory deficit
Recurrent laryngeal palsy	Vagus (CN-X)	• Hoarse voice • Unilateral vocal cord paralysis on laryngoscopy • Structural lesion in the lower neck or upper chest is often identified, especially as a tumor.
Pure lesions of the accessory (CN-XI) and hypoglossal (CN-XII) nerves are uncommon in routine practice, and are usually seen in the setting of multiple lower cranial neuropathies from chronic meningitis (e.g., fungal and neoplastic) and with brainstem stroke.		

Cranial Nerve Dysfunction

APPROACH TO ATAXIA	
Definition of ataxia	• Ataxia is poor coordination in the absence of paralysis. • It can affect gait, limbs, and/or trunk.
Common causes of ataxia	• Gait ataxia is often caused by stroke or alcoholism. Inherited ataxias are rare. • Unilateral limb ataxia is usually due to stroke or tumor affecting the basal ganglia, cerebellum, and/or brainstem. • Bilateral limb ataxia can be due to brainstem stroke, or other lesion, multiple sclerosis, inherited ataxia, or other brainstem or basal ganglia lesion.
Difference between gait and limb ataxia?	• Gait ataxia is manifest only when walking. • Limb ataxia is manifest when testing each limb while not standing. • Gait and limb ataxia may coexist with many disorders.
Differentiation of weakness from ataxia	• Weakness may produce ataxia, so intact muscle strength must be assured. • Weakness causing poor coordination mainly affects proximal muscles, whereas cerebellar and other causes produce distal or entire limb incoordination.
Type of Ataxia	**Features**
Sensory ataxia	• Sensory loss may produce ataxia, which can be confused with cerebellar ataxia. • Marked difference in limb ataxia with eyes open and closed suggests sensory ataxia, whereas cerebellar ataxia is affected in both circumstances. • Peripheral polyneuropathy and dorsal column deficits are considered.
Cerebellar ataxia	• Gait ataxia is broad-based. • Limb ataxia is worsened as the limb reaches the target, as with finger-nose-finger testing, the terminal movement of the finger oscillates more than during transit between targets. • A wide range of degenerative, neoplastic, vascular, and toxic causes of cerebellar ataxia are considered.
Frontal lobe ataxia	• Gait ataxia with small steps. Can be confused with parkinsonism. • Stiffness may be present without tremor or cogwheel rigidity. • Can be seen with mass or destructive lesions of the frontal lobes • Degenerative conditions also are considered.

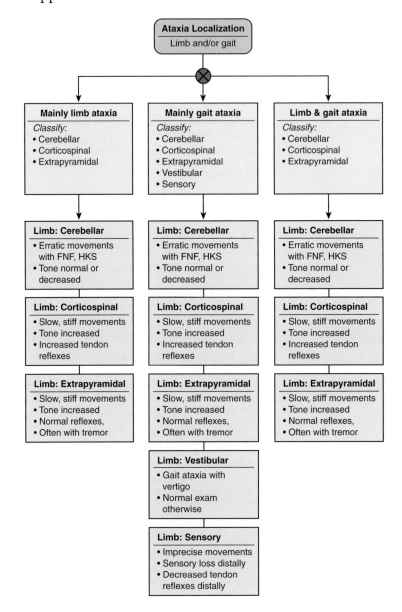

Ataxia Localization
Limb and/or gait

Mainly limb ataxia
Classify:
• Cerebellar
• Corticospinal
• Extrapyramidal

Mainly gait ataxia
Classify:
• Cerebellar
• Corticospinal
• Extrapyramidal
• Vestibular
• Sensory

Limb & gait ataxia
Classify:
• Cerebellar
• Corticospinal
• Extrapyramidal

Limb: Cerebellar
• Erratic movements
  with FNF, HKS
• Tone normal or
  decreased

Limb: Cerebellar
• Erratic movements
  with FNF, HKS
• Tone normal or
  decreased

Limb: Cerebellar
• Erratic movements
  with FNF, HKS
• Tone normal or
  decreased

Limb: Corticospinal
• Slow, stiff movements
• Tone increased
• Increased tendon
  reflexes

Limb: Corticospinal
• Slow, stiff movements
• Tone increased
• Increased tendon
  reflexes

Limb: Corticospinal
• Slow, stiff movements
• Tone increased
• Increased tendon
  reflexes

Limb: Extrapyramidal
• Slow, stiff movements
• Tone increased
• Normal reflexes,
• Often with tremor

Limb: Extrapyramidal
• Slow, stiff movements
• Tone increased
• Normal reflexes,
• Often with tremor

Limb: Extrapyramidal
• Slow, stiff movements
• Tone increased
• Normal reflexes,
• Often with tremor

Limb: Vestibular
• Gait ataxia with
  vertigo
• Normal exam
  otherwise

Limb: Sensory
• Imprecise movements
• Sensory loss distally
• Decreased tendon
  reflexes distally

LOCALIZATION AND DIAGNOSIS OF GAIT ATAXIA		
Location	Findings	Causes
Cerebrum	• Stiff gait width is usually narrow-based.	• Multiple sclerosis • Stroke
Brainstem	• Gait that is usually narrow-based but could also be broad-based • Tone is often increased.	• Stroke • Tumor • Central pontine myelinolysis • Multiple sclerosis
Cerebellum	• Broad-based gait with lurching movements • Tone may be normal or decreased.	• Alcohol • Stroke • Tumor • Multiple sclerosis
Spinal cord	• Stiff gait with narrow or broad stance • Corticospinal tract findings with increased DTRs and up-going plantar responses	• Spondylosis • Transverse myelitis • B_{12} deficiency • Tumors • Multiple sclerosis
Peripheral nerve	• Signs of neuropathy with sensory deficit, decreased distal tendon reflexes • Gait difficulty without other neurologic deficits • Proprioception is affected.	• Diabetes • Other metabolic disturbance • Cancer, as a remote effect of from chemotherapy • Heavy metals • Immune-mediated (esp. MMN, CIDP)
Vestibular system	• Gait difficulty with vertigo • No other neurologic deficit, including coordination and cranial nerve function	• Vestibular neuronitis • Meniere's disease • Acoustic neuroma

LOCALIZATION AND DIAGNOSIS OF LIMB ATAXIA		
Location	Findings	Causes
Cerebrum	• Lesions of the cortex produce weakness and incoordination of the contralateral limb(s). • Subcortical lesions can produce coordination deficit without prominent weakness.	• Stroke • Multiple sclerosis • Tumors • Infections—abscess or encephalitis • Trauma
Brainstem	• Lesions of the brainstem usually produce cranial nerve dysfunction and weakness in addition to limb ataxia. • Gait ataxia coexists.	• Stroke • Infection (brainstem encephalitis) • Multiple sclerosis • Central pontine myelinolysis
Cerebellum	• Appendicular ataxia affecting the same same side as the lesion • Gait may not be affected if the lesion is confined to the cerebellar hemisphere.	• Stroke • Tumors • Multiple sclerosis • Paraneoplastic syndromes
Spinal cord	• Corticospinal tract signs, which are usually bilateral • Gait is usually affected as well.	• Transverse myelitis • Multiple sclerosis • Trauma • Cord infarction • B_{12} deficiency
Peripheral nerve	• Weakness is more common than limb ataxia.	• Plexus injuries, usually from trauma • Limb ataxia is uncommon with single nerve injuries.

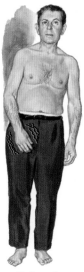

Unilateral
involvement;
blank facies;
affected arm in
semiflexed position
with tremor; patient
leans to unaffected
side

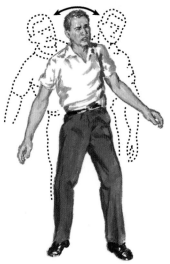

Wide-based gait of midline
cerebellar tumor or other lesion

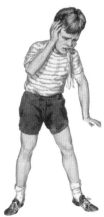

Child with ataxia,
wide gait,
tendency to fall,
headache, and
vomiting

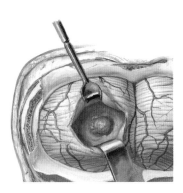

Dissection showing
cystic tumor of
cerebellum with
nodule

APPROACH TO EPISODIC DISORDERS	
Approach to episodic disorders	• Get a good history to help determine which is the most likely category. • Perform tests as needed to accurately diagnose the cause.
Types of disorders	• Syncope • Seizure • Transient ischemic attack • Migraine • Narcolepsy/cataplexy

Type of Episode	Features
Syncope	• Episodic unconsciousness due to cerebral hypoperfusion • Causes can be cardiac arrhythmia, cerebrovascular disease, orthostatic hypotension or sustained hypotension, increased intracranial pressure, vasovagal syncope.
Seizure	• Episodic neurologic disturbance due to generation of electrical discharges • Seizures can be generalized or partial (focal). • Motor manifestations are variable from generalized tonic/clonic activity to absence without any motor symptoms. • Seizures can be idiopathic or associated with structural abnormality of the brain.
Transient ischemic attack	• Episodic neurologic deficit due to transient focal ischemia • Symptoms and signs depend on the location. Common symptoms are focal weakness or sensory loss, incoordination and dizziness, loss of vision in one eye or one hemifield, and loss of speech.
Migraine	• Episodes of headaches that may be associated with neurologic symptoms, such as an aura • The aura usually preceded the pain, but they can be contemporaneous.
Narcolepsy/cataplexy	• *Narcolepsy*—sleep disorder with excessive daytime sleepiness. May show sleep attacks. • *Cataplexy*—attacks of paralysis with preservation of cognition and respiratory function. Associated with narcolepsy.

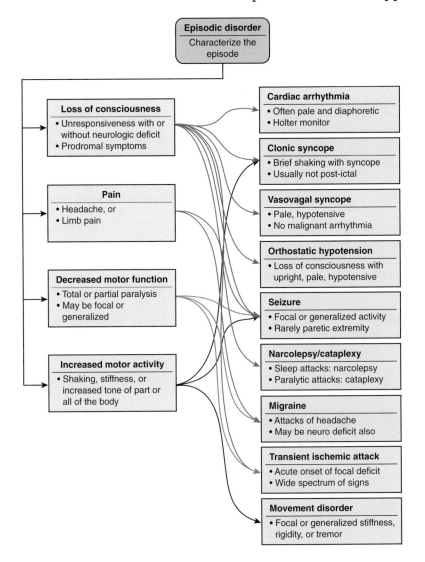

TESTS USED FOR EVALUATION		
Test	**Indication**	**Results and Interpretation**
ECG	Possible cardiac arrhythmia	• Routine ECG often does not detect arrhythmias. • May show signs of acute or previous ischemic change or abnormal conduction pathways.
Prolonged cardiac monitoring	Possible cardiac arrhythmia	Helpful if positive for arrhythmia, but even prolonged monitoring cannot eliminate cardiac causes unless the epoch of recording captures a spell.
EEG	Possible seizure	Epileptiform activity on the EEG is consistent with seizure activity, but absence does not rule out seizure.
Tilt-table testing	Possible orthostasis, when routine BP examination is inconclusive	Detailed testing is helpful for diagnosis of orthostatic hypotension.
MRI with MRA	Possible mass lesion or vascular occlusive disease, either of which may affect CNS perfusion pressure	Determination of mass lesion or arterial insufficiency as causes of episode
Echocardiogram	Possible cardiac contractility defect or outflow obstruction. Possible valvular abnormality.	Seldom are results surprising if ECG and cardiac examinations are normal, but can show some significant abnormalities in old and young, which may predispose to syncope.

DIAGNOSIS OF EPISODIC DISORDERS AND SYNCOPE		
Disorder	**Features**	**Diagnosis**
Cardiac arrhythmia	• Sudden loss of consciousness • May have chest pain, but often no cardiac symptoms	• ECG • Long-term cardiac monitoring, using a Holter or event monitor, may need to be initiated.
Seizure	• Episodic loss of awareness, focal jerking of an extremity, of loss of consciousness • May be associated with generalized tonic/clonic activity	• Clinical diagnosis on the basis of symptoms. • EEG can confirm inter-ictal or ictal activity in many, but not all, patients. MRI is done to look for focal structural lesion.
Vasovagal syncope	• Loss of consciousness, associated with reduction in systemic blood pressure not related to posture • May be precipitated by emotion.	• Clinical diagnosis, and may be difficult to definitively establish this diagnosis. • Orthostasis and arrhythmia always have to be considered.

Disorder	Features	Diagnosis
Clonic syncope	• Syncope from almost any cause can be associated with brief jerking of the extremities after the episode.	• Clinical diagnosis, based on history and possible observation • Not all jerking is seizure activity.
Orthostatic hypotension	• Light-headedness or loss of consciousness when the patient arises to stand • More likely in patients with Parkinson's disease and on some medications	• Measurement of blood pressure in laying, sitting, and standing states • Tilt-table testing

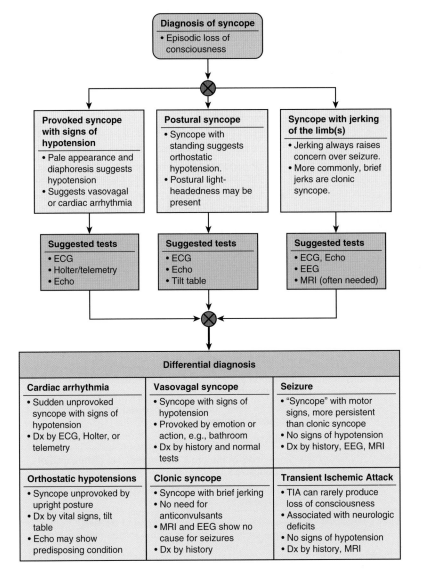

Episodic Disorders: Approach

DIAGNOSIS OF SEIZURES	
Type of seizures	• *Generalized*—seizure begins in subcortical circuits so that the seizure is generalized from the onset. • *Partial*—seizure begins from a focus, which may be due to a focal structural lesion. Note: Details of individual types are discussed below and in the section on *Disorders: Seizures*
Features suggesting a seizure	• Shaking of one or more extremities during the episode (but some can occur with nonseizure activity as well) • Confusion after the event (post-ictal period)
Features that suggest an episode is not a seizure	• Lack of pulse during the event • Marked paleness and other signs of hypotension during an event • Events are precipitated by standing (suggests orthostasis). • Events are precipitated by stress (suggests pseudoseizure or vasovagal syncope).
Studies performed on patients with suspected seizures	• MRI to look for a focal structural lesion. Performed on most patients. • EEG to characterize the seizure type. Note that EEG may be normal between seizures. • LP performed for some patients with new-onset seizures that may be due to infection or meningeal tumor. • Long-term video—EEG monitoring performed when the diagnosis is in doubt after routine evaluation. Recording of an event with video, EEG, ECG, and other parametric data can make a definitive diagnosis.

TYPES OF SEIZURES	
Types of Seizure	**Features**
GENERALIZED SEIZURES	
Absence	• Episodic loss of responsiveness without major motor symptoms • Predominantly in children although may continue to adult life • No post-ictal suppression
Generalized tonic/clonic	• Unresponsiveness associated with shaking of the arms and legs. Incontinence can occur. • Often an initial tonic phase followed by clonic phase that progressively slows • Post-ictal suppression
Myoclonic	• Single jerks of the arms and/or legs. No disturbance of consciousness. • Can be seen with other seizure types including generalized tonic/clonic
Secondarily generalized	• Generalized seizure due to spread of discharge from a focus. A simple partial or complex partial seizure may lead to the generalized seizure.

Types of Seizure	Features
PARTIAL SEIZURES	
Simple partial	• Focal motor or (rarely) sensory symptoms of one limb or one side of the body
	• Due to a cortical focus, usually resulting from a structural lesion
Complex partial	• Wide variety of behaviors, all of which include disturbance of consciousness
	• Due to a focus usually in the temporal or frontal lobe, often associated with a focal structural lesion

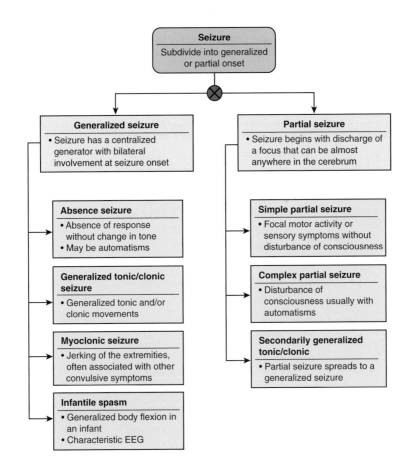

HEADACHE	
Definition	• Pain in the head and related structures, with a myriad of possible causes • As always, history and physical examination are the most important parts of the evaluation.
Diagnosis of headache	• *Primary headaches* have no clearly identifiable underlying cause, whereas *secondary headaches* arise from another existing and identifiable disease process. • The diagnosis of a primary headache syndrome can be considered if none other is found and if other diagnostic criteria are met. • In general, new-onset headaches associated with neurologic dysfunction are worrisome for underlying brain lesions or disease processes, whereas chronic stereotypical headaches without associated fixed abnormalities on neurologic exam usually represent benign primary headache syndromes.
Approach to evaluation	• Initial investigation of headache seeks to diagnose and manage any underlying pathology. • Evaluation is most important for patients with new-onset headache or the "worst headache of their life."
Initial headache evaluation	• History and general physical examination • Neurologic examination • Blood tests: CMP, CBC, TSH, ANA, ESR • Brain imaging with CT or MRI is often needed.
Important causes of secondary headache	• Space-occupying intracranial lesion • Cancer of the head and/or neck • Arteritis/vasculitis • Hypoxia or hypercarbia • Ruptured or leaking intracranial aneurism • Head trauma • Systemic or CNS infection • Medications • Toxins • Ocular, ear, or sinus infection/inflammation • Abnormalities in intracranial pressure, whether too high or too low
Danger signs in headache	• Sudden onset of severe headache (thunderclap headache) • Headache associated with abnormalities in neurologic examination • New headache onset after age 50 • Headache worst upon wakening or waking one up from sleep • Headache with fever • "Worst headache of my life" description • Headache no longer responds to medication as before • Headache worse at night

Initial Headache Evaluation

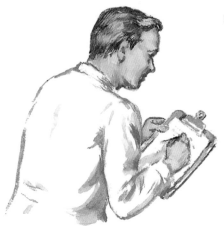

History
(from patient
and family,
with emphasis
on onset
and timing)

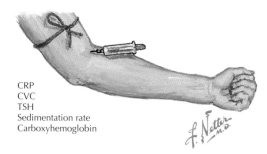

· Elevated
sedimentation
rate

CRP
CVC
TSH
Sedimentation rate
Carboxyhemoglobin

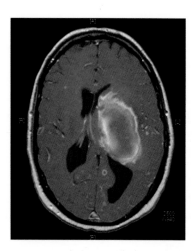

The most important part of the diagnosis of
headache syndromes is a complete history.
This is followed by a careful exam
concentrating on identification of serious
causes of headache. When needed, imaging
and/or blood work is ordered. Diagnostic
studies are needed, especially if the patient
has headaches that are atypical or refractory
to treatment or if there are abnormalities
on examination.

PRIMARY HEADACHE SYNDROMES	
Common primary headache syndromes	**After secondary causes of headache have been satisfactorily ruled out, the diagnosis of benign primary headache syndromes can be considered.**
Migraine	• Moderate-to-severe pain • Throbbing quality of pain • Tendency to be worse on one side than the other • Nausea and or vomiting • Worsened by activity • Duration of hours to days • Photophobia, phonophobia, osmophobia may be cited. • Strong family history of headache may be cited. • Recurrent episodic headaches • 10%–15% of cases are preceded by 10–45 minutes of aura. • More common in women than men by a 3 : 1 ratio • About 28 million people in the United States affected, only 50% diagnosed • Second most common reason cited for missed work days • Aura precedes headache in only 10%–15% of cases. • Diagnosis assumes other causes of headache have been excluded. • Over-the-counter analgesics are often ineffective.
Tension-type headache	• Dull, constant pain • More often occipital, hatband-like and bilateral, or generalized • Not worsened by activity • No sex predominance • Mild-to-moderate severity • Over-the-counter analgesics often effective at least temporarily. • Diagnosis assumes other causes of headache have been excluded.
Cluster headache	• Very severe to extreme pain • Unilateral, periorbital, sharp, and/or intense stabbing sensation • Agitation—patient prefers to walk around rather than lie still • Tendency to occur in "clusters" of attacks over several days to weeks • Duration of 30 minutes to two hours on average • Male preponderance of 5 : 1 • Ipsilateral lacrimation, conjunctival injection, mydriasis, or miosis may be present. • Nausea not typically present. • Usually resolves quickly with inhalation of 100% oxygen (can be diagnostic)

Indomethacin-responsive syndromes	There are a few primary headache syndromes that seem to respond preferentially to administration of indomethacin. The reason for this is unknown.
Hemicrania continua	• Moderate-to-severe pain • Unilateral and typically sharp and/or throbbing sensation • Duration of three weeks or more • Mild-to-moderate nausea and/or phonophobia often cited • Assumes underlying neurologic disease is excluded
Paroxysmal hemicrania	• Also known as "ice pick pains" • Very sharp and brief pain • Can occur in different locations over the head
Neuralgiform headache	The neuralgiform syndromes comprise a separate group of head pain apart from the other primary headache syndromes. In trigeminal and glossopharyngeal neuralgia, the pain generating structure is known, if not the pathophysiology. Treatment approach is therefore different. Investigation should include MRI brain imaging.
Trigeminal neuralgia	• Lancinating, sharp, electrical paroxysmal, recurrent pain in the distribution of one or more trigeminal nerve branches • Can occur spontaneously or be triggered by various stimuli • Can often be triggered by tactile stimuli near the painful area • Can be triggered by eating, drinking, brushing teeth, applying makeup • Multiple attacks per day are common. • No fixed neurologic deficit, apart from hyperalgesia and dysesthesia • Typically confined to one branch of the trigeminal nerve
Glossopharyngeal neuralgia	• Lancinating and/or sharp or deep pain in the hypopharyngeal area • Can be associated with dysguesia

Causes of Headache

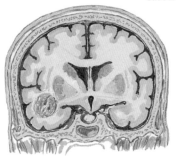

Tumor

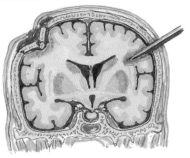

Trauma
(depressed fracture,
penetrating wound

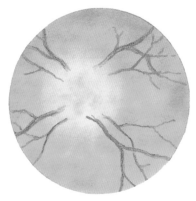

Papilledema may be caused
by increased intracranial
pressure secondary to
rupture of cerebral aneurysm

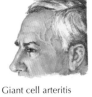

Intracerebral aneurysm.
Spasm in distal vessel

Giant cell arteritis

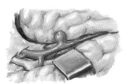

Medication

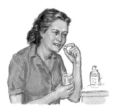

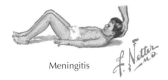

Meningitis

WEAKNESS	
Definition	• Loss of strength or voluntary motor power • May be associated with fatigue
Establishing the diagnosis	• Careful attention to the pattern, onset, distribution, and progression of weakness enables a generation of differential diagnoses. • As always, history and physical exam are by far the most powerful and important diagnostic tests.
Differentiating features	• Acute versus chronic • Static versus dynamic • Location • Time of onset and duration • Associated symptoms: pain, sensation loss, incoordination, paresthesias • Presence or absence of muscle atrophy • Muscle tone changes • Myalgia, fasciculations, or cramps • Effect of exercise on weakness: fatigue with exercise versus improvement with exercise (warm-up phenomenon)
Neurologic localizations for weakness	• Upper motor neuron • Brain • Spinal cord (corticospinal tracts) • Lower motor neuron (anterior horn cell) • Peripheral nerve • Axonal loss • Demyelination with conduction block • Neuromuscular junction • Presynaptic • Postsynaptic • Muscle

Grading muscle weakness	• Many methods and grading scales exist. Choose a favorite method and strive to apply it consistently.
	• For cranial nerves, a simple percentage of normal will suffice to grade weakness, with 100% considered normal.
	• For appendicular weakness, the familiar Medical Research Council (MRC) system may be the most common. In this scale:
	  • MRC 5 is normal.
	  • MRC 4 is the ability to resist gravity and resistance.
	  • MRC 3 is the ability to move a joint against gravity but not resistance.
	  • MRC 2 is the ability to move a joint with gravity removed.
	  • MRC 1 is a flicker or trace of contraction.
	  • MRC 0 is no movement at all.

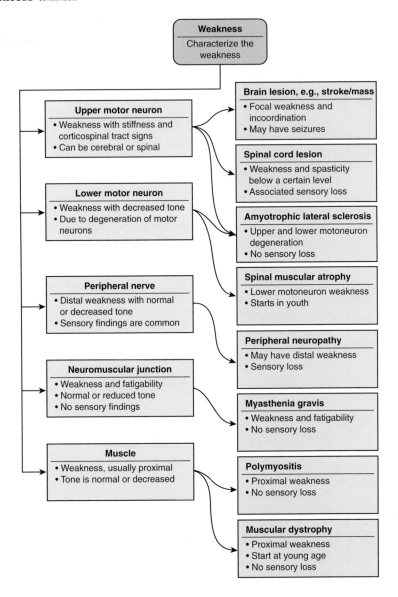

GENERAL PATTERNS OF WEAKNESS	
Upper Motor Neuron	**Weakness due to Dysfunction of Upper Motor Neurons in the Brain or Descending Corticospinal Tracts can be Focal, Generalized, or Unilateral**
Acute onset	Acute onset of focal or unilateral weakness is strongly suggestive of stroke, in the absence of trauma.
Gradual onset	• Suggestive of a space-occupying lesion, either in the cranium or spinal canal • Movements are stiff and clumsy, and reflexes are typically exaggerated. This is called spasticity. • Pathological reflexes, e.g., Babinski or Hoffmann, may be noted. • Gradual onset of generalized spastic weakness can also arise from a number of causes—general, nutritional, and infectious. Depending upon the site of the lesion, other neurologic functions may be affected. The presence and pattern of abnormalities allows localization of the lesion within the neuraxis.
Weakness caused by lesions in or near the motor cortex	• Accompanied by a gross clumsiness and lack of control of specific individual muscles not explainable by cerebellar ataxia or sensory loss. • Clumsiness disproportionate to weakness can suggest a cortical origin of weakness. • Reflexes are generally increased in the area of the weakness.
Weakness arising from spinal cord dysfunction	• Spinal cord lesions usually produce bilateral weakness though unilateral weakness can occur, especially with intraparenchymal lesions. • Spinal cord dysfunction is often suspected by its association with other signs of spinal cord dysfunction, such as bowel/bladder control changes, pinprick, and/or proprioceptive loss below a certain level, or in the case of a hemicord lesion, loss of pinprick sensation on the side opposite to that of the weakness. • Reflexes are normal above the level of the lesion and increased below the level of the lesion.
Lower Motor Neuron	**Lower Motor Neuron Lesions can Produce Weakness that is Focal or Generalized**
Weakness due to dysfunction of the anterior horn cell	• This usually is noted in the setting of motor neuron disease, and is relatively uncommon. • Suggestive features include: prominent fasciculations, atrophy, cramping, and variable changes in reflexes depending on the degree of associated involvement of upper motor neurons, such as seen in amyotrophic lateral sclerosis. • Although cramping is common, pain is usually absent. • The distribution of weakness is typically very asymmetric in onset and severity. Electrophysiologic testing with EMG is a helpful adjunct to the physical examination. • Reflexes are lost or decreased in proportion to the muscle weakness, in the absence of coexistent upper motor neuron dysfunction (as with ALS). • Electrophysiological testing with EMG is a helpful adjunct to the physical examination.

GENERAL PATTERNS OF WEAKNESS–cont'd	
Weakness due to injury or dysfunction in a specific spinal root	• This is quite common. • Nerve roots in the cervical and lumbar spine are frequently injured by herniated intervertebral discs. • This typically results in pain radiating in the distribution of the root and weakness in muscles supplied by the root. • Aggravation of pain by traction on the nerve root is frequent.
Peripheral Nerve	**Weakness Arising from Peripheral Nerve Lesions can be Focal, Multifocal, or Generalized**
Weakness due to focal lesions	• In the case of a focal, single nerve lesion, weakness is found only in the muscles supplied by that particular nerve, distal to the site of injury. • Sensory loss in the distribution of the affected nerve is quite helpful in confirming clinical suspicion of a focal nerve lesion. • Lesions of nerve plexuses can be extremely difficult to diagnose because of the complexity of neuroanatomy and varied presentations. Diagnostic clues gleaned from a carefully taken history combined with detailed electrophysiologic studies assist in making the appropriate diagnosis. In general, sensory, and motor dysfunction in a region of an arm or leg is noted, which does not conform to a pattern of radicular or peripheral nerve involvement.
Weakness due to multifocal lesions	• In multifocal peripheral nerve conditions, e.g., mononeuritis multiplex, multiple nerves are affected. This condition is asymmetric by definition. Sensory loss typically parallels loss of motor function with respect to the affected nerves.
Weakness due to generalized lesion	• Generalized peripheral neuropathy is a common cause of weakness. In the case of length-dependent axonal neuropathy, e.g., diabetic neuropathy, weakness is typically symmetric and worst distally, improving gradually as the examiner tests more proximal muscles. Reflexes are decreased or absent, more so distally than proximally. Painful dysesthesias and burning sensations accompanied by sensory loss more distally complete the clinical picture. Pain is usually moderate and more bothersome than the weakness. In the case of demyelinating neuropathy, weakness and sensory loss are typical, and pain is less common and often absent. Weakness and loss of reflex is typically worse distally than proximally.
Neuromuscular Junction	

- The hallmarks of weakness caused by neuromuscular junction dysfunction are variability and fatigability. The distribution of weakness is usually proximal greater than distal, often with prominent ocular and craniofacial weakness, including ptosis.
- There is no pain or sensory loss.
- Diaphragmatic weakness leading to respiratory failure can occur.
- Appendicular weakness is usually symmetric, and ocular muscle weakness is usually asymmetric.
- Exercise of weak muscles makes them even weaker and can be an important diagnostic clue. Reflexes are variably affected.

GENERAL PATTERNS OF WEAKNESS–cont'd
Muscle

- Weakness caused by muscle disease is typically of gradual onset and symmetric.
- Myalgia is variable.
- Weakness is usually worse proximally and reflex loss parallels the degree of weakness.
- Muscle cramps are less common than with motor neuron disease, and fasciculations are usually absent.

CUTANEOUS SENSATION ABNORMALITIES	
Types of abnormalities	• *Sensory loss*—decreased sensation to an appropriate stimulus • *Paresthesias*—abnormal spontaneous sensation, often described as a "pins-and-needles" sensation • *Dysesthesias*—similar to paresthesias, but due to touch or other stimuli. A form of misperception of a stimulus. • *Pain*—pain of neural origin can be burning, stinging, lancinating, or combinations of these. Burning pain is usually involving small-diameter nerve fibers. Stinging and lancinating pains are usually involving large-diameter nerve fibers.
Keys to diagnosis of sensory deficits	• Characterize the deficit. • Localize the deficit. • Determine what pathologies could produce this deficit.
Pearls of sensory localization	• Sensory loss of the entire side of the body is usually of thalamic origin. • Sensory loss over part of one limb is seldom of central origin, and suggests a peripheral neuropathic process. • Sensory loss that precisely splits the midline, including vibration, is usually nonphysiologic, i.e., not due to organic disease.

Tests to Diagnose Peripheral Sensory Deficits	
TEST	**UTILITY**
Nerve conduction study (NCS)	• Uses electrical stimuli to measure conduction velocities of motor and sensory nerves in the arms and legs • Most sensitive for detecting damage to the myelin sheath producing slowed or blocked conduction.
Electromyography (EMG)	• Uses needle electrodes to assess electrical properties of muscles • Most sensitive for detecting damage to the nerve axons or direct damage to the muscles as in myopathies
Magnetic resonance imaging (MRI)	• Performed on the arm or leg for identification of tumor or other mass lesion affecting a peripheral nerve • Performed on the head or spine for diagnosis of inflammatory, infiltrating, or vascular lesions of the brain, spinal cord, or nerve roots

Electromyography (EMG)

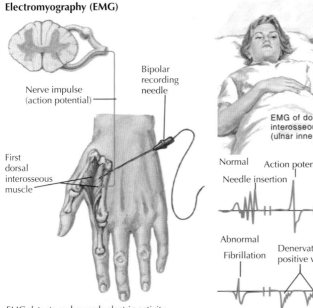

Nerve impulse (action potential)

Bipolar recording needle

First dorsal interosseous muscle

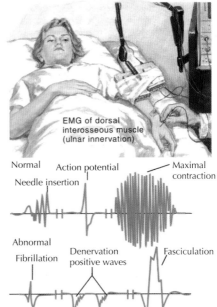

EMG of dorsal interosseous muscle (ulnar innervation)

Normal

Action potential

Needle insertion

Maximal contraction

Abnormal

Fibrillation

Denervation positive waves

Fasciculation

EMG detects and records electric activity or potentials within muscle in various phases of voluntary contraction

Compression–induced denervation produces abnormal spontaneous potentials

Nerve conduction studies

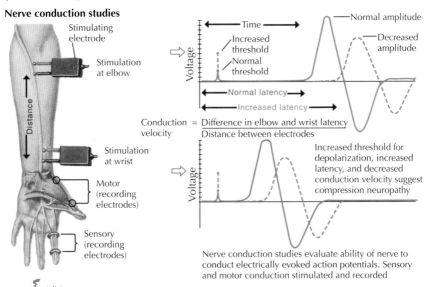

Stimulating electrode

Stimulation at elbow

Distance

Stimulation at wrist

Motor (recording electrodes)

Sensory (recording electrodes)

Time

Normal amplitude

Increased threshold

Decreased amplitude

Normal threshold

Normal latency

Increased latency

$$\text{Conduction velocity} = \frac{\text{Difference in elbow and wrist latency}}{\text{Distance between electrodes}}$$

Increased threshold for depolarization, increased latency, and decreased conduction velocity suggest compression neuropathy

Nerve conduction studies evaluate ability of nerve to conduct electrically evoked action potentials. Sensory and motor conduction stimulated and recorded

JOHN A. CRAIG—MD

IMPORTANT DISORDERS OF CUTANEOUS SENSATION		
Disorder	Features	Diagnosis
Median neuropathy–Carpal tunnel syndrome	• Loss of sensation and often pain on the median side of the palm • May be weakness of median-innervated muscles, including abductor pollicis brevis	• NCS shows slowed motor and/or sensory nerve conduction of the median nerve at the wrist. • EMG may show denervation of the abductor pollicis brevis.
Ulnar neuropathy–entrapment at the elbow	• Loss of sensation and often pain on the ulnar side of the hand, palmar and dorsal surface. • Weakness may be present in the ulnar-innervated intrinsic muscles of the hand, including interossei	• NCS shows slowed ulnar motor nerve conduction across the elbow. • EMG may show denervation present in the ulnar-innervated hand intrinsic muscles.
Hemisensory loss	• Loss of sensation and often pain on one entire side of the body • Usually due to thalamic damage from stroke or mass lesion	• MRI of the head is performed to look for thalamic lesion. If this is negative, the cervical spine should be studied.
Loss of sensation below a certain spinal level	• Loss of sensation beginning at a spinal level. At the interface between normal and abnormal sensation, there is a transition that often is not distinct. • Motor deficit and extensor plantar responses are common, but not invariable. • Hyper-reflexia below the lesion is common, even without weakness.	• MRI of the spine covering the level of the transition. If negative, MRI of the spine and brain above the transition may be warranted. If negative, LP may be needed to again, look for infection and multiple sclerosis.
Meralgia paresthetica–damage to the lateral femoral cutaneous nerve	• Loss of sensation on the lateral thigh, often with pain in the area • Pain with dysesthesias is often present. • No weakness or reflex abnormalities are present.	• This is a clinical diagnosis; tests play a limited role in diagnosis. • NCS can be done of this nerve, but is often technically difficult.

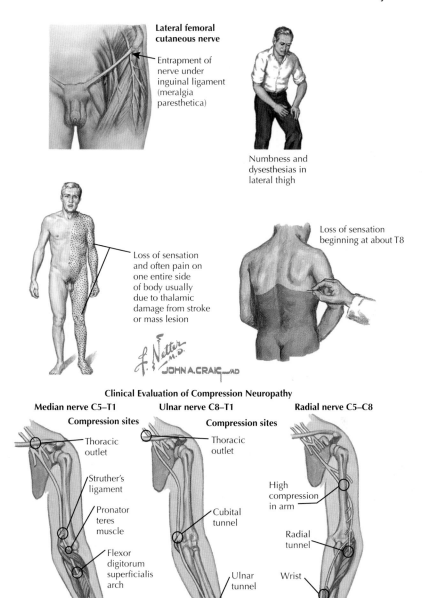

Lateral femoral cutaneous nerve

Entrapment of nerve under inguinal ligament (meralgia paresthetica)

Numbness and dysesthesias in lateral thigh

Loss of sensation and often pain on one entire side of body usually due to thalamic damage from stroke or mass lesion

Loss of sensation beginning at about T8

Clinical Evaluation of Compression Neuropathy

Median nerve C5–T1

Compression sites

Thoracic outlet

Struther's ligament

Pronator teres muscle

Flexor digitorum superficialis arch

Carpal tunnel

Sensory distribution

Ulnar nerve C8–T1

Compression sites

Thoracic outlet

Cubital tunnel

Ulnar tunnel

Sensory distribution

Radial nerve C5–C8

High compression in arm

Radial tunnel

Wrist

Sensory distribution

Motor and sensory functions of each nerve assessed individually throughout entire upper extremity to delineate level of compression or entrapment

Carpal Tunnel Syndrome

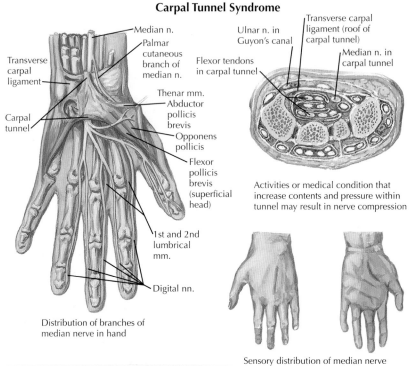

Median n.

Palmar cutaneous branch of median n.

Transverse carpal ligament

Carpal tunnel

Thenar mm.
Abductor pollicis brevis
Opponens pollicis
Flexor pollicis brevis (superficial head)

1st and 2nd lumbrical mm.

Digital nn.

Ulnar n. in Guyon's canal

Transverse carpal ligament (roof of carpal tunnel)

Flexor tendons in carpal tunnel

Median n. in carpal tunnel

Activities or medical condition that increase contents and pressure within tunnel may result in nerve compression

Distribution of branches of median nerve in hand

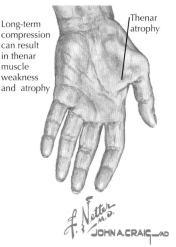

Sensory distribution of median nerve

Long-term compression can result in thenar muscle weakness and atrophy

Thenar atrophy

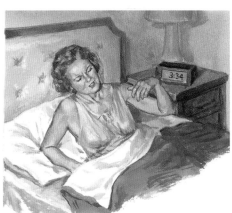

Patient awakened by tingling, pain, or both in sensory distribution of median nerve

Sensation: Cutaneous Sensory Deficit

VISION DEFICITS	
Types of abnormalities	• Visual loss in part or all of one field • Unilateral or bilateral deficits
Keys to localization	• Loss of vision in one eye suggests a lesion of the optic nerve. • Congruous visual field defect of both eyes suggests a lesion behind the optic chiasm in the occipital cortex or radiations. • Incongruous visual field losses in the two eyes suggest a lesion at or near the optic chiasm; this includes bitemporal and binasal hemianopias.
Visual Finding	**Lesion Localization**
Loss of vision in one eye	Lesion of the optic nerve
Congruous visual loss in both eyes	Lesion behind the optic chiasm
Incongruous visual loss in both eyes	Lesion near or at the optic chiasm
Bitemporal hemianopia	Chiasmal lesion
Binasal hemianopia	Chiasmal or perichiasmal lesion
Macular sparing homonymous hemianopia	Occipital lobe sparing the occipital pole, typical of PCA infarct
Superior quadrant defect	Temporal lobe, affecting Meyer's loop
Inferior quadrant defect	Parietal lobe, affecting optic radiations

IMPORTANT CAUSES OF VISUAL FIELD LOSS		
Disorder	**Clinical Features**	**Diagnosis**
Optic neuritis	• Loss of vision in one or both eyes • Can occur as an isolated entity or as part of multiple sclerosis	• MRI • LP
Temporal arteritis	Temporal headache may lead to unilateral or bilateral visual loss	• Elevated ESR • Temporal artery biopsy may show inflammation.
MCA infarction	• Homonymous hemianopia • Usually hemiparesis	• CT is performed urgently. • MRI is more sensitive for acute ischemia.
PCA infarction	Homonymous hemianopia, sparing the macula, which is supplied by the MCA	• CT is performed urgently. • MRI is more sensitive for acute ischemia.
Pituitary tumor	Junctional scotoma—incongruous visual field loss	• MRI

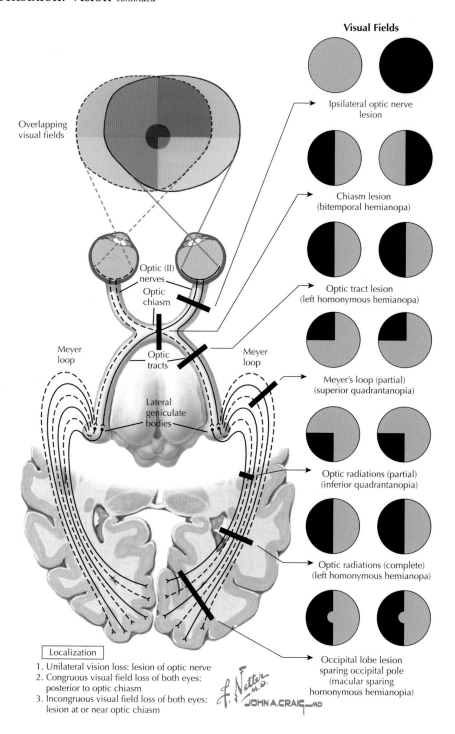

Visual Fields

Overlapping visual fields

Ipsilateral optic nerve lesion

Chiasm lesion (bitemporal hemianopa)

Optic tract lesion (left homonymous hemianopa)

Optic (II) nerves

Optic chiasm

Meyer loop

Optic tracts

Meyer loop

Meyer's loop (partial) (superior quadrantanopia)

Lateral geniculate bodies

Optic radiations (partial) (inferior quadrantanopia)

Optic radiations (complete) (left homonymous hemianopa)

Occipital lobe lesion sparing occipital pole (macular sparing homonymous hemianopia)

Localization
1. Unilateral vision loss: lesion of optic nerve
2. Congruous visual field loss of both eyes: posterior to optic chiasm
3. Incongruous visual field loss of both eyes: lesion at or near optic chiasm

JOHN A. CRAIG—AD

DIAGNOSIS OF TREMOR		
Types of tremor	• Essential tremor • Parkinsonism • Physiologic tremor • Cerebellar tremor	
Clinical Entities	**Clinical Features**	**Diagnosis**
Essential tremor	• Tremor at 5–8 Hz, with action affecting • No tremor at rest	• Diagnosed by clinical features • Otherwise normal exam
Parkinsonism	• Tremor at 4–5 Hz, most prominent at rest • Associated rigidity, bradykinesia, and loss of postural reflexes	• Diagnosed by clinical features • Associated motor and gait findings
Physiologic tremor	• Tremor with action and posture, exacerbated by hyperadrenergic states	• Diagnosed by clinical features
Cerebellar tremor	• Tremor at about 3 Hz with action • Associated with other signs of cerebellar dysfunction • Tremor is most prominent as the limb approaches the target.	• Diagnosed by clinical features • MRI to look for tumors, infarction, other lesions of the cerebellum • Genetic testing may be needed for cerebellar ataxias.

Parkinsonism

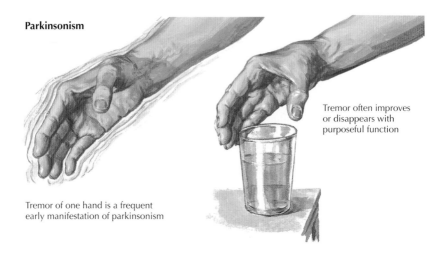

Tremor often improves or disappears with purposeful function

Tremor of one hand is a frequent early manifestation of parkinsonism

Rest Tremor

Usually called parkinsonian tremor, occurs in a limb that is not voluntarily activated. It is suppressed with voluntary movement. It may appear as "pill rolling."

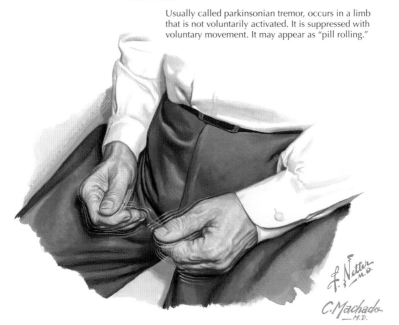

DIAGNOSIS OF RIGIDITY AND STIFFNESS		
Types of rigidity	• Extrapyramidal akinetic syndromes • Spasticity • Syndromes of continuous muscle fiber activity	
Syndromes	**Clinical Features**	**Causes**
Extrapyramidal akinetic syndromes	• Increased tone in both extensor and flexor muscles • Cogwheel rigidity—a stop/go to passive limb movement	• Parkinson's disease • Other parkinsonian syndromes, including PSP, MSA, and striatonigral degeneration • Drug-induced parkinsonism • Vascular parkinsonism
Spasticity	• Rigidity, especially of extensor and antigravity muscles • Other signs of corticospinal tract dysfunction, including hyperreflexia and extensor plantar responses	• Stroke • Multiple sclerosis • B_{12} deficiency and other metabolic dysfunctions • Spinal cord damage from any cause
Syndrome of continuous muscle fiber activity	• Rare conditions producing stiffness that is of lower motor neuron or other peripheral cause • Not a central lesion • Stiffness of the muscles without other sign of corticospinal or extrapyramidal dysfunction	• Stiff person syndrome • Neuromyotonia (Isaac's syndrome)

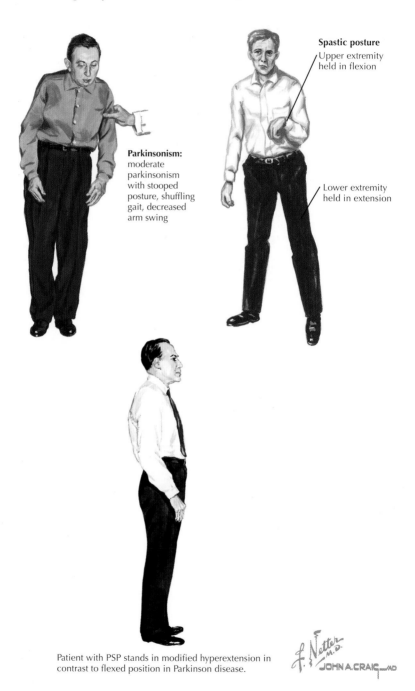

Parkinsonism: moderate parkinsonism with stooped posture, shuffling gait, decreased arm swing

Spastic posture
Upper extremity held in flexion

Lower extremity held in extension

Patient with PSP stands in modified hyperextension in contrast to flexed position in Parkinson disease.

HYPERKINETIC DISORDERS: DYKINESIAS (ATHETOSIS, CHOREA) BALLISM, AND DYSTONIA	

Definition	Hyperkinetic disorders are characterized by excessive movement.
	
	 • Dyskinesia is the global term referring to certain types of involuntary movements, except tremor. Two forms are athetosis and chorea:
	
	  • Athetosis is a writhing movement.
	
	  • Chorea is a rapid movement.
	
	 • Ballism is violent flinging movement.
	
	 • Dystonia is an abnormal posture created by contraction of muscle groups.

Presentation	Clinical Findings	Diagnostic Possibilities
Dyskinesias	• Repetitive movements which are typically stereotyped. May involve face (orobuccal dyskinesia), legs, or arms. • Differs from chorea in that the movements are not random with somewhat of a rhythm.	• Tardive dyskinesia is seen especially with neuroleptic use. • Parkinson's disease patients may develop dyskinesias with dopaminergic therapy.
Athetosis	• Slow, writhing involuntary movements • A form of dyskinesia	• Structural lesions of the basal ganglia, including infarction, tumor, infections, and vascular malformations
Chorea	• Rapid involuntary movements • A form of dyskinesia	• Similar as for athetosis • Huntington's disease
Ballism	• Violent, flinging movements of usually one side • Considered a type of chorea	• Damage to the subthalamic nucleus, usually infarction • Hemorrhage, tumor, and infections are possible causes.
Dystonia	• Action-induced dystonia is posturing and writhing movements induced by movement. • Dystonia at rest may involve neck muscles or limbs.	• Idiopathic • Inherited • Drugs, especially dopaminergic agents for parkinsonism, some anticonvulsants, and calcium-channel blockers

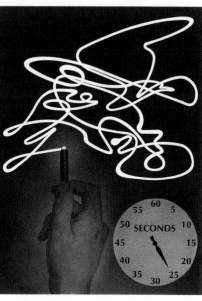

Huntington disease
Middle-aged person; mental deterioration, grimacing, choreiform movements

Sydenham chorea: spontaneous uncoordinated movements demonstrated by electric penlight held in patient's hand

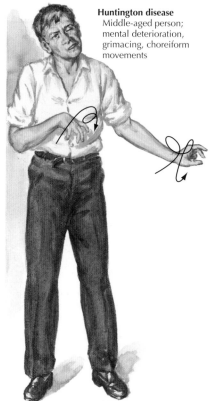

Untreated torticollis in 12-year-old boy. Thick, fibrotic, tendon-like bands have replaced sternocleidomastoid muscle, making head appear tethered to clavicle. Two heads of left sternocleidomastoid muscle prominent

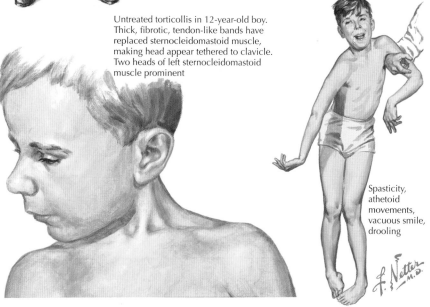

Spasticity, athetoid movements, vacuous smile, drooling

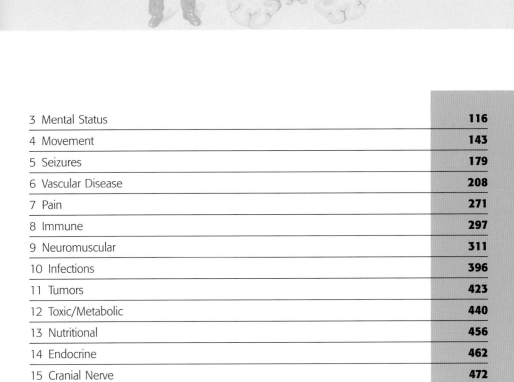

Disorders

DEMENTIA OVERVIEW	

Common features of dementia	• Memory loss of at least 6 months duration
	• Other cognitive difficulty, including any of:
	  • Aphasia, usually incomplete
	  • Spatial disorientation
	  • Calculation difficulty

Findings that suggests a specific diagnosis	• *No noncognitive symptoms or signs*: Alzheimer's disease (AD) > frontotemporal disease (FTD), pseudodementia, mild cognitive impairment (MCI) • *Parkinsonism*: dementia with Lewy bodies (DLB) > NPH > VaD • *Disinhibition, obsessive-compulsive behavior*: FTD • *Ataxia, urinary incontinence*: normal pressure hydrocephalus (NPH) > VaD • *Depression*: Pseudodementia > AD, FTD > DLB • *Focal or multifocal neurologic deficits*: VaD
Test	**Diagnostic Implications**
Neuropsych testing	• Performed when needed to differentiate cognitive changes with aging, pseudodementia, cortical dementia (e.g., AD), or subcortical dementia (DLB)
MRI brain	• Imaging study-of-choice for most patients. Can show mass lesions, infarctions (VaD), regional atrophy (FTD) or general (AD) atrophy, or hydrocephalus (NPH).
CT brain	• Performed if MRI cannot be done. Can show major infarctions (VaD), hydrocephalus (NPH), or most mass lesions.
PET scan	• Can show regional changes typical of AD, FTD, VaD, but may be normal early in the disease
Electroencephalogram (EEG)	• Seldom needed for dementia, only if prion disease or seizure is suspected
Lumbar Puncture	• Seldom needed for dementia, only if infection or NPH is suspected
Labs	• Can identify thyroid disorder, B_{12} deficiency, vascular risk factors, or metabolic abnormalities

Diagnosis	Summary of Features
Cognitive changes with aging	• Normal aging produces changes in recall, multitasking, language, and access time. Studies are normal including neuropsych testing.
Mild cognitive impairment (MCI)	• Memory and cognitive changes that do not meet criteria for dementia • Many of these patients progress to dementia, usually AD.
Pseudodementia	• Cognitive changes due to depression or anxiety, superimposed on cognitive changes with aging • Diagnosed by neuropsych testing. Other studies are normal.
Alzheimer's disease (AD)	• Cognitive deficit without other signs is usually AD. Can be sporadic or familial. • Imaging shows atrophy or is normal. Neuropsych testing shows cortical deficit.
Frontotemporal dementia (FTD)	• Dementia with frontal lobe findings including obsessive and compulsive features, disinhibition • Differentiated by neuropsych testing. Positron emission tomography (PET) scan can also differentiate. MRI may show regional atrophy suggesting the diagnosis.
Dementia with Lewy Bodies (DLB)	• Parkinsonism plus dementia. Can look like the combination of AD and PD, but is neither. • Essentially equivalent to the dementia that can develop later with Parkinson's disease (PD).
Vascular dementia (VaD)	• Focal or multifocal infarctions can produce dementia, which can advance in a stepwise fashion or progressively.
Normal pressure hydrocephalus (NPH)	• The triad is dementia, ataxia, and urinary incontinence, although all three are not always present. • Suspected when CT or MRI shows ventriculomegaly. Confirmation is required.

ALZHEIMER'S DISEASE (AD)	
Description	• Degenerative disease characterized by progressive dementia, with other neurologic functions being relatively unaffected • Most common cause of dementia
Pathophysiology	• Neurodegenerative disease with probable genetic and environmental contributions • Cholinergic projections from the substantia innominata are particularly affected, although other neurons and other transmitter systems are affected as well.
Clinical findings	• Memory loss with other signs of cognitive dysfunction. Errors in short-term memory, calculations, judgment, construction, or other spheres are typical. • Motor, coordination, gait, and reflex functions are normal, at least during the mild-to-moderate stages.
Laboratory studies	• MRI and CT are normal or only show atrophy. PET may show biparietal hypometabolism, but is rarely done. • LP is normal, but rarely done. LP is indicated if the patient has signs of infection or demyelination or a brief duration of cognitive difficulty. • Laboratory studies are normal, including CMP, CBC, B_{12}, folate, ANA, ESR, TSH, and FT4.
Diagnosis	• Clinical diagnosis is based on dementia without other causes having been identified. • Imaging and labs do not show another cause for the dementia. • PET scan may show classic findings, but is not always positive, and is seldom needed.
Differential diagnosis	• *Frontotemporal dementia and other degenerative dementias.* Presence of motor or prominent behavioral deficits suggests these. • *Vascular dementia.* Focal or multifocal deficits and imaging findings of multiple infarctions suggests this diagnosis. • *Mild cognitive impairment.* Neuropsych testing is diagnostic. • *Pseudodementia.* Neuropsych testing is diagnostic. • *Cognitive changes with aging.* Neuropsych testing is diagnostic.
Management	• Cholinesterase inhibitors improve cognition and behavior for many patients. They may have some neuroprotective effect on slowing degeneration, but this is not proved. This is mainly for patients with mild to moderate disease. These agents include donepezil, rivastigmine, and galantamine. • Memantine is an NMDA receptor antagonist that improves cognition and behavior for some patients with moderate to severe disease. • Neuroleptics are occasionally needed for patients with psychosis, although cholinesterase inhibitors can also help. • Antidepressants are often used for coexistent depression, and they can also help with behavioral difficulties. Selective serotonin reuptake inhibitors (SSRIs) are most commonly used.

ALZHEIMER'S DISEASE (AD)—cont'd	
Management *cont'd*	• Benzodiazepines are occasionally used for agitation, but can exacerbate cognitive difficulty.
Clinical course	• Progressive decline is expected over years. • Total care is inevitable unless the patient succumbs to some other illness.

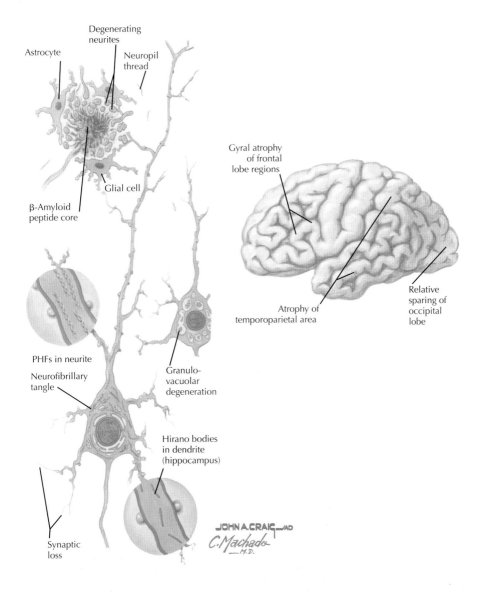

Degenerating neurites

Astrocyte

Neuropil thread

Gyral atrophy of frontal lobe regions

Glial cell

β-Amyloid peptide core

Relative sparing of occipital lobe

Atrophy of temporoparietal area

PHFs in neurite

Neurofibrillary tangle

Granulo-vacuolar degeneration

Hirano bodies in dendrite (hippocampus)

JOHN A. CRAIG—AD
C. Machado
—M.D.

Synaptic loss

MILD COGNITIVE IMPAIRMENT (MCI)	
Description	• Memory loss, but does not meet the criteria for dementia
	• Leads to dementia in many patients, but not all. The type of dementia is usually AD.
Pathophysiology	• Mild memory difficulty due to aging changes plus the possibility of incipient degeneration
Clinical findings	• Memory loss that is out of the ordinary for age
	• Normal motor, coordination, and gait examinations
Laboratory studies	• Labs include chemistries, CBC, B_{12}, thyroid functions, and are usually normal.
	• MRI or CT is normal.
	• Neuropsychologic testing is often needed and is diagnostic.
Diagnosis	• Clinical findings of memory loss, but without meeting the criteria for dementia
	• Neuropsych testing usually confirms this diagnosis when a patient is being evaluated for dementia versus cognitive changes due to aging.
Differential diagnosis	• *AD and other dementias.* Criteria for dementia are not met with MCI, although patients may ultimately progress to one of these disorders.
	• *Depression/pseudodementia.* Memory difficulty is due to affective disturbance, rather than organic dementia. Neuropsych testing can be diagnostic.
	• *Cognitive changes with aging* (see next table)
	• *Baseline low intellectual function.* Neuropsych testing is diagnostic.
Management	• Cholinesterase inhibitors and vitamin supplementation are used by some, but effectiveness in reducing progression to dementia is not proven.
	• Follow-up evaluation is needed to see if the patient progresses to dementia.
	• Vascular risk-factor reduction may reduce progression to frank dementia.
Clinical course	• Some patients progress to dementia, usually AD.
	• The percentage is debatable, between 30%–70%.

COGNITIVE CHANGES WITH AGING	
Description	• This is not a disorder, but rather the normal cognitive changes that occur through middle and senior years. • Patients may notice these changes and ask to be evaluated for dementia.
Pathophysiology	• Normal aging. There is neuronal loss over years. • Cognitive changes evolve over decades, which is somewhat counterbalanced by the increased database gained through lifelong learning.
Clinical findings	• Alterations in concentration, multitasking, and naming are especially affected. • Access time for information increases with advancing age.
Laboratory studies	• Normal, but usually are not needed • Imaging is normal or shows age-appropriate atrophy. • Neuropsych testing is often needed.
Diagnosis	• Neuropsych testing is performed for patients concerned about memory and often shows no dementia, but rather cognitive changes with aging. When this is seen, further diagnostic testing is not needed.
Management	• Reassurance is important. • Patient should be seen for follow-up to determine if they progress to dementia.
Clinical course	There is no greater chance for these patients to develop dementia than there is for the general population, but because dementia is common, a subset of these patients will eventually deteriorate.

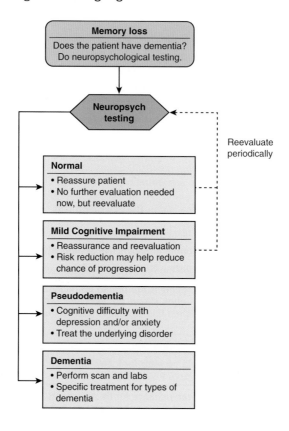

Memory loss

Does the patient have dementia?
Do neuropsychological testing.

Neuropsych testing

Reevaluate periodically

Normal
- Reassure patient
- No further evaluation needed now, but reevaluate

Mild Cognitive Impairment
- Reassurance and reevaluation
- Risk reduction may help reduce chance of progression

Pseudodementia
- Cognitive difficulty with depression and/or anxiety
- Treat the underlying disorder

Dementia
- Perform scan and labs
- Specific treatment for types of dementia

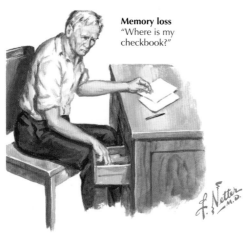

Memory loss
"Where is my checkbook?"

DEMENTIA WITH LEWY BODIES (DLB)	
Description	• Dementia with parkinsonism is the most common presentation. • Clinically appears to be the combination of Parkinson's disease (PD) plus AD, but it is neither.
Pathophysiology	• Neurodegenerative disease with cortical and subcortical degeneration • Some overlap with AD in pathology. Lewy bodies are seen in the cerebral cortex.
Clinical findings	• Dementia, plus signs of parkinsonism • Psychosis is common. • Parkinsonism is indistinguishable from PD, and includes tremor, rigidity, bradykinesia, and loss of postural reflexes. Gait is shuffling and posture is stooped.
Laboratory studies	• CT and MRI are normal or show atrophy. • Routine laboratory studies are normal.
Diagnosis	Criteria include dementia along with two of the following three clinical findings: • Fluctuating cognition or level of consciousness • Visual hallucinations • Parkinsonian motor signs • Often has psychosis, delusions, or hallucinations early in the course
Differential diagnosis	• *Alzheimer's disease.* Lacks the gait and motor deficit. • *Parkinson's disease.* Lacks dementia, although there may be mild cognitive changes. • *Normal pressure hydrocephalus.* Ataxia and dementia, but without rigidity and cogwheeling. Imaging shows increased ventricular size.
Management	• Cognitive dysfunction is treated with cholinesterase inhibitors. • Psychotic features are treated with atypical neuroleptics. • Parkinsonism treatment same as for PD, but dopaminergic treatment may exacerbate the psychotic features.
Clinical course	• Progressive deterioration is expected. Cholinesterase inhibitors can help the cognitive dysfunction, and dopaminergic agents can improve the movement disorder, but worsening is inevitable over years. • Psychotic features can make use of dopaminergic agents difficult. Atypical neuroleptics may be needed.

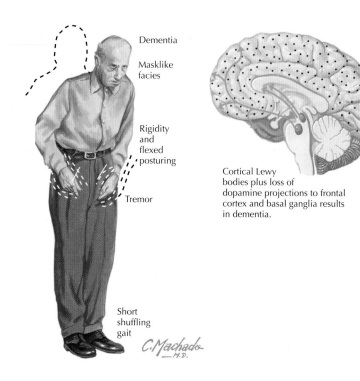

Dementia

Masklike facies

Rigidity and flexed posturing

Tremor

Short shuffling gait

Cortical Lewy bodies plus loss of dopamine projections to frontal cortex and basal ganglia results in dementia.

FRONTOTEMPORAL DEMENTIA (FTD)	
Description	• Group of degenerative diseases with involvement of both frontal lobes • Temporal lobe involvement may be asymmetric. • Pick's disease is the prototypic disorder. • Primary progressive aphasia (PPA) is a less common subset of FTD.
Pathophysiology	• Neurodegenerative disease with involvement of bilateral frontal lobes and temporal lobes • Specific neuropathology depends on the entity. Pick's disease is characterized by argentophilic neuronal inclusions (Pick bodies) • Some cases are inherited and may be related to chromosome 17.
Clinical findings	• Behavioral disorder and dementia • Disinhibition and overactivity indicative of frontal lobe dysfunction. Inappropriate sexuality often is seen. Occasionally, withdrawn and apathetic behavior is seen early. • Progresses to apathy and muteness • PPA initially presents with language difficulty, with other cognitive deficits developing later.
Laboratory studies	• Lab and cerebrospinal fluid (CSF) are normal. • MRI and CT may show frontal and temporal lobe atrophy with cortical predominance. • PET may show specific hypometabolism in the frontal and temporal regions.
Diagnosis	• Clinical features of behavioral and cognitive changes with atrophy in frontal and temporal distribution • May be misdiagnosed as AD. FTD is much less common and has prominent behavioral abnormalities earlier than in AD. • Neuropsych testing can aid differentiation. • Speech pathololgy evaluation can help with diagnosis of PPA.
Differential diagnosis	• *Alzheimer's disease.* Dementia, but with less behavioral change exhibited. • *Vascular dementia.* Dementia with multifocal neurologic deficits, including motor deficits, not expected with FTD. • *Normal pressure hydrocephalus.* Dementia with frontal lobe signs can develop. The ataxia and incontinence argue against FTD. Imaging differentiates these.
Management	• There are no medicines that have been proven effective for functional improvement of FTD or PPA. • SSRIs are effective medications for some of the obsessive and depressive symptoms. • Atypical neuroleptics also are used for behavioral abnormalities. • Cholinesterase inhibitors are of little value, although an occasional patient may respond.
Clinical course	• Progressive deterioration is expected; however, improvement in behavior can occur with SSRIs. • Treatment does not stop the degeneration. • PPA progresses to muteness. Cognitive changes appear to develop, although cognitive testing in the presence of marked language deficit is difficult.

Lobar Dementias

Frontotemporal dementias (FTDs)

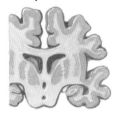

Atrophy of frontal and/or
temporal areas

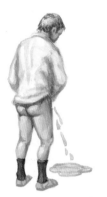

Bizarre, uninhibited
socially inappropriate
behavior

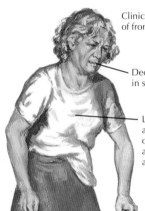

Clinical features
of frontal lobe variant

Decrease
in speech

Loss of
awareness
of personal
appearance
and hygiene

Oral fixation:
increased eating
causes weight
gain

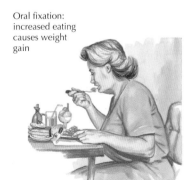

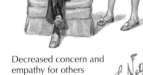

Decreased concern and
empathy for others

VASCULAR DEMENTIA (VAD)	
Description	• Progressive or stepwise dementia due to multiple infarctions • Vascular changes may precipitate a degenerative cascade, which can look like a degenerative dementia.
Pathophysiology	• Multiple infarctions affecting cortical and/or subcortical regions • Progressive deterioration in cognitive and other neurologic functions
Clinical findings	• Progressive dementia, often with stepwise worsening • Patients almost always have vascular risk factors. • Motor and coordination deficits are seen in addition to the cognitive changes. • This usually is a subcortical dementia, meaning that the pathology affects subcortical white matter, as opposed to AD, which is a cortical dementia.
Laboratory studies	• CT and MRI show multiple infarcts, which may be cortical or subcortical. • Labs are usually normal. Vascular risk factors may be identified on labs, such as hyperlipidemia, homocysteinemia, elevated CRP, or antiphospholipid antibody. These studies are performed on patients with suspected vascular dementia. • Vascular imaging may be needed, including carotid and cardiac ultrasound, to look for a source of the multiple infarctions.
Diagnosis	• Based on dementia with subcortical features plus signs of CNS and/or non-CNS vascular disease • Imaging shows multiple infarctions. Note that MRI in elderly and some middle-aged patients may show multiple abnormalities on T2 and FLAIR imaging that look like microinfarcts, but these are not always relevant, and do not, by themselves, make the diagnosis of vascular dementia.
Differential diagnosis	• *Alzheimer's disease.* Dementia without focal findings, including motor or gait deficits. Neuropsych testing results usually suggest cortical dementia. • *Frontotemporal dementia.* Dementia without focal findings, including motor and gait. Imaging differentiates, showing lobar atrophy rather than multifocal infarctions. • *Normal pressure hydrocephalus.* Dementia with ataxia and incontinence is a typical triad. Imaging shows increased ventricular size rather than global atrophy. Cisternography usually differentiates as well. • *Brain tumor.* Confusion with headache and papilledema are common. Onset is faster than with VaD. Imaging shows mass lesion.
Management	• Cholinesterase inhibitors may be helpful for treatment of the cognitive decline. • Neuroleptics occasionally are needed for behavioral changes. • Antithrombotic therapy and risk reduction often are used in an attempt to slow progression. • Vitamin supplementation occasionally is used, although evidence of effectiveness is incomplete.

VASCULAR DEMENTIA (VAD)—cont'd	
Clinical course	• Progressive decline is expected. • Progression may be slowed by controlling vascular risk factors. • Risk of non-neurologic vascular events is increased, including MI and PAD.

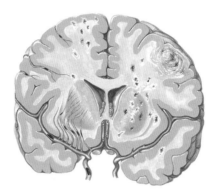

Cerebrovascular disease results in multiple small cortical and subcortical infarcts.

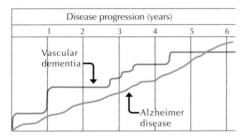

Clinical progression. Vascular dementia exhibits abrupt onset and stepwise progression in contrast to gradual onset and progression of Alzheimer disease.

NORMAL PRESSURE HYDROCEPHALUS (NPH)	
Description	• Disorder of CSF circulation resulting in a triad of dementia, ataxia, and incontinence • Not all elements of the triad are apparent.
Pathophysiology	• Progressive increase in ventricular size • Cause usually is not known. Increased CSF pressure may produce increased ventricular size, which is then compensated with reduction in CSF pressure to the normal range.
Clinical findings	• Gait difficulty typically develops first, followed by dementia, then urinary incontinence. • No focal neurologic deficits are seen.
Laboratory studies	• Routine labs are normal. • CT and MRI show increased ventricular size out of proportion to cortical atrophy.
Diagnosis	• CT and MRI findings must exist to suggest the diagnosis, although these imaging studies are not confirmatory. • Radionucleotide cisternography shows reflux of tracer into the ventricles. • Removal of CSF may result in clinical improvement, which can be helpful diagnostically. • Laboratory studies for other reversible causes are negative.
Differential diagnosis	• *Alzheimer's disease.* Progressive dementia without ataxia. • *Frontotemporal dementia.* Progressive dementia with disinhibition and other frontal lobe signs. Ataxia is not expected early in the disease. • *Vascular dementia.* Dementia with stepwise progression. Multifocal findings on exam. Imaging shows multifocal infarctions, rather than ventriculomegaly as seen with NPH. • *Parkinson's disease.* Memory deficit is common with PD, and progresses to dementia in some. Stooped posture, rigidity, bradykinesia, and tremor suggest PD rather than NPH.
Management	• Placement of shunt to drain CSF into the peritoneal cavity can result in clinical improvement in dementia and ataxia. • LP with CSF drainage can produce short-term improvement, but is not a long-term solution.
Clinical course	• Without treatment, progression is expected. • With treatment, most patients show some improvement, but patients do not become normal. • Complications of shunting have to be considered, including stroke, hemorrhage, seizures, and infection. Shunts may require revision.

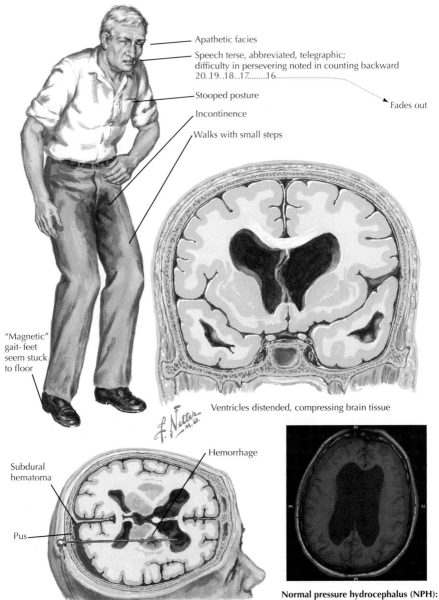

Apathetic facies

Speech terse, abbreviated, telegraphic; difficulty in persevering noted in counting backward 20.19..18..17.......16............

Fades out

Stooped posture

Incontinence

Walks with small steps

"Magnetic" gait- feet seem stuck to floor

Ventricles distended, compressing brain tissue

Hemorrhage

Subdural hematoma

Pus

Shunting may reduce size of ventricles and relieve symptoms but may cause hemorrhage along cannula tract, brain edema, subdural hematoma, and infection

Normal pressure hydrocephalus (NPH): The triad is dementia, ataxia, and urinary incontinence, though not all patients have all symptoms. Diagnosis is suspected by increased ventricular size on CT or MRI

TRANSIENT GLOBAL AMNESIA (TGA)	
Description	• Episodic loss of memory without other neurologic deficits • Deficit is not attributable to TIA, seizure, or migraine.
Pathophysiology	• Unknown. May be related to migraine, vascular insufficiency without occlusion, or regional suppression of electrical activity.
Clinical findings	• Occurs in middle-aged or elderly. Presents with loss of memory for several hours to 24 hours. • During the episode, patient has both anterograde and retrograde memory loss, often repeating questions and demonstrating persistent disorientation. • Complete recovery of memory is expected, but the patient is amnesic for much of the time of the transient amnesia. • Examination shows no language or other neurologic deficit during or after the episode—only memory loss during the event.
Laboratory studies	• MRI is normal with TGA. This is in contrast to transient ischemic attack (TIA), where up to 40% of patients will show abnormalities on diffusion-weighted imaging. • Routine laboratory studies are normal. B_{12} level and thyroid function tests are commonly ordered. • Vascular imaging studies are indicated if TIA is considered, but is seldom needed for patients with classic TGA.
Diagnosis	Clinical diagnosis, with a number of pertinent negatives, including: • No neurologic deficits on exam • No language difficulty—only the content was abnormal • No abnormalities on imaging or lab
Differential diagnosis	• *Transient ischemic attack.* Episodic neurologic deficit that can be motor, sensory, or language. Confusion in the absence of other signs is unlikely to be TIA. • *Seizure.* Episodic loss of awareness or major motor activity. The level of functioning is much lower during a seizure than TGA. • *Migraine.* Confusion can develop at the onset in a patient with migraine. However, this tends to occur in younger patients and is associated with headache. • *Psychogenic amnesia.* Inconsistencies in mental status testing argue in favor of a psychogenic cause for the amnesia. Psychological testing may be needed.
Management	• No treatment is needed for most patients. • Patients with vascular risk factors who could have had a TIA should be treated appropriately, including antithrombotic agents and other risk reduction as indicated.
Clinical course	• TGA does not recur in most patients. • In those occasional patients with recurrent TGA, there may be an increased likelihood for persistent cerebral ischemic disease or dementia.

Amnesia

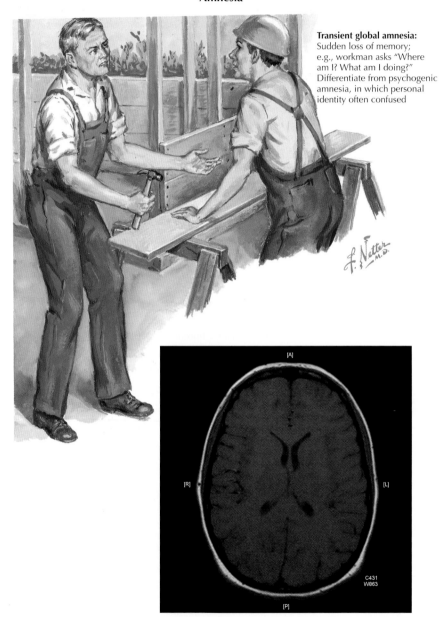

Transient global amnesia:
Sudden loss of memory;
e.g., workman asks "Where
am I? What am I doing?"
Differentiate from psychogenic
amnesia, in which personal
identity often confused

Transient global amnesia:
Loss of memory for up to 24 hours which is not due to infarction
or hemorrhage. The patient has no focal deficits during the episode,
so the cognitive deficit may not be immediately obvious to coworkers.
This patient has forgotten his task and purpose. The MRI of the brain
is normal.

METABOLIC ENCEPHALOPATHY	
Description	Mental status change due to abnormalities in electrolytes, sugar, or other metabolic disorder

Pathophysiology	• Multiple metabolic abnormalities can cause encephalopathy.
	• Often, there are multiple simultaneous abnormalities.
	• Common causes are:
	  • Renal failure
	  • Hepatic failure
	  • Fluid-electrolyte disorder

Clinical findings	• Confusion, with behavioral abnormalities including agitation, apathy, and symptoms of delirium • No focal findings are seen.

Laboratory studies	• Multiple causes can be identified on lab testing. Some of the abnormalities are:
	  • Sodium ↑ or ↓
	  • Glucose ↑ or ↓
	  • Ammonia ↑
	  • Carbon dioxide ↑ (especially in patients with chronic obstructive pulmonary disease [COPD])
	  • Calcium ↑

Diagnosis	• Measurement of multiple metabolic parameters is performed for patients with encephalopathy of unknown cause. • Imaging with MRI or CT often is performed.
Differential diagnosis	• *Stroke.* Infarction can produce mental status change, but usually with focal findings. PCA infarction can produce mental status change with hemianopia, which could be missed on examination. No paralysis develops. • *Intracerebral hematoma.* Hemorrhage is more likely in some patients with metabolic derangements, especially renal and hepatic failure. • *CNS infection.* Patients at risk for metabolic encephalopathy also are often predisposed to meningitis or encephalitis, and these need to be considered. Patients with marked encephalopathy may not show meningeal signs. Fever and increased white blood cells are not always present.
Management	• Management of the metabolic derangement • Avoidance of drugs that could contribute to the encephalopathy
Clinical course	• Improvement is expected when the metabolic derangement is treated. • Recurrence is common in patients who are susceptible to metabolic encephalopathy, especially those with hepatic and renal insufficiency.

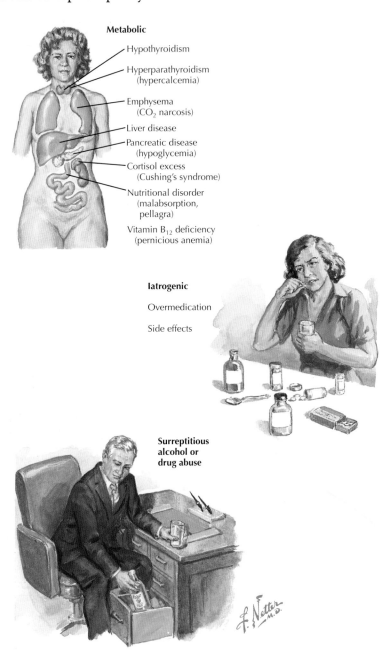

Metabolic

Hypothyroidism

Hyperparathyroidism
(hypercalcemia)

Emphysema
(CO_2 narcosis)

Liver disease

Pancreatic disease
(hypoglycemia)

Cortisol excess
(Cushing's syndrome)

Nutritional disorder
(malabsorption,
pellagra)

Vitamin B_{12} deficiency
(pernicious anemia)

Iatrogenic

Overmedication

Side effects

**Surreptitious
alcohol or
drug abuse**

WERNICKE'S ENCEPHALOPATHY	
Description	Neurologic symptoms of confusion, ataxia, and ocular motor defects due thiamine deficiency
Pathophysiology	• Thiamine deficiency is most commonly seen in malnourished alcoholics. • Patients with AIDS and cancer are also at risk for Wernicke's encephalopathy.

Clinical findings	Ocular motor deficits are important diagnostically and include:
	  • Horizontal nystagmus
	  • Defective abduction of either eye
	  • Mental status changes, including confusion and agitation.
	  • Ataxia affects gait more than limbs.

Laboratory studies	• Laboratory studies are nondiagnostic. However, patients with Wernicke's are more likely to have electrolyte derangements and hepatic failure. • Imaging is normal, but should be done to look for tumor, infection, hemorrhage, and infarction. • LP may be needed to look for chronic infection.
Diagnosis	• Clinical findings. There are no diagnostic lab tests. • Imaging and routine labs are performed to look for other diagnoses.
Differential diagnosis	• *Infections.* Chronic meningitis or encephalitis should be considered. • *Subdural hematoma.* Hemorrhage can present with all of the findings of Wernicke's encephalopathy without other focal signs.
Management	• Thiamine replacement • Nutritional supplementation • Magnesium administration often is needed. • Patients should be encouraged to use services that could help to prevent recurrence, including drug and alcohol rehabilitation programs, e.g., Alcoholics Anonymous.
Clinical course	• Many patients with Wernicke's encephalopathy progress to Korsakoff's psychosis without treatment. Improvement can occur with treatment. • Risk for recurrence exists with continued malnutrition.

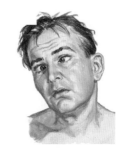

Wernicke's syndrome

Ophthalmoplegia
(6th nerve palsy)
↓
Confusion
↓
Coma
↓
Death

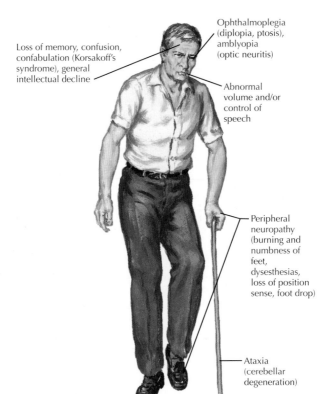

Loss of memory, confusion, confabulation (Korsakoff's syndrome), general intellectual decline

Ophthalmoplegia (diplopia, ptosis), amblyopia (optic neuritis)

Abnormal volume and/or control of speech

Peripheral neuropathy (burning and numbness of feet, dysesthesias, loss of position sense, foot drop)

Ataxia (cerebellar degeneration)

Plus other systemic involvement: liver disease, pancreatitis, gastritis, osteoporosis

HYPOXIC-ISCHEMIC ENCEPHALOPATHY (HIE)	
Description	• Mental status change due to global loss of oxygen (hypoxia or anoxia) or loss of perfusion (ischemia) • This entity does not include focal ischemic damage (stroke).
Pathophysiology	• Loss of perfusion usually is due to hypotension. This can be from arrhythmia, vasodilation, blood loss, aortic dissection, or orthostasis. • Loss of oxygenation can be from loss of perfusion or from reduction in blood oxygen from pulmonary failure. • Increased CO_2 associated with COPD can additionally contribute to mental status changes.
Clinical findings	• There is a wide spectrum of deficits, from mild confusion to agitation to coma. • Increased duration or severity of hypoxia results in increased deficit. • Myoclonus, seizures, and muscle spasms can develop as a consequence of the hypoxia. • After an episode of hypoxia, patients may initially show improvement, only to show a late deterioration, within 1–2 weeks after the episode.

Laboratory studies	Routine labs are unrevealing, unless there was other organ damage due to the hypoxia, e.g., renal or hepatic. CT and MRI may be normal. Later, development of white matter changes is especially seen in patients with persistent deficits.
	
	EEG can show a variety of patterns:
	  • Suppression and diffuse slowing have indeterminate, prognostic implications.
	  • Alpha coma and burst-suppression pattern indicate a poor prognosis for good neurologic recovery.

Diagnosis	Clinical diagnosis with encephalopathy after an episode of syncope or cardiac arrest. An occasional patient with encephalopathy may be recovering from an unwitnessed episode of hypoxia.
Differential diagnosis	• *Stroke.* Patients may develop confusion and seizure-like activity from stroke, although the examination usually shows definite focal signs. Either hemorrhage or infarction can result in abrupt mental status change. • *Metabolic encephalopathy.* Confusion and myoclonus occur without other focal signs. Onset is more gradual than with HIE.
Management	Supportive care only. Good medical management can allow for recovery, but no treatment hastens recovery. Other organ damage, hyperthermia, and blood pressure dysregulation may impede recovery.
Clinical course	• Improvement is common, but not invariable. • Short duration of hypoxia and general good health can allow for excellent recovery with little or no deficit. However, cerebral edema leading to brain death or the persistent vegetative state can result from severe hypoxia.

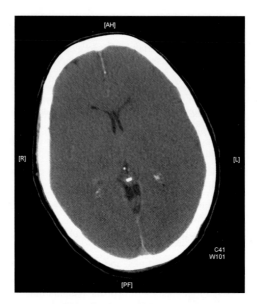

Hypoxic-ischemic encephalopathy (HIE):
CT of the brain showing loss of normal
grey-white differentiation.

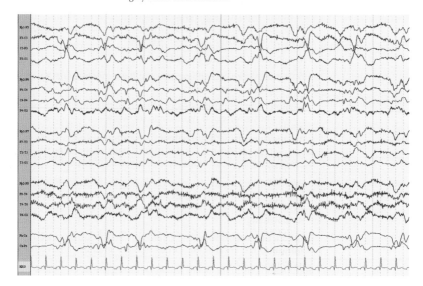

HIE: EEG of the same patient showing rhythms which are slow and disorganized.

TOXIC ENCEPHALOPATHY	
Description	• Mental status changes due to toxic effects of agents • Medications, illicit drugs, or chemicals can be causes.

Pathophysiology	The list of medicines that can produce toxic encephalopathy is huge. Some of the more important agents are:
	  • Sedative hypnotics
	  • Anticonvulsants (especially at high levels)
	  • Antidepressants
	  • Analgesics
	  • Neuroleptics

Clinical findings	• Confusion with varying manifestations, including agitation or apathy • No focal findings develop from toxic encephalopathy.
Laboratory studies	• Drug screen may show the offending agent, although overdoses of many commonly used medications will not be revealed. • Imaging with CT or MRI is often needed to look for structural lesions. • LP may be needed if CNS infection is considered.
Diagnosis	• Clinical diagnosis is suggested by the subacute onset of confusion without focal findings. • Diagnosis is supported by drug screen, drug level, or historical information indicating toxic effect. • Absence of other medical causes is essential, including stroke, intracerebral hemorrhage, or other metabolic derangement.
Differential diagnosis	• *Metabolic encephalopathy.* Can look just like toxic encephalopathy, so metabolic evaluation is needed. • *Stroke.* Can produce mental status changes, although there also are usually focal findings. • *Chronic hypoxia or hypercarbia.* Patients with COPD can show confusion, which can resemble toxic encephalopathy, including agitation.
Management	• Supportive care is essential. • Removal of the offending agent by dialysis is sometimes needed, although the body's metabolism seldom makes this necessary.
Clinical course	Improvement is expected, unless there is a complication from hypoxia or some other insult.

Agitation

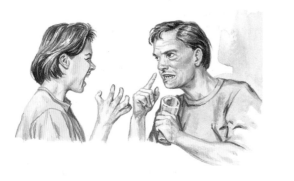
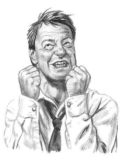

Apathy

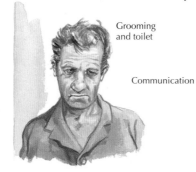

Grooming
and toilet

Communication

Dressing

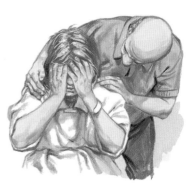

PSYCHIATRIC CAUSES OF MENTAL STATUS CHANGE	
Description	Confusion, coma, or other cognitive changes due to psychiatric disturbance rather than organic encephalopathy
Pathophysiology	• Psychiatric causes fall into several categories. Most are subconscious and the patient is not trying to fool the examiner. In a few cases, the difficulty is intentional (malingering). • Psychiatric disturbances producing cognitive disturbances include psychosis, catatonia, conversion disorder, and depression.
Clinical findings	• Patients may have disturbance of cognitive function, which could suggest organic encephalopathy or seizure. The range of alteration of consciousness includes memory loss to dementia to coma. • Pseudodementia is a cognitive change resembling dementia, but due to depression or other psychiatric cause. • Conversion disorder can produce unresponsiveness that may resemble coma, but the patient lacks the changes in posture, appearance, and reflex responses which would characterize coma. There are a number of exam findings that help to distinguish psychogenic unresponsiveness from coma. • Psychosis can occur in an isolated fashion or as part of an organic encephalopathy. Therefore, when psychosis is present it is not always clear whether the psychosis is primary or secondary.
Laboratory studies	• Routine labs are normal. • Imaging is normal. • EEG is normal, which is a helpful factor in differentiating organic encephalopathy from psychogenic unresponsiveness or psychosis. • Neuropsych testing often is needed in addition to careful examination for accurate diagnosis.
Diagnosis	• Psychogenic unresponsiveness is determined by exam showing that the patient is able to internalize commands and make movements, but does not do so due to subconscious or conscious factors. • Imaging, blood, and EEG often are performed to rule out other reversible causes. Thiamine deficiency should always be considered.
Differential diagnosis	• *Seizures.* Can resemble psychogenic unresponsiveness. Patients in absence status or complex partial status may be unresponsive, yet have no overt signs of epileptiform activity on examination. EEG is required to be certain of this diagnosis. • *Paralysis due to acquired disorder or medication.* Can produce unresponsiveness with a normal EEG. However, respiratory function usually is affected.

PSYCHIATRIC CAUSES OF MENTAL STATUS CHANGE—cont'd	
Management	• Psychiatric consultation should be considered, since many of these disorders require significant psychiatric expertise. Neuroleptics often are required for psychosis.
	• Psychiatric counseling is needed for most patients with conversion disorder. However, a caring and thoughtful physician can sometimes give the patient the support and assistance they need to prevent a return to the same psychiatric state.
Clinical course	Most patients improve after their event, although many will subsequently have further episodes.

OVERVIEW OF MOVEMENT DISORDERS	
Important disorders	• Parkinson's disease and related degenerative diseases • Secondary parkinsonism • Essential tremor • Chorea and athetosis • Dystonia • Ballism
Disorder	**Summary of Clinical Features**
Parkinson's disease (PD)	• Rigidity, bradykinesia, postural instability in varying amounts • Often asymmetric especially at onset • Tremor that is more prominent at rest, increases with gait, and decreases with voluntary movement • No other cause is identified

Secondary parkinsonism	Parkinsonian features due to a specific cause such as:
	  • Medications including some neuroleptics
	  • Infarctions
	  • Toxins
	May be less likely to exhibit tremor than patients with PD

Progressive supranuclear palsy (PSP)	• Parkinsonian features associated with supranuclear gaze palsy • Posture characterized by neck extension rather than flexion
Dementia with Lewy bodies (DLB)	• Parkinsonism plus dementia. Onset of the dementia and movement disorder within 1 year is DLB, whereas onset of dementia more than 1 year after the parkinsonian symptoms is usually called Parkinson's disease with dementia (PDD), but this can be considered the same condition. • No other cause is identified.

Multiple system atrophy (MSA)	• Parkinsonism plus other symptoms in varying combination
	• The additional findings can be:
	  • Orthostatic hypotension
	  • Cerebellar ataxia
	  • Corticospinal tract abnormalities

Essential tremor (ET)	• Postural and action tremor without any other signs of movement disorder • Often familial
Dystonia	• Abnormal focal or regional muscle tone often producing abnormal posture • Can be primary or secondary
Chorea and athetosis	• Spontaneous movements that can be writhing (athetosis) or more rapid (chorea) • Can be primary or secondary
Ballism	• Violent flinging movement, usually unilateral (hemiballismus) • Clinical diagnosis of acute onset of movement disorder, usually due to stroke

ESSENTIAL TREMOR (ET)	
Description	• Action and postural tremor without other signs of movement disorder
Pathophysiology	• Idiopathic • Familial predisposition in the majority of patients
Clinical findings	• Action and postural tremor of about 5–8 Hz affecting the arms • Action tremor means "with activity of the limb," such as moving the arms for finger-nose-finger testing or a routine activity such as eating. • Postural tremor means while holding an active posture, as with holding the arms in front of the body. • No other motor defect or other neurologic deficit is present.
Laboratory studies	• Normal imaging • Normal laboratory studies
Diagnosis	• Clinical features. Action and postural tremor without other clinical findings. • Positive family history supports the diagnosis. • There are no diagnostic tests for ET.
Differential diagnosis	• *Parkinsonism.* PD and other parkinsonian disorders often have tremor, but this mainly is a resting tremor and is associated with other signs of the movement disorder. • *Hyperthyroidism.* Hyperthyroid states produce tremor that is worse with action. Thyroid function tests are abnormal. • *Physiologic tremor.* Everyone has some mild tremor with fine movements, and this is increased with fatigue, illness, fright, and other hyperadrenergic states.
Management	• Primidone (low-dose) or beta-blockers (e.g., propranolol) are the first-line therapy for most patients. • Propranolol is sometimes used on a prn basis rather than as a scheduled dose. • Other drugs that may help some patients include clonazepam, gabapentin, and topiramate. • Botox injection is helpful for some patients with hand tremor that interferes with fine activity. • Surgical treatments include deep brain stimulation and thalamotomy, but these are rarely indicated.
Clinical course	• ET gradually worsens over years. • Development of other neurologic deficits is not expected. • Early treatment does not alter the course of the condition.

Essential Tremor (ET)

Typically bilateral, this movement disorder is the most common. It may be accentuated with goal-directed movement of the limbs. Essential tremor affects the hands and facial musculature (in this order of prevalence). Most common presentation is the association of hand tremor and tremor in cranial musculature.

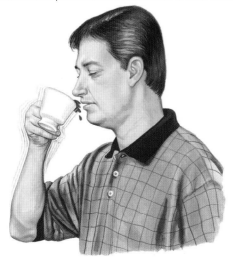

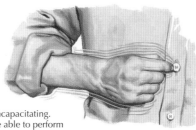

ET is considered benign, it can become incapacitating. In the severe forms the patient may not be able to perform essential daily activities, such as drinking from a cup or dressing.

A useful clinical clue is that alcohol temporarily alleviates the symptoms.

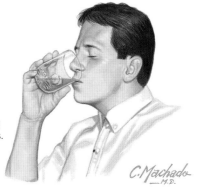

PARKINSON'S DISEASE (PD)	
Description	• Neurodegenerative disease producing tremor, incoordination, and gait deficits • Second most common cause of tremor (first is essential tremor)
Pathophysiology	• Degeneration of projections from the substantia nigra to the basal ganglia • Unknown trigger of the neuronal degeneration
Clinical findings	• Tremor that is most prominent at rest, decreased by action, and increased by walking • Stooped posture with a narrow stance • Gait is shuffling with narrow base, short steps, decreased arm swing, and festination. • Tone is increased in limb muscles with rigidity and cogwheeling.
Laboratory studies	• CT and MRI show no significant abnormalities. • Blood and urine tests are negative.
Diagnosis	• Clinical diagnosis with any combinations of rigidity, bradykinesia, resting tremor, and loss of postural reflexes • Imaging and labs do not reveal another cause.
Differential diagnosis	• *Other parkinsonian syndromes, such as PSP, MSA.* Typical parkinsonian symptoms are combined with other features, such as orthostatis or peripheral neuropathy. • *Drug-induced parkinsonism.* Parkinsonism induced by neuroleptic or another drug. Cannot be distinguished clinically—have to diagnose by course after discontinuation of the offending agent. • *Vascular parkinsonism.* Multiple cerebral infarctions can produce a clinical picture similar to PD. Imaging shows the vascular disease. • *Normal pressure hydrocephalus.* Ataxia, dementia, and urinary incontinence. Some increased tone is seen, but not the cogwheeling of parkinsonism. No tremor is expected.

Management	• Maintenance of activity is crucial.
	• Drug classes available include:
	  • Anticholinergics
	  • Dopamine agonists
	  • Levodopa
	  • Catechol-O-methyl transferase (COMT) inhibitors
	  • Monoamine oxidase inhibitors
	  • Dopamine-releasing agents
	• Tremor is treated mainly with anticholinergic drugs such as trihexyphenidyl.
	• Dopamine agonists and levodopa are also somewhat effective.
	• Rigidity and bradykinesia are treated with dopamine agonists or levodopa. Both classes can be used together for patients with moderate to advanced disease.

PARKINSON'S DISEASE (PD)—cont'd	
	• Age of the patient influences drug selection. Young patients are usually started on dopamine agonists, whereas older patients are treated with levodopa. • Levodopa is given in combination with carbidopa, which reduces the systemic adverse effects of the levodopa. • COMT inhibitors prolong the action of levodopa by inhibiting metabolism. • Levodopa/carbidopa combinations are supplied in three formulations: regular release, sustained release, and in combination with entacapone (COMT inhibitor)
Clinical course	• PD is a progressive disease, resulting in increased disability over time. • Drugs have a symptomatic effect. • Protective effects of agents are mild, if present at all. • Patients develop more fluctuations and over time response to medicines decrease.

Clinical signs of Parkinson's Disease

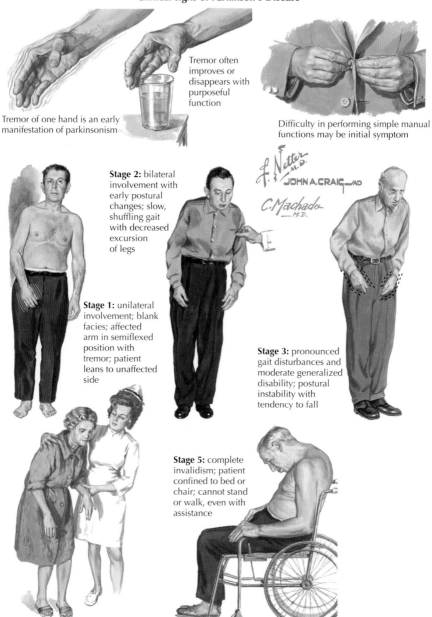

Tremor of one hand is an early manifestation of parkinsonism

Tremor often improves or disappears with purposeful function

Difficulty in performing simple manual functions may be initial symptom

Stage 2: bilateral involvement with early postural changes; slow, shuffling gait with decreased excursion of legs

Stage 1: unilateral involvement; blank facies; affected arm in semiflexed position with tremor; patient leans to unaffected side

Stage 3: pronounced gait disturbances and moderate generalized disability; postural instability with tendency to fall

Stage 5: complete invalidism; patient confined to bed or chair; cannot stand or walk, even with assistance

Stage 4: significant disability; limited ambulation with assistance

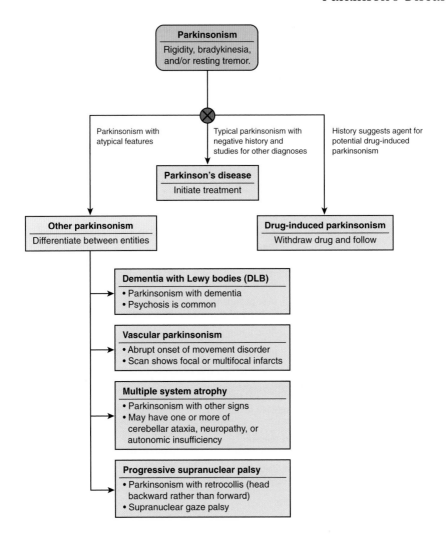

Parkinsonism

Rigidity, bradykinesia, and/or resting tremor.

Parkinsonism with atypical features

Typical parkinsonism with negative history and studies for other diagnoses

History suggests agent for potential drug-induced parkinsonism

Parkinson's disease

Initiate treatment

Other parkinsonism

Differentiate between entities

Drug-induced parkinsonism

Withdraw drug and follow

Dementia with Lewy bodies (DLB)
- Parkinsonism with dementia
- Psychosis is common

Vascular parkinsonism
- Abrupt onset of movement disorder
- Scan shows focal or multifocal infarcts

Multiple system atrophy
- Parkinsonism with other signs
- May have one or more of cerebellar ataxia, neuropathy, or autonomic insufficiency

Progressive supranuclear palsy
- Parkinsonism with retrocollis (head backward rather than forward)
- Supranuclear gaze palsy

4 Drug Treatment of Parkinson's Disease

DRUG TREATMENT OF PARKINSON'S DISEASE	
Clinical Scenario	**Treatment Guidelines**
Tremor	• Anticholinergic agents are the first line of therapy for most patients. • Dopamine agonists and levodopa are also effective as a second line.
Rigidity and bradykinesia	• Levodopa, especially for older patients • Dopamine agonists, especially for younger patients • Combination of levodopa and agonists are used for more severe disease.
Fluctuations	• Change from immediate release to sustained release levodopa. • Add COMT inhibitor or MAOB inhibitor to levodopa preparation. • Replace levodopa preparations with dopamine agonists.
Drug-induced dyskinesias	• Reduce the dose of the dopaminergic agent. • May reduce the dose of levodopa and replace it with dopamine agonist for fewer dyskinesias. • Amantadine may reduce dyskinesias in some patients.
Loss of effectiveness of dopaminergic regimen	• Increase the dose of the dopaminergic agent. • Combine the use of levodopa with a dopamine agonist.

Drug Class	**Commonly Used Agents**	**Drug Use**
Levodopa	• Regular release levodopa/carbidopa • Sustained release levodopa/carbidopa • Levodopa/carbidopa with entacapone	• Used alone or in combination with dopamine agonists for rigidity and bradykinesia • First-line therapy for many older patients
Dopamine agonists	• Ropinerole • Pramipexole • Pergolide	• Used alone or in combination with levodopa agents for rigidity, bradykinesia, and to a lesser extent— tremor • First-line therapy for many young patients
Anticholinergics	• Trihexyphenidyl • Benztropine	• Used mainly for tremor
Dopamine releasers	• Amantadine	• Promotes dopamine release • Used for mild disease • Reduces drug-induced dyskinesias in patients treated with high doses of other dopaminergic agents

Drug Class	Commonly Used Agents	Drug Use
COMT inhibitors	• Entacapone • Tolcapone	• Tolcapone seldom used • Inhibits breakdown of levodopa • Used for fluctuations • Always given with levodopa no benefit by themselves
MAO Inhibitors	• Selegiline • Rasagiline	• Used for long-duration therapy • May have a mild neuroprotective effect

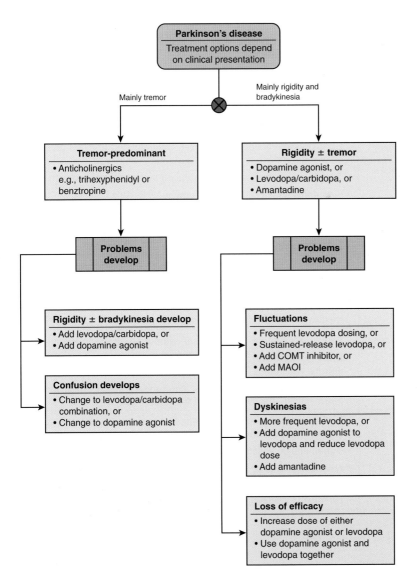

DRUG-INDUCED PARKINSONISM	
Description	• Parkinsonian features due to medications, usually neuroleptics
Pathophysiology	• Alteration in dopamine transmission due to certain drugs. • The most common offending drugs are neuroleptics, with an emphasis on older drugs. • Atypical neuroleptics have a much lower incidence of drug-induced extrapyramidal disorders, including parkinsonism and tardive dyskinesia.
Drugs that may produce parkinsonism	• Neuroleptics, especially older agents • Methyldopa (antihypertensive) • Metoclopromide (for gastric motility and nausea) • Prochlorperazine (phenothiazine antiemetic) • Flunarizine (calcium-channel blocker) • Amiodarone (antiarrhythmic agent that occasionally causes tremor, rarely associated with parkinsonism) • Valproate (antiepileptic with multiple other uses that occasionally causes a tremor that can be mistaken for parkinsonism)
Clinical findings	• All of the features of Parkinson's disease shown. Drug-induced parkinsonism cannot be definitively differentiated from PD on clinical grounds. • Tremor is less likely with drug-induced parkinsonism than with PD. • Symptoms initially are more symmetric with drug-induced parkinsonism than with PD.
Laboratory studies	• Imaging is normal. • Labs are normal.
Diagnosis	• Diagnosis is suspected by clinical findings and the absence of other causes on examination, plus a history of precipitant drug use. • All patients with parkinsonism should be asked about their medication history, including discontinued drugs.
Differential diagnosis	• *Parkinson's disease.* Parkinsonism without an offending agent. • *Other parkinsonian syndromes.* Parkinsonism with other signs of deficits, which may include orthostatis or neuropathy. • *Normal pressure hydrocephalus.* Can produce ataxia similar to parkinsonism, but without all of the limb findings.
Management	• Withdrawal of the offending agent. The patient should be followed to determine whether the extrapyramidal symptoms improve. • Dopaminergic agents often are not needed. • Amantadine can be used if there is incomplete improvement. • Follow-up is needed to look for development of idiopathic Parkinson's disease.

DRUG-INDUCED PARKINSONISM—cont'd	
Clinical course	• Most patients improve after withdrawal of the drug, within days to weeks.
	• Benefit is seen within 2–3 months in the vast majority of patients.
	• Some patients eventually are found to have idiopathic Parkinson's disease, which was unmasked by the offending drug. The drug did not cause PD.

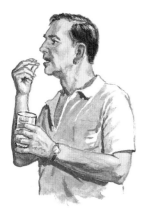
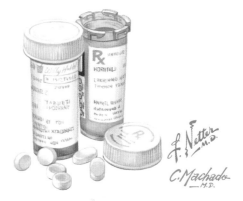

SECONDARY PARKINSONISM	
Definition	• Parkinsonism due to a cause other than idiopathic Parkinson's disease

Pathophysiology	• Other degenerative diseases:
	  • Progressive supranuclear palsy
	  • Striato nigral degeneration
	  • Dementia with Lewy bodies
	  • Multiple-system atrophy
	  • Corticobasal degeneration
	  • Drug-induced parkinsonism
	  • Vascular parkinsonism
	  • Post hypoxic parkinsonism
	  • Post encephalitic parkinsonism
	  • Head injuries
	• Many of these disorders are discussed elsewhere in the book.

Clinical findings	• Rigidity, bradykinesia • Gait disorder with shuffling, narrow-based gait • Tremor may be present, but is less prominent than with idiopathic PD. • Cognitive dysfunction is more common with secondary parkinsonism than in PD.
Laboratory studies	• Imaging is normal. • Blood tests are normal.
Diagnosis	• Clinical features, with historical or examination signs of precipitating disorders • Normal imaging and labs
Differential diagnosis	• *Parkinson's disease.* Rigidity, bradykinesia, and tremor, without the additional signs of these related disorders. • *Normal pressure hydrocephalus.* Can present with ataxia, but imaging shows increased ventricular size.

Management	Management of the offending cause (if possible):
	  • Withdrawal of a causative drug
	  • Treatment of infection, if present
	  • Secondary prevention of vascular disease
	  • Treat the symptoms with the same medications and according to the same guidelines as for PD.

Clinical course	• Depends on the cause. Drug-induced parkinsonism has a good prognosis for improvement. • Parkinsonism due to head injury or vascular disease may not be progressive.

Parkinson Disease: Anatomy with Biochemical Pathways

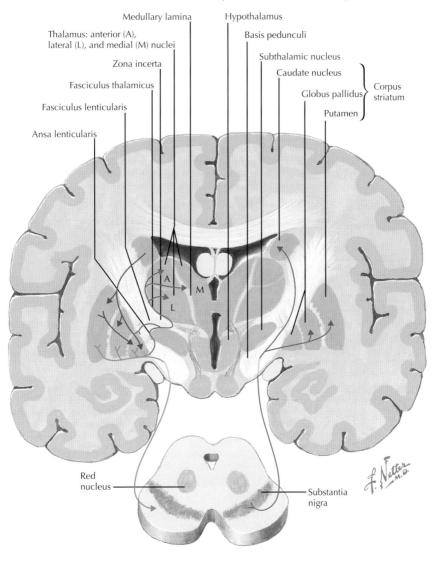

Medullary lamina

Thalamus: anterior (A), lateral (L), and medial (M) nuclei

Zona incerta

Fasciculus thalamicus

Fasciculus lenticularis

Ansa lenticularis

Hypothalamus

Basis pedunculi

Subthalamic nucleus

Caudate nucleus

Globus pallidus

Putamen

Corpus striatum

Red nucleus

Substantia nigra

—— Cholinergic
—— γ-Aminobutyric acid (GABA)
—— Dopaminergic
—— Unknown

PROGRESSIVE SUPRANUCLEAR PALSY (PSP)	
Description	• Disorder with parkinsonism, but with different degenerative pattern and clinical features • Formerly called Steele-Richardson-Olszewski syndrome
Pathophysiology	• Degenerative condition of unknown etiology
Clinical findings	• Parkinsonism with rigidity, bradykinesia, and ataxia with falling • Supranuclear gaze palsy. Difficulty with vertical eye movements, both saccadic and pursuit. This means that with voluntary gaze, there is impairment in eye movements, whereas with reflexive gaze (such as manually tilting the head) there is relative preservation of eye movement. This is distinct from nuclear lesions, where there would be impaired ocular motor function with both reflexive and voluntary movements. • Dystonia of neck and shoulder muscles is common. • Facial expression and backwards head tilt can give a characteristic appearance that can be recognized immediately. • Dysarthria is common.
Laboratory studies	• Routine laboratory studies are normal. • MRI usually shows no abnormalities. Subtle changes in midbrain and ventricular architecture usually are not noticed by radiologists.
Diagnosis	• Clinical features of parkinsonism with retrocollis strongly suggests the diagnosis. • Absence of other etiologies identified on labs and imaging
Differential diagnosis	• Parkinson's disease • Multiple system atrophy
Management	• Parkinsonism may be treated with dopaminergic agents, although the response usually is lacking. A good response is some evidence in favor of PD rather than PSP. • Anticholinergic agents occasionally are a benefit in combination with dopaminergic agents, and they also may help sialorrhea. • SSRIs and TCAs can be helpful, independently of their antidepressant effect. • Botox injections are occasionally used for neck rigidity, and rarely for sialorrhea.
Clinical course	• Gradual worsening is expected. • Patients usually die of complications from immobility, including pneumonia.

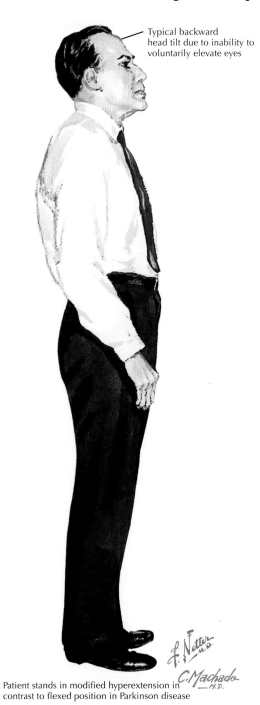

Typical backward head tilt due to inability to voluntarily elevate eyes

Patient stands in modified hyperextension in contrast to flexed position in Parkinson disease

MULTIPLE SYSTEM ATROPHY (MSA)	

Description	• MSA is a group of disorders that are characterized by CNS and autonomic disturbance.
	• Elements traditionally have been olivopontocerebellar atrophy (OPCA), striatonigral degeneration, and MSA with orthostatic hypotension. These are now renamed:
	  • MSA-P (prominently parkinsonism)
	  • MSA-C (predominantly cerebellar)
	  • MSA-A (predominantly autonomic)
	• Almost any combination of deficits relative to these regions can develop, but these are the most prominent.

Pathophysiology	• Neurodegenerative disease of unknown etiology

Clinical findings	• **MSA-P**—Striatonigral degeneration:
	  • Parkinsonism with rigidity, bradykinesia, instability
	  • Postural hypotension, urinary incontinence, male erectile dysfunction are common.
	• **MSA-C**—Olivopontocerebellar atrophy:
	  • Cerebellar ataxia
	  • Corticospinal tract signs, including hyperreflexia and abnormal plantar responses
	  • Dysarthria
	• **MSA-A**—MSA with orthostatic hypotension (Shy-Drager syndrome):
	  • Symptoms of parkinsonism and/or cerebellar ataxia with autonomic deficits, including orthostatic hypotension, which may be severe
	  • Three types are parkinsonian, cerebellar, and combined. This classification describes the most prominent type of associated motor deficit.

Laboratory studies	• Routine laboratory studies are normal. • MRI may show atrophic changes in the cerebellum and pons.
Diagnosis	• Clinical diagnosis supported by imaging findings • Special autonomic testing may be needed.
Differential diagnosis	• *Parkinson's disease.* Movement disorder without prominent autonomic deficits, although some orthostatic hypotension is seen. • *Normal pressure hydrocephalus.* Ataxia without the parkinsonian signs seen with MSA.
Management	• Parkinsonian symptoms may be treated with dopaminergic agents, although the effectiveness of these interventions is limited. • Orthostatic hypotension can be managed with selected drugs, including fludrocortisone or midodrine. Liberalization of salt intake may help. Because some patients have supine hypertension, there commonly is a difficult balance between this supine hypertension and the orthostatic hypotension.
Clinical course	• These are all progressive diseases. • Medications and physical measures may result in some functional improvement, but do not alter the course of the disease.

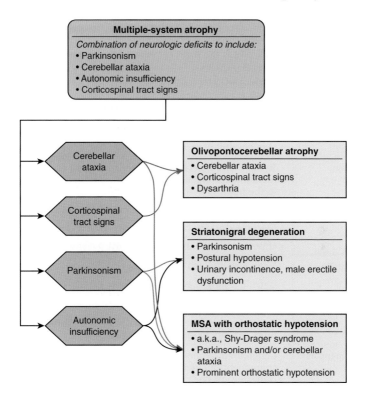

TORTICOLLIS (CERVICAL DYSTONIA, TORSION DYSTONIA, SPASMODIC TORTICOLLIS)	
Description	• Torticollis is the most common of the dystonias, affecting the cervical muscles. • Afflicted patients have turning and/or tilting of the head.
Pathophysiology	• Idiopathic for many patients. Thought to be due to circuit abnormalities in the basal ganglia without a structural lesion in most patients. • May develop as a result of trauma
Clinical findings	• Twisting of the neck to one side is the most common manifestation. Variants are tilting to one side, either to the back or to the front. • Muscles exhibiting the contraction are hypertrophied. • Dystonia changes outside of the cervical region are not seen. • Onset is after the age of 30 in most patients.
Laboratory studies	• Normal routine lab and imaging • Genetic testing is available for some genetic dystonias.
Diagnosis	• Clinical diagnosis of the abnormal posture • Supportive negative tests. Cervical spine imaging is indicated in most patients to look for a structural lesion.
Differential diagnosis	• *Generalized dystonia*. Dystonic posturing of the neck can be a component of a generalized dystonia. Torticollis has only craniocervical findings.
Management	• Anticholinergic medications, including trihexyphenidyl or benztropine • Botox injections are effective for many patients and are a first-line treatment for many patients. • Dopamergic agents may be tried in refractory cases. • Surgical options include deep brain stimulation; however, this is rarely performed.
Clinical course	• Gradually worsens, although patients may be stable for years. • Clinical improvement may give the impression of remission, but this does not persist.

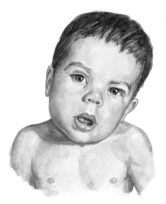

Child with muscular torticollis. Head tilted to left with chin turned slightly to right because of contracture of left sternocleidomastoid muscle. Note facial symmetry (flattening of left side of face)

Untreated torticollis in 12-year-old boy. Thick, fibrotic, tendon-like bands have replaced sternocleidomastoid muscle, making head appear tethered to clavicle. Two heads of left sternocleidomastoid muscle prominent

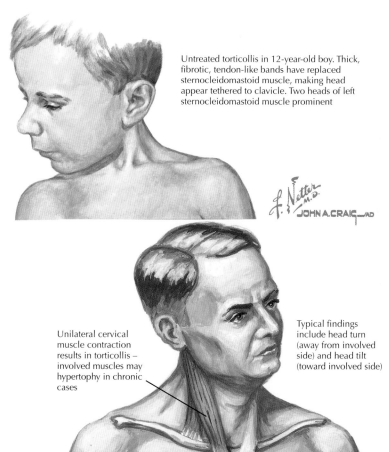

Unilateral cervical muscle contraction results in torticollis – involved muscles may hypertophy in chronic cases

Typical findings include head turn (away from involved side) and head tilt (toward involved side)

HUNTINGTON'S DISEASE	
Description	• Autosomal dominant degenerative disease characterized by motor and cognitive changes • Chorea, behavioral abnormalities, and dementia are typical.
Pathophysiology	• Genetic disorder, inherited as autosomal dominant • Expansion of a trinucleotide repeat in the DNA coding for Huntingtin
Clinical findings	• Onset is at any age, usually 30s to 40s. • Chorea, which is initially mild then worsens, with more violent movement development. • Rigidity and bradykinesia, suggestive of parkinsonism, may develop later. Dystonia may also develop. • Behavioral abnormalities are common in early stages, including personality change, depression, and psychosis. • Dementia develops later than the behavioral changes. Has the appearance of a subcortical dementia.
Laboratory studies	• Genetic testing can be performed for patients or unaffected family members, although there are numerous implications to consider before testing asymptomatic people. • Imaging shows caudate atrophy, altering the appearance of the frontal horns. • Routine labs are normal.
Diagnosis	• Clinical diagnosis is sufficient for many patients with fully developed disease. • Genetic testing can be performed for confirmation of the clinical diagnosis. • Note that presymptomatic testing is available, but should not be performed without genetic and psychological counseling being offered.
Differential diagnosis	• *Benign chorea.* Chorea that tends to be hereditary. Not associated with dementia, behavioral disturbance, or other motor deficits. • *Multiple sclerosis.* Can produce progressive ataxia and other motor deficits in this age group (30s to 40s).
Management	• *Chorea.* Diazepam, clonazepam, valproate, or neuroleptics can be tried. • *Behavior.* SSRIs, VPA, and neuroleptics are used. • *Psychosis.* Neuroleptics are used, with atypical neuroleptics being favored. • *Dementia.* Choinesterase inhibitors and memantine may be helpful, but further study is needed. • *Rigidity.* Dopaminergic agent as used for PD, although these may exacerbate psychosis. • *Genetic counseling* should be given, with family educated about the inheritance.
Clinical course	• *Progressive condition.* No treatment alters the course of the disease. • Symptomatic treatment of the movement disorder is helpful for many patients.

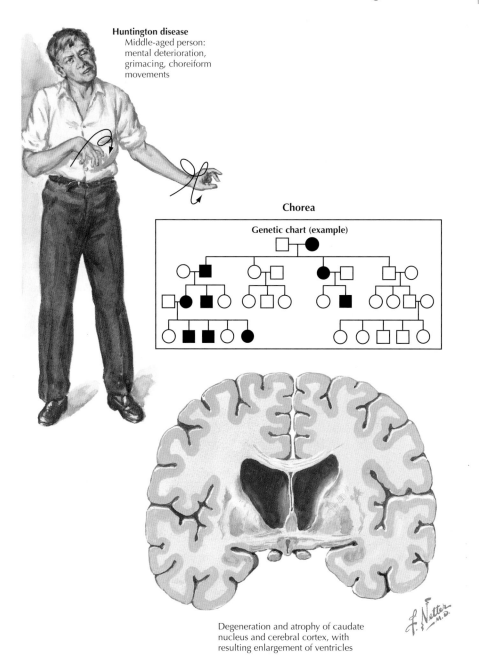

Huntington disease
Middle-aged person: mental deterioration, grimacing, choreiform movements

Chorea

Genetic chart (example)

Degeneration and atrophy of caudate nucleus and cerebral cortex, with resulting enlargement of ventricles

4 | Wilson's Disease

WILSON'S DISEASE	
Description	• Disorder of copper metabolism, with impaired elimination with usage of ceruloplasmin • Presents with parkinsonian signs plus cognitive, eye, and fingernail abnormalities
Pathophysiology	• Deficiency of ceruloplasmin and decreased copper elimination • Copper accumulation produces brain, eye, bone, and subungual abnormalities. • Autosomal recessive inheritance
Clinical findings	• Movement disorder begins in young adult life with rigidity and bradykinesia suggestive of PD. • Poor coordination; dysarthria; and rest, postural, or action tremor • Neuropsychiatric disturbances, including behavioral disorders, mood disturbance, cognitive decline, and/or psychosis • Eye findings, including Kayser-Fleischer rings—green-brown corneal discoloration (present in more than 90%). Also, can have cataracts, which have a distinctive appearance (sunflower cataract). • Skeletal abnormalities, including osteoporosis
Laboratory studies	• Decreased serum ceruloplasmin (>98% of patients) • Decreased serum copper (>80% of patients) • Increased copper excretion in the urine (about 80%) • Osteoporosis (about 80%) • MRI shows abnormalities on proton density-imaging in the basal ganglia. Lesions are much less common in treated patients (44% versus virtually all untreated patients)
Diagnosis	• Clinical diagnosis, with confirmation by copper studies listed above. • The eye findings are strongly suggestive.
Differential diagnosis	• *Parkinson's disease* and related neurodegenerative diseases. • *Multiple sclerosis.* Can produce progressive ataxia, but the bone, eye, and nail findings would not be expected. MS also produces multiple white matter changes not seen in Wilson's disease.
Management	• Copper chelating agents are used • Some advocate zinc and pyridoxine supplementation • Dietary copper restriction
Clinical course	• Progression is expected, although treatment may result in improvement in clinical findings and imaging.

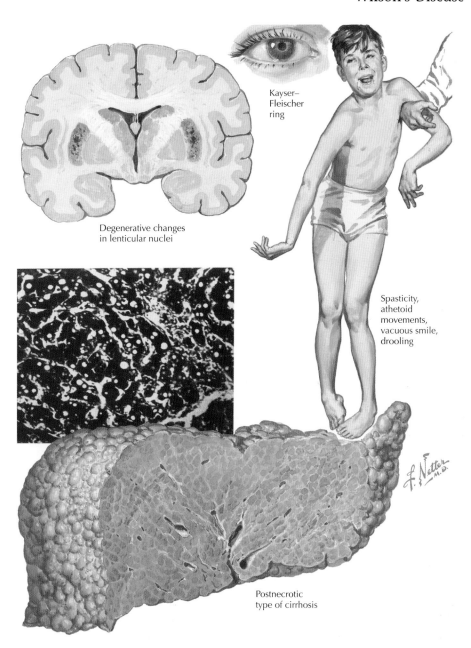

Kayser–
Fleischer
ring

Degenerative changes
in lenticular nuclei

Spasticity,
athetoid
movements,
vacuous smile,
drooling

Postnecrotic
type of cirrhosis

CORTICOBASAL DEGENERATION	
Description	• Neurodegenerative disease characterized by parkinsonism, which initially is strongly unilateral • Distinguishing feature is the "alien hand" syndrome.
Pathophysiology	• Degenerative disease of unknown etiology • Degeneration is both cortical and subcortical.
Clinical findings	• Parkinsonism features, including rigidity and bradykinesia, which are initially unilateral, but eventually become bilateral • Gait ataxia is present early and progresses to immobility over time. • Dysphagia is common. • Dystonia and myoclonus often develop, which helps to distinguish from PD. • Apraxia of limb movement is common. The limb may make complex movements without voluntary command—the so-called "alien hand" syndrome. • Cognitive disturbance is seen later in the course, as well as the appearance of frontal lobe syndrome. Memory loss is seen, but disinhibition, perseveration, and other frontal lobe findings predominate.
Laboratory studies	• MRI and CT show no specific findings, serving only to rule out other disorders, such as hydrocephalus, vascular disease, and tumor. • Routine labs are normal. Labs performed to look for other diagnoses include B_{12} level, ceruloplasmin, thyroid function tests, and RPR.
Diagnosis	• Clinical features of unilateral parkinsonism, with associated myoclonus and apraxia • The alien hand syndrome is suggestive.
Differential diagnosis	• Parkinson's disease and related diseases, especially PSP and striatonigral degeneration • Normal pressure hydrocephalus. Imaging differentiates. • Frontal lobe damage due to mass lesion or infarction. Imaging is diagnostic.
Management	• Dopaminergic agents often are used, although they usually are not effective. • SSRIs are commonly used for depression associated with the disorder. • Myoclonus may be treated with benzodiazepines, such as clonazepam.
Clinical course	• Progressive condition. Deterioration is expected. With time, the extrapyramidal symptoms become bilateral, more symmetric, and more disabling. • Cognitive deterioration develops later in the course.

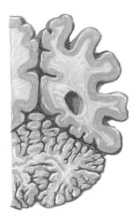

Contralateral asymmetric
atrophy of parietal lobe

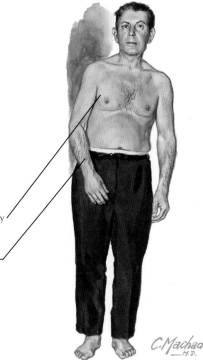

Apraxia may inhibit everyday
activities such as dressing

Stiff, jerky limb posturing

Patient may exhibit "alien
limb" phenomenon in limb
contralateral to cortical
atrophy

CENTRAL PONTINE MYELINOLYSIS (CPM)	
Description	• Metabolic disorder resulting in demyelination most prominent in the pons • Rapid correction of hyponatremia is the prototypic cause. • Spastic quadriplegia and bulbar dysfunction are typical.
Pathophysiology	• Rapid reversal of hyponatremia predisposes to CPM, although it can develop with metabolic problems in the absence of rapid reversal. • Demyelination occurs in the white matter of the pons, with lesser degrees of higher cerebral demyelination occasionally developing. The demyelination is thought to be due to osmotic damage.
Clinical findings	• Weakness with spasticity of the arms and legs, bulbar weakness, and gaze difficulty develop over a few days • Preceding marked metabolic derangements have almost always been present.
Laboratory studies	• MRI shows demyelinating changes most prominent in the basis pontis. White matter changes higher in the hemispheres occasionally can coexist, but raises the possibility of alternative diagnoses. • Routine labs show metabolic derangements predating the neurologic symptoms, especially hyponatremia. Other osmotic disturbances can predispose to CPM.
Diagnosis	• Clinical features of progressive corticospinal tract and bulbar dysfunction • MRI evidence of demyelination in the basis pontis
Differential diagnosis	• *Acute disseminated encephalomyelitis.* Rapidly progressive motor, sensory, and cognitive deficits sometimes associated with fever, head and neck pain, and/or seizures. • *Multiple sclerosis.* Relapsing/remitting focal deficits that may include quadriplegia if spinal cord affected. No metabolic abnormalities are seen. MRI appearance if of multifocal lesions • *Brainstem stroke.* Acute onset of quadriplegia and brainstem dysfunction. No predisposing metabolic derangement. More acute onset than CPM.
Management	• Electrolyte abnormalities should be judiciously corrected, which can lower the risk for development of CPM. • No treatment for the demyelination is effective. • Improvement may occur, and prolonged support and physical therapy may result in recovery of much function.
Clinical course	• Progresses over a few days, then recovery of some function may take weeks and months.

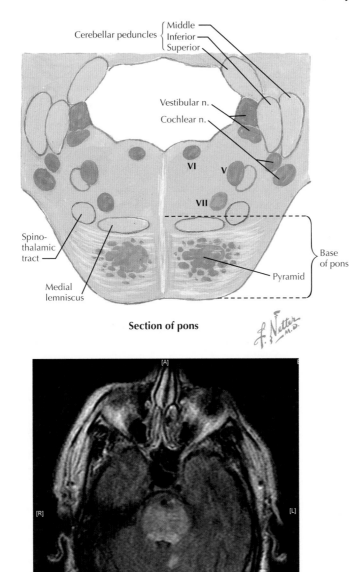

Cerebellar peduncles { Middle / Inferior / Superior

Vestibular n.

Cochlear n.

VI   V

VII

Spino-thalamic tract

Medial lemniscus

Pyramid

Base of pons

Section of pons

Central pontine myelinolysis (CPM): MRI showing pontine hyperintensity. The anatomic diagram shows the structures involved with the lesion.

DYSTONIA	
Description	• Movement disorder characterized by sustained contraction of muscles with resultant abnormal posture
Pathophysiology	• Primary or idiopathic dystonias are frequently genetic. There is no structural deficit. • Secondary dystonias are due to a variety of neurologic disorders, with trauma being a common cause. • Drug-induced dystonia should always be considered, including levodopa, neuroleptics, metoclopramide, some anticonvulsants, and some calcium channel-blocking agents.
Clinical findings	• Abnormal posture, twisting of the head or limbs • Dystonic posturing often is provoked by movement, writing, and walking. • Affected muscles often show hypertrophy.
Laboratory studies	• Normal routine laboratory studies • Imaging usually is normal. Tumors, stroke, and trauma may produce abnormalities on CT or MRI.
Diagnosis	• Clinical diagnosis of the abnormal posture due to contraction of muscles without paralysis. • Imaging and laboratory studies may show a cause of secondary dystonia; however, patients with primary dystonia have negative studies. • Drugs as listed above should be considered and eliminated if possible. • Ceruloplasmin should be checked for Wilson's disease.
Differential diagnosis	• *Spasticity.* Stiffness of one limb or one side may occur from damage to the corticospinal tract. This is associated with pathologic reflexes and defective movement of the affected muscles. Corticospinal dysfunction is not seen with dystonia. • *Seizure.* Tonic seizure may produce twisting of the body. This is episodic, however, and there is no abnormal posture or tone during routine exam. • *Paroxysmal dystonia.* A rare episodic dystonia that is treated with carbamazepine or other antiepileptic drug. • *Torticollis.* Torsion dystonia is a form of focal dystonia.
Management	• Botox injections commonly are used for focal dystonias. For many patients, this is the treatment of choice, but should only be performed by trained and experienced physicians. • Medicines for dystonia can be helpful, but may produce sedation. Some of the drugs used include anticholinergic agents such as trihexyphenidyl, antispasticity agents such as baclofen, benzodiazepines such as clonazepam, dopamergic agents such as combination carbidopa/levodopa (Sinemet), or the catecholamine depleter tetrabenazine. • Deep brain stimulation also is being studied.
Clinical course	• Most patients respond to medical treatment or Botox injections. Refractory patients will consider newer agents and surgical procedures. • Progression of symptoms is limited for most patients.

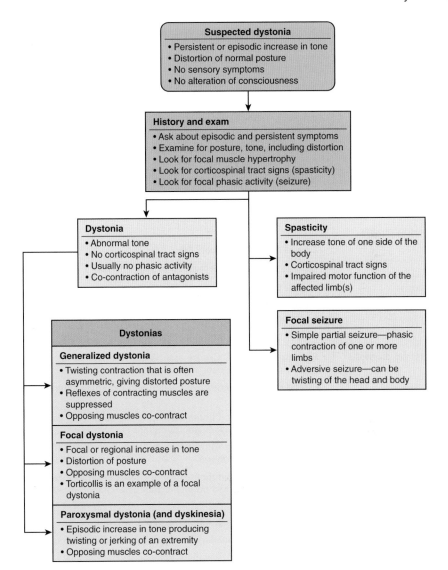

Suspected dystonia
- Persistent or episodic increase in tone
- Distortion of normal posture
- No sensory symptoms
- No alteration of consciousness

History and exam
- Ask about episodic and persistent symptoms
- Examine for posture, tone, including distortion
- Look for focal muscle hypertrophy
- Look for corticospinal tract signs (spasticity)
- Look for focal phasic activity (seizure)

Dystonia
- Abnormal tone
- No corticospinal tract signs
- Usually no phasic activity
- Co-contraction of antagonists

Spasticity
- Increase tone of one side of the body
- Corticospinal tract signs
- Impaired motor function of the affected limb(s)

Focal seizure
- Simple partial seizure—phasic contraction of one or more limbs
- Adversive seizure—can be twisting of the head and body

Dystonias

Generalized dystonia
- Twisting contraction that is often asymmetric, giving distorted posture
- Reflexes of contracting muscles are suppressed
- Opposing muscles co-contract

Focal dystonia
- Focal or regional increase in tone
- Distortion of posture
- Opposing muscles co-contract
- Torticollis is an example of a focal dystonia

Paroxysmal dystonia (and dyskinesia)
- Episodic increase in tone producing twisting or jerking of an extremity
- Opposing muscles co-contract

TARDIVE DYSKINESIA (TD)	
Description	• Movement disorder with repetitive movement of the mouth and tongue or limbs • Related to use of neuroleptics in most, but not all, patients
Pathophysiology	• Related to changes in dopamine transmission affecting the basal ganglia in many patients, although alternative pathways also may be involved • Neuroleptics are the most common cause. Atypical neuroleptics are less likely to produce this.
Clinical findings	• Repetitive movements of the tongue and facial muscles and/or movements of the extremities • Movements can be briefly suppressed.
Laboratory studies	• Routine labs are normal. • CT and MRI are unremarkable. • Genetic testing may be needed to look for HD.
Diagnosis	• Clinical features of dyskinesias • Absence of parkinsonian features, dementia, or other signs of neurologic deterioration • History of exposure to a drug that would predispose to TD
Differential diagnosis	• *Parkinson's disease.* Can be associated with dyskinesias, although usually due to treatment with dopaminergic agents. • *Essential tremor.* Tremor with action and with maintaining posture. Commonly familial. • *Huntington disease.* Chorea and/or rigidity associated with behavioral abnormalities and dementia. • *Sydenham's chorea.* Chorea in association with rheumatic fever, usually seen in childhood. • *Senile chorea.* Uncommon cause of chorea in seniors. No history of neuroleptic use and no intellectual deterioration to suggest Huntington's.
Management	• Discontinuation of the offending agent, where possible • If a neuroleptic is needed, an atypical agent should be used. • Increasing doses of dopamine antagonists occasionally is used, although this should be avoided, if possible. • There are a number of other unproved treatments, although these should usually be used by neurologists.
Clinical course	• Most patients improve with discontinuation of the offending agent. • Transient worsening can sometimes develop after discontinuation of neuroleptics, with later improvement.

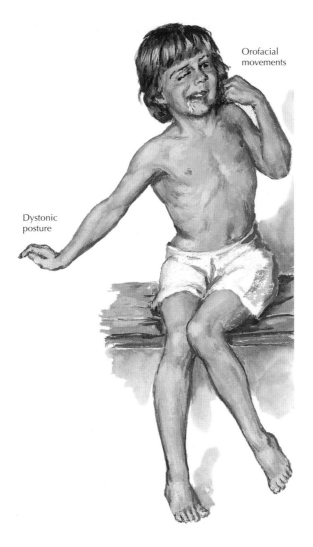

Orofacial
movements

Dystonic
posture

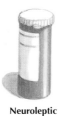

Neuroleptic

ATHETOSIS, CHOREA, AND BALLISM	
Athetosis and Chorea	
Description	• Involuntary movements of the extremities, either unilateral or bilateral • These entities are considered together because they are on a continuum.
Pathophysiology	• Lesion of the basal ganglia that can be structural or degenerative • Mass lesion, infarction, and genetic defects are most common.
Clinical findings	• *Athetosis.* Slow, writhing, involuntary movements. • *Chorea.* More rapid movements of the digits and extremities. • Presence of other deficits depends on the etiology. • *Senile chorea.* Chorea without other findings in elderly patients. • *Sydenham's chorea.* Chorea as a component of a post-streptococcal infection syndrome and seen with behavioral disorders.
Laboratory studies	• Routine labs are normal. • Imaging with MRI or CT usually is normal, although with unilateral symptoms, structural lesion of the basal ganglia can be seen—infarction, hemorrhage, tumor, infection, vascular malformation.
Diagnosis	• Clinical features of writhing or faster movements, or a combination of the movements. • Bilateral symptoms are more likely to be idiopathic and genetic. • Unilateral symptoms are more likely to be due to a structural lesion. Acute onset suggests infarction or hemorrhage.
Differential diagnosis	• *Essential tremor.* Tremor with action or holding posture that looks very different from chorea. • *Partial seizure.* Focal jerking that has a stereotyped appearance and is usually less complex than the movements of athetosis and chorea.
Management	• Neuroleptics commonly are used. Both older and atypical neuroleptics have been tried. • Dopamine-depleting agents (e.g., reserpine) occasionally are used. • Benzodiazepines and other sedative hypnotics are tried. • Gabapentin is helpful for some patients. • Tetrabenazine is helpful for some patients, although this is not available in the United States.
Clinical course	• Prognosis depends on cause. Senile chorea is slowly progressive. Structural lesions that cannot be cured will be associated with persistent, though not progressive, chorea. Chorea due to infarction or hemorrhage usually improves, although persistent neurologic deficit is common.

ATHETOSIS, CHOREA, AND BALLISM—cont'd	
Ballism (Hemiballismus)	
Description	• Wild-flinging involuntary movements of the extremities • Most common manifestation is hemiballismus—one-sided ballism.
Pathophysiology	• Lesion of the subthalamic nucleus, most commonly infarction
Clinical findings	• Involuntary violent flinging movements of one side of the body • Often has an acute onset • Incapacitates the patient. Patients may injure themselves on the bedrails.
Laboratory studies	• MRI may show lesion in the subthalamic nucleus, although lesion elsewhere in the basal ganglia can rarely present as hemiballismus. • Routine labs are normal or show nonspecific abnormalities.
Diagnosis	• Clinical appearance is diagnostic. The only question is the etiology of the lesion. • Imaging may show an area of infarction in the region of the subthalamic nucleus.
Differential diagnosis	• When symptoms are purely one-sided (hemiballismus), there is little differential diagnosis. • *Partial seizures.* Jerking of one side of the body can be an uncommon manifestation of simple partial seizures.
Management	• Neuroleptics commonly are used, with both typical and atypical agents used. • Gabapentin is sometimes used. • Sedatives including benzodiazepines and barbiturates have been used, but these are not typically first-line.
Clinical course	• Hemiballismus due to subthalamic nucleus infarction typically improves with or without treatment. Treatment does not alter the completeness of recovery, but often is necessary for comfort of the patient and family.

4 Myoclonus

MYOCLONUS	
Description	• Brief, single jerks of all or part of the body • Myoclonus does not interfere with cognitive function, although the cause might.
Pathophysiology	• There are numerous potential causes. • In the hospital, generalized myoclonus usually is due to metabolic derangements such as hepatic or renal failure, or due to the sequelae of a hypoxic episode. • In the office, essential myoclonus and juvenile myoclonus epilepsy are the most common causes.
Clinical findings	• *Postanoxic myoclonus.* Jerking of the body within hours after a significant anoxic episode, such as respiratory or cardiac arrest. Myoclonus can be synchronous or asynchronous. The jerks are single, with a varying interval between them. Cognitive function is severely impaired. With improvement in mental status, the myoclonus may persist. • *Juvenile myoclonic epilepsy.* Myoclonus that is associated with generalized seizures. • *Essential myoclonus.* Uncommon disorder characterized by multifocal jerks without other neurologic deficit, although focal dystonias in some kindreds have been reported. Myoclonus disappears in sleep. Not all patients have a positive family history. • *Metabolic myoclonus.* Patients with hepatic or renal failure may have generalized or multifocal myoclonus, which can be positive (where there is a jerk) or negative (where a limb holding a posture suddenly releases tone).
Laboratory studies	• Normal routine labs • Imaging is normal for patients with essential myoclonus, juvenile myoclonic epilepsy (JME), and metabolic myoclonus. Patients with anoxic myoclonus may have normal imaging or develop anoxic changes, such as loss of gray/white differentiation and edema. • EEG is sometimes done to look for seizures.
Diagnosis	• Clinical features, which are best observed by the clinician rather than being based on history • Examination for other movement disorders is performed.
Differential diagnosis	• *Asterixis.* A lapse of posture that can be repetitive, giving a flapping appearance. This commonly is seen in liver disease, and is a form of negative myoclonus. • *Myoclonic seizure.* Myoclonus can be associated with seizures, as in JME, and the differentiation is onset at a young age, the presence of seizures in addition to the myoclonus, and a specific pattern on the EEG.

MYOCLONUS—cont'd	
Management	• A variety of drugs have been used, including benzodiazepines, barbiturates, valproate, and levetiracetam.
Clinical course	• Prognosis depends on cause.
	• Anoxic myoclonus usually improves, although some patients will still have myoclonus even after their cognitive function has improved. This can be a significant detriment to motor rehabilitation.
	• JME is a life-long disorder that continues to require treatment.
	• Essential myoclonus requires life-long treatment, but usually does not result in prominent neurologic disability.

Essential Myoclonus

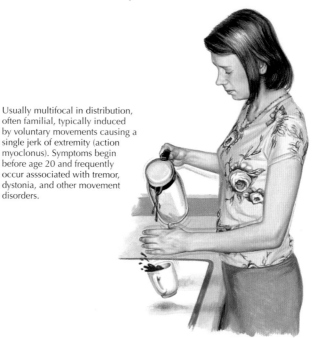

Usually multifocal in distribution, often familial, typically induced by voluntary movements causing a single jerk of extremity (action myoclonus). Symptoms begin before age 20 and frequently occur asssociated with tremor, dystonia, and other movement disorders.

Post-Anoxic Myoclonus

A variety of stimuli such as noise, light, and touch can provoke this type of myoclonus in multiple areas of the body.

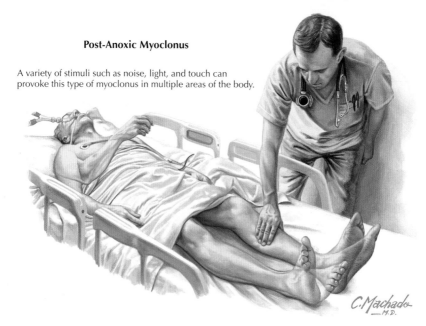

OVERVIEW OF SEIZURES	
Generalized	• Generalized seizures start within the depths of the brain and involve the entirety of the cerebral hemispheres at about the same time. • The seizure may involve one region more than another, e.g., frontal.
Partial	• Partial seizures start within a cortical focus. Note that the focus may not always be seen on imaging and may not always produce electroencephalogram (EEG) changes on scalp recordings.

Generalized Seizures	Features
Absence	• Episodic loss of awareness without major motor activity • There is no aura, no post-ictal confusion, or somnolence. • EEG shows 3/sec spike-wave pattern. • Onset is in childhood, although seizures can persist into adult life. • About 40% of patients also have generalized tonic/clonic seizures.
Generalized tonic/clonic	• Major motor seizures with stiffening (tonic phase) and shaking (clonic phase) • Patients are unresponsive during the seizure, and have post-ictal confusion and usually drowsiness. • EEG shows spike-wave discharges of varying frequency. EEG typically is obscured by muscle and movement artifacts during the seizure.
Myoclonic	• Brief jerks that do not interfere with consciousness plus generalized seizures • EEG usually shows a fast (4–5/sec) spike-wave pattern.

Partial Seizures	Features
Simple partial	• Focal jerking of one extremity or one side is the most common. There is no disturbance of consciousness. • EEG shows focal spikes over the contralateral hemisphere.
Complex partial	• Disturbance of consciousness with or without motor activity is typical of complex partial seizures. • EEG shows focal spikes over the frontal or temporal lobes. Some foci are too deep to be seen without the use of depth or subdural strip electrodes.
Secondarily generalized	• Focal seizures can spread to involve the remainder of the brain. This is called secondarily-generalized because it starts focal and becomes generalized. This is as opposed to primary generalized seizures, where the entirety of the brain is involved from the onset.
Seizure versus epilepsy	• *Seizure* is a single event. • *Epilepsy* is having recurrent unprovoked seizures. Not all patients with seizures have epilepsy—either they have a single event or they have provoked events (e.g., head injury or alcohol withdrawal).

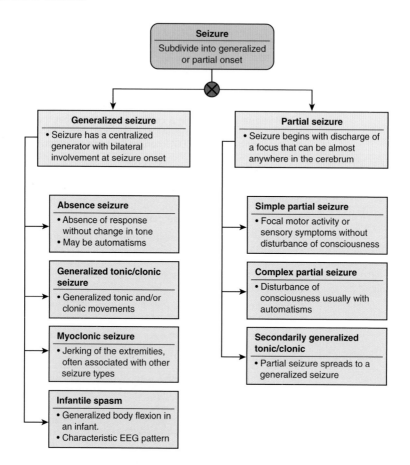

SEIZURE SYMPTOMS AND SIGNS	
Aura	• Consists of symptoms that herald the onset of a seizure • Likely represents the earliest phase of abnormal synchronous epileptiform activity • Common auras are sensory, including dysesthesias, and positive visual phenomena.
Tonic activity	• Stiffening of the extremities, either on one side or both sides, with generalized seizures • May be followed by clonic activity
Clonic activity	• Rhythmic shaking of an extremity on one or both sides of the body • Can sometimes precede the clonic phase of a seizure
Myoclonic activity	• Brief jerks that do not disturb consciousness • Myoclonus can be focal, multifocal, or generalized. • Myoclonus can occur with or without seizures.
Loss of consciousness	• Expected in patients with generalized seizures of all types • Not associated with disturbance of consciousness during the brief myoclonus, but associated seizures are linked with impaired consciousness • *Simple partial seizures* are not associated with disturbance of consciousness, and the foci usually are in the frontal, parietal, or occipital region. • *Complex partial seizures* are associated with disturbance of consciousness, and usually are due to foci in the temporal or frontal lobes.
Automatism	• Automatic stereotyped movements that occur in some people with absence and partial seizures • *Common automatisms* are lip smacking, chewing, eye blinking, and picking at clothes or at the air. • *Complex automatisms* are more common with complex partial seizures than with absence epilepsy.
Post-ictal symptoms	• Confusion, sedation, lethargy, and sometimes agitation follow a seizure in the post-ictal period. • Absence of post-ictal symptoms is present with absence seizures and often with pseudoseizures (psychogenic seizures).

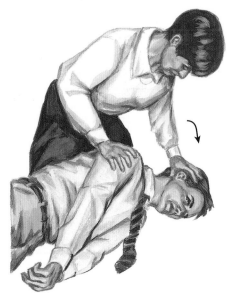

Help person lie down and roll onto side to help avoid aspiration

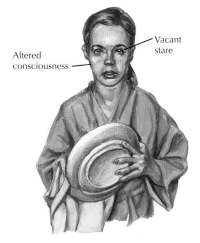

Altered consciousness

Vacant stare

Patient may unconsciously continue preictal activity

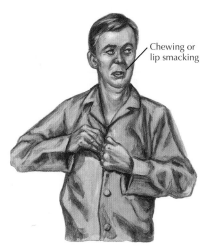

Chewing or lip smacking

Repetitive, seemingly purposeful activity such as dressing and undressing or fumbling with buttons

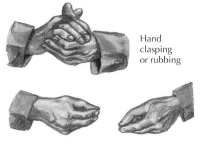

Hand clasping or rubbing

Pill-rolling movements

JOHN A.CRAIG—AD

GENERALIZED SEIZURES	
Description	• Involve the entirety of the cerebral cortex. Seizures may start generalized or become generalized after a focal onset.
Pathophysiology	• The entirety of the cerebral cortex is involved in generalized seizures. • *Primary generalized seizures* involve the entirety of the cortex from the onset. • *Secondary generalized seizures* start with a partial seizure, which spreads to the entirety of the cortex.

Clinical findings	• Neurologic exam usually is normal unless the seizure is due to a defect, such as mass, infarct, infection, hypoxia, or other insult.
	• The most common manifestations of generalized seizures include:
	  • Generalized *tonic/clonic* seizures
	  • Absence seizures
	  • Myoclonic seizures
	  • Infantile spasms

Laboratory studies	• MRI and CT are normal for most patients. Imaging is most likely to be abnormal if the neurologic exam is abnormal, or if the generalized seizure is secondarily generalized. • Labs are normal unless metabolic disturbance is the cause of the seizure, e.g., disorder of sodium, calcium, magnesium, glucose, renal function, and hepatic function.
Diagnosis	• Clinical findings are key, i.e., generalized *tonic/clonic* activity or absence (loss of responsiveness without loss of tone). • EEG may be normal between seizures (interictal) but should show epileptiform activity at the beginning of a seizure, and suppression and slowing following a seizure (post-ictal). Ictal EEG may be obscured by movement and muscle artifact.
Differential diagnosis	• *Pseudoseizure.* Patients may have generalized shaking, which looks like a generalized seizure not due to abnormal brain activity. Unresponsiveness without motor activity resembling absence seizure also can be a pseudoseizure. • *Complex partial seizure.* Unresponsiveness without motor activity or loss of tone can be a complex partial seizure and can resemble absence seizure.
Management	• A variety of medications are effective for generalized seizures. • Generalized tonic/clonic seizures usually are treated with phenytoin, carbamazepine, or valproate, as well as some of the newer anticonvulsants. • Absence seizures usually are treated with ethosuximide, valproate, or lamotrigine.
Clinical course	• Most patients have control of seizures with anticonvulsant therapy and self-care. • Patients with secondary generalized seizures are less likely to have control than those with primary generalized seizures.

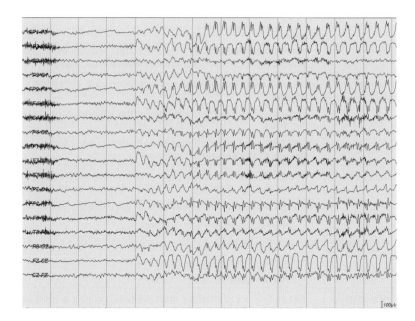

Absence seizure: Rhythmic 3/second spike-wake discharge typical or absence seizure, a form of primary generalized epilepsy

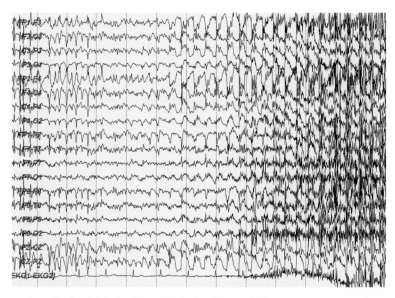

Generalized tonic/clonic seizure: Rapid polyspike-wave discharge seen in a patient with generalized tonic/clonic seizures

PARTIAL SEIZURES	
Description	• Seizures that originate from a defined cortical focus • The seizure activity involves only part of the brain, at least initially.
Pathophysiology	• One or more foci of epileptiform activity may exist in patients with partial seizures. • Some foci are due to focal observable structural lesions, including tumors, developmental abnormalities, hamartomas, neural migration abnormalities, vascular anomalies, infarctions, infections, trauma, mesial temporal sclerosis, and others. • Other foci are due to circuit abnormalities, which cannot be discerned even on microscopic examination.

Clinical findings	• Can have a variety of presentations. Simple and complex are the main categories, with the latter affecting consciousness:
	  • *Simple partial seizures* are characterized by focal sensory or motor symptoms, including dysesthesias, shaking, turning, twisting, or dystonic posturing.
	  • *Complex partial seizures* are characterized by alteration of consciousness, often with automatisms. These seizures may resemble absence seizures but with more complex automatisms.

Laboratory studies	• Magnetic resonance imaging (MRI) and computed tomography (CT) are more likely to be abnormal with partial seizures than with generalized seizures. MRI is the most sensitive test for structural lesion. Mesial temporal pathology may be missed unless specifically looked for. • Routine labs usually are normal. • EEG usually is abnormal with partial seizures, although some patients may have normal interictal or even ictal EEGs if the seizure's focus is deep to the scalp.
Diagnosis	• Clinical features supported by EEG abnormalities during the ictal or interictal period. • Imaging may be abnormal, which would be supportive but not diagnostic of partial seizures. • Routine labs typically are normal.
Differential diagnosis	• *Absence seizures.* Staring spells of absence seizures can be mistaken for complex partial seizures. • *Dystonia.* Movement disorders such as dystonia and dyskinesias can be mistaken for partial seizures.
Management	• A wide variety of medications are used for partial seizures, as outlined on the pages for simple partial seizures and complex partial seizures. • Surgery is needed for some patients with partial seizures who do not have total control of seizures with medicines.
Clinical course	• Most patients have control of their seizures with medications. • Control with medication is less likely with partial seizures than with generalized seizures.

Simple Partial Seizures

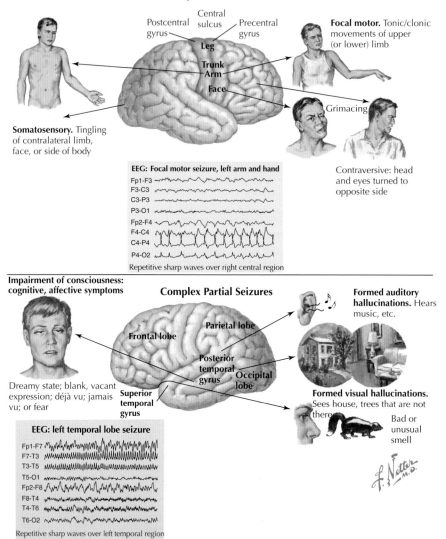

Postcentral gyrus — Central sulcus — Precentral gyrus

Leg
Trunk
Arm
Face

Focal motor. Tonic/clonic movements of upper (or lower) limb

Grimacing

Somatosensory. Tingling of contralateral limb, face, or side of body

Contraversive: head and eyes turned to opposite side

EEG: Focal motor seizure, left arm and hand

Fp1-F3
F3-C3
C3-P3
P3-O1
Fp2-F4
F4-C4
C4-P4
P4-O2

Repetitive sharp waves over right central region

Impairment of consciousness: cognitive, affective symptoms

Complex Partial Seizures

Parietal lobe
Frontal lobe
Posterior temporal gyrus
Occipital lobe
Superior temporal gyrus

Dreamy state; blank, vacant expression; déjà vu; jamais vu; or fear

Formed auditory hallucinations. Hears music, etc.

Formed visual hallucinations. Sees house, trees that are not there

Bad or unusual smell

EEG: left temporal lobe seizure

Fp1-F7
F7-T3
T3-T5
T5-O1
Fp2-F8
F8-T4
T4-T6
T6-O2

Repetitive sharp waves over left temporal region

ABSENCE EPILEPSY	
Description	• Absence seizures are primary generalized seizures characterized by unresponsiveness without loss of postural tone. • EEG shows characteristic 3/sec spike-and-wave pattern
Pathophysiology	• Absence seizures are idiopathic, with a genetic contribution. • True absence seizures do not develop from structural lesions.
Clinical findings	• Patients present with episodes of unresponsiveness without loss of postural tone. Patient remains upright and stares, and cannot be stimulated out of the event. • There is no aura before the seizure. • Automatisms are common, including licking lips or fumbling an object the patient was holding. These are more common with increased duration of seizure. • Episodes are provoked by hyperventilation. • There is no post-ictal confusion or drowsiness. • Onset is in childhood, although it can persist into adult life. • Some patients will develop generalized tonic/clonic seizures, as many as 40%.
Laboratory studies	• CT and MRI are normal. Although commonly ordered, the chance of finding a structural lesion with a typical absence epilepsy history is very low. • Routine laboratory studies are normal. • EEG shows 3/sec spike-and-wave discharge. Clinical seizures and EEG discharges are provoked by hyperventilation. The finding of discharges on routine EEG is so common, that a lack of them raises questions in the diagnosis.
Diagnosis	• Clinical history of staring spells • No abnormalities on examination or on imaging • EEG findings of typical 3/sec spike-and-wave discharge
Differential diagnosis	• *Inattention.* Children may stare, and be suspected as having absence seizures, especially by teachers. The automatisms and absence of responsiveness during the episode argues against this. • *Complex partial seizures.* Some patients with CPS may have staring spells that can resemble absence seizures. These patients tend to be adults rather than children, have more prominent automatisms that are not so duration-dependent, and have post-ictal confusion or alteration in consciousness.
Management	• Ethosuximide and valproate are the most commonly used agents for treatment of absence seizures. Lamotrigine also is used. A number of other newer anticonvulsants are being used.
Clinical course	• There are no long-term neurologic deficits associated with absence epilepsy. • Most patients (60%–80%) have remission of absence seizures.

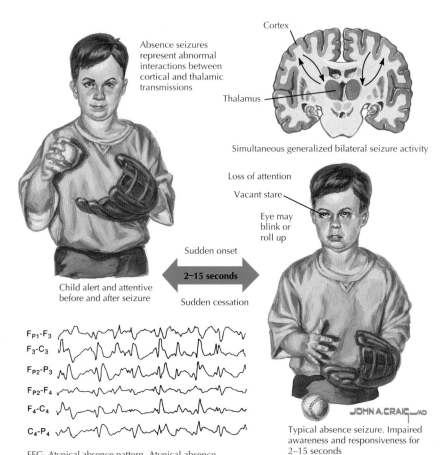

Absence seizures represent abnormal interactions between cortical and thalamic transmissions

Cortex

Thalamus

Simultaneous generalized bilateral seizure activity

Loss of attention

Vacant stare

Eye may blink or roll up

Sudden onset

2–15 seconds

Child alert and attentive before and after seizure

Sudden cessation

Typical absence seizure. Impaired awareness and responsiveness for 2–15 seconds

JOHN A. CRAIG—AD

EEG. Atypical absence pattern. Atypical absence seizures may be associated with mental retardation and tonic or atonic seizures

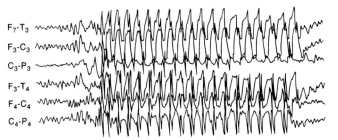

EEG. Typical absence pattern

GENERALIZED TONIC/CLONIC SEIZURES	
Description	• Major motor seizures, characterized by shaking and stiffening of the extremities • Generalized seizure discharges are seen on the EEG.
Pathophysiology	• Synchronous electrical discharge develops within deep regions of the brain. Circuits involving the cortex are entrained with the discharge resulting in synchronous activation of the cerebral cortex. • The seizure discharge eventually stops by incompletely understood cellular and intercellular systems.
Clinical findings	• The seizure usually begins with stiffening of the extremities (tonic phase), which is usually extensor. There may be a flexor component—especially of the arms—early in the seizure. • Shaking of the arms and legs develops, which is synchronous. • Loss of consciousness is always a feature of generalized tonic/clonic seizures. • Post-ictal somnolence and confusion is expected. Agitation occasionally occurs in the post-ictal period.
Laboratory studies	• MRI usually is normal. • EEG may be normal in the inter-ictal period or show brief bursts of generalized spikes. EEG during the seizure shows generalized spikes, although the EEG may be obscured by movement artifact, making detection of the spikes impossible except at the very beginning of the seizure. EEG after the seizure is suppressed and slower than normal EEG. • Labs are normal. • LP usually is normal, unless the generalized seizure is a manifestation of meningitis or encephalitis.
Diagnosis	• GTC seizures are suspected when a patient presents with generalized tonic/clonic activity. This is a clinical diagnosis. • EEG confirmation seizure activity is occasionally performed during the seizure. Inter-ictal abnormalities on EEG are more common with partial seizures than generalized seizures.
Differential diagnosis	• *Pseudoseizures.* Patients with pseudoseizures most commonly have episodes that resemble generalized tonic/clonic seizures, although there are some clinical differences. • *Clonic syncope.* Patients with arrhythmia or other causes of syncope with cerebral hypoperfusion or hypoxia can have brief shaking associated with the syncope. This easily can be mistaken for generalized tonic/clonic seizure activity.
Management	• Many drugs are available for generalized tonic/clonic seizures. Older drugs include phenytoin, valproate, and carbamazepine. • Many newer drugs also are helpful, although they have not been studied in generalized seizures as in depth as they have been for partial seizures. • Vagal nerve stimulation is seldom used for generalized seizures.
Clinical course	• Seizure can be controlled with medicines in most patients, although there are some individuals who have persistent seizures despite maximal medical therapy.

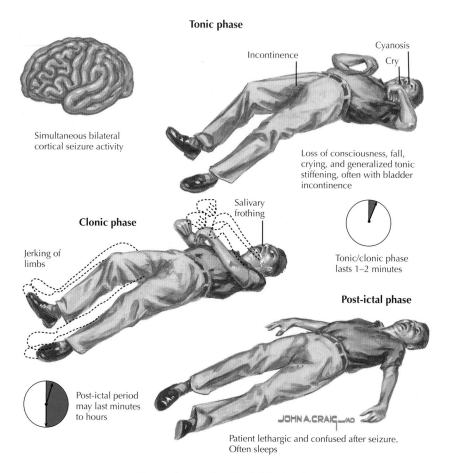

Tonic phase

Simultaneous bilateral cortical seizure activity

Incontinence

Cyanosis
Cry

Loss of consciousness, fall, crying, and generalized tonic stiffening, often with bladder incontinence

Clonic phase

Salivary frothing

Jerking of limbs

Tonic/clonic phase lasts 1–2 minutes

Post-ictal phase

Post-ictal period may last minutes to hours

Patient lethargic and confused after seizure. Often sleeps

JOHN A.CRAIG—AD

Stages of generalized tonic/clonic seizure

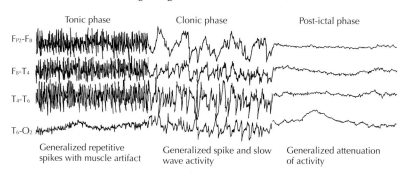

Tonic phase	Clonic phase	Post-ictal phase

F_{P2}-F_8

F_8-T_4

T_4-T_6

T_6-O_2

Generalized repetitive spikes with muscle artifact

Generalized spike and slow wave activity

Generalized attenuation of activity

PSEUDOSEIZURES	
Description	• Clinical seizure activities that are not due to epileptiform discharge, but rather a manifestation of a conversion disorder or malingering • Sometimes called "non epileptic" seizures
Pathophysiology	• Conversion disorder is the most common cause, where there is a subconscious drive for a variety of reasons. Some of the reasons are attention, escape from an adverse situation, or control over others. • Malingering is the cause in a minority of cases. Some of the reasons are seeking of disability or attention, or compensation in litigation.

Clinical findings	• Clinical seizure activity can have a variety of manifestations. These include episodes that look like generalized tonic/clonic seizures and absence seizures.
	• Features that suggest pseudoseizures rather than epileptic seizures are:
	  • Back and forth rocking
	  • Pelvic thrusting
	  • Bicycle movements of the legs
	  • Retained consciousness with an apparent generalized seizure
	  • Directed violence against an individual
	  • Absence of a post-ictal period
	  • Warning signs that cause the patient to call family or nurse before the seizure
	• These findings do not definitively indicate pseudoseizure but are generally suggestive.

Laboratory studies	• MRI and CT are normal. • Routine labs are normal. • EEG is normal during a pseudoseizure, although there may be muscle and movement artifact that would likely obscure the background. • Long-term video-EEG monitoring may be needed for differentiation.
Diagnosis	• Clinical features and EEG are supportive of the diagnosis of pseudoseizures. • Pseudoseizures and epileptic seizures are coexistent in some patients, so the presence of pseudoseizures does not rule out epileptic seizures.
Differential diagnosis	• *Epileptic seizures.* Genuine seizures may be bizarre, and have the appearance of pseudoseizures. Also, partial seizures with foci in certain areas (e.g., supplementary motor) may have epileptic seizure activity without abnormalities on scalp EEG. • *Cardiac arrhythmia.* Arrhythmia may be associated with loss of responsiveness and shaking that may look like seizure activity. The absence of spike-wave pattern on the EEG might suggest pseudoseizure, although the electrocardiogram (ECG) would show the arrhythmia.

PSEUDOSEIZURES	
Management	• Withdrawal of anticonvulsants is performed for most patients with pseudoseizures, although one would want to be quite sure that there were not coexistent epileptic seizures.
	• Psychological consultation should be recommended and ongoing support for resolution of the psychological issues that predisposed to the pseudoseizures.
Clinical course	Most patients improve with treatment; however, ongoing support is needed to address the underlying causes.

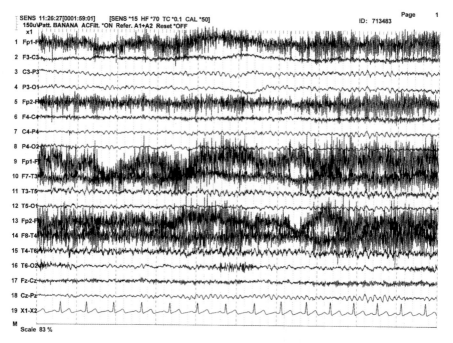

Pseudoseizure: EEG during a clinical seizure without EEG abnormality. The EEG background is normal and the fast activity is muscle artifact.

JUVENILE MYOCLONIC EPILEPSY (JME)	
Description	• A generalized epilepsy that begins in childhood and is associated with brief jerks plus generalized seizures • Seizures can be generalized tonic/clonic and/or absence.
Pathophysiology	• JME is an idiopathic disorder. No structural cause is identified. • There is a genetic predisposition. Patients with JME have increased incidences of family members with epilepsy.
Clinical findings	• Brief myoclonic jerks • Generalized seizures, most likely after awakening, in the morning. Can have generalized tonic/clonic, or less commonly, absence seizures. • Intellect is normal. • Neurologic exam is normal.
Laboratory studies	• MRI and CT are normal. • Routine labs are normal. • EEG shows fast (4–6/sec) spike-and-wave, or polyspike-and-wave discharge in the interictal state. Prolonged discharges are seen with seizures. Absence seizures in patients with JME show the 3/sec spike-and-wave pattern.
Diagnosis	• Clinical history of myoclonus with generalized seizures suggests JME. • EEG provides supportive evidence if a fast spike-and-wave pattern is seen. • Examination, including intellectual function, should be normal.
Differential diagnosis	• *Generalized tonic/clonic seizures.* These can occur without myoclonus. • *Absence seizures.* These rarely can have associated myoclonus, and in this case, myoclonus occurs immediately prior to the absence (myoclonic absence).
Management	• Valproate and lamotrigine are the most commonly used agents. • Monotherapy is used for most patients.
Clinical course	• Many patients have control of seizures with medication; however, some individuals will continue to have seizures despite medications. • Most patients with JME do not "outgrow" seizures, and will continue to need anticonvulsants throughout adult life.

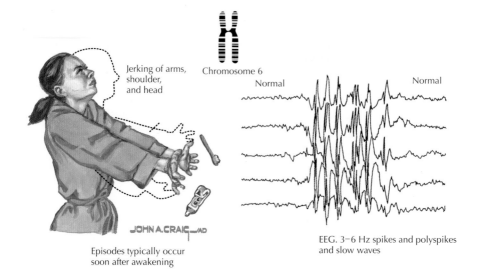

Jerking of arms, shoulder, and head

Chromosome 6

Normal

Normal

JOHN A. CRAIG—AD

Episodes typically occur soon after awakening

EEG. 3–6 Hz spikes and polyspikes and slow waves

SIMPLE PARTIAL SEIZURES (SPS)	
Description	• Seizure of focal origin, producing elementary motor or sensory symptoms • Differentiated from complex partial by absence of disturbance of consciousness
Pathophysiology	• Usually due to a focal structural lesion
Clinical findings	• Focal motor activity is the most common, including: • Focal clonic activity • Turning of the head/body to one side (versive seizure) • Dystonic posturing • Focal sensory symptoms, e.g., dysesthesias • Normal examination
Laboratory studies	• Imaging may show focal structural lesion, which can be of almost any etiology. Most common are encephalomalacia from stroke or trauma, tumor, vascular malformation, and developmental abnormality. • Normal routine labs • EEG may show focal discharge during the seizure activity.
Diagnosis	• Clinical features of focal motor activity associated with focal epileptiform activity on EEG • Exam is usually normal; however, there could be focal signs associated with a focal structural lesion that causes the simple partial seizures.
Differential diagnosis	• *Dystonia.* Twisting of the head and neck and posturing of one or more extremities is characteristic of dystonia. The dystonic movements are constant rather than episodic. Also, patients with dystonia can still make voluntary movements superimposed on the involuntary movements, unlike partial seizures. • *Spasticity.* Stiffness of one or more extremities due to spasticity is characterized by tonic activity and reduction in voluntary use of the extremity. The constancy of the contraction differentiates the spasticity from seizure activity, which could also be tonic, but is more likely to be episodic. • *Torsion dystonia.* Torsion dystonia is characterized by abnormal twisting of the head and neck. This can have the appearance of a simple partial seizure, but is constant, rather than episodic. The arm is not affected.
Management	• A variety of anticonvulsants are used for simple partial seizures. Phenytoin is classically used, but carbamazepine, valproate, and many of the newer anticonvulsants often are used. • Seizure surgery is sometimes needed for patients with simple partial seizures.
Clinical course	• Many patients have control of seizures through medication. Some patients will require more than one medication. • Seizure surgery is sometimes effective for selected patients with simple partial seizures.

Partial Motor and Somatosensory Seizures

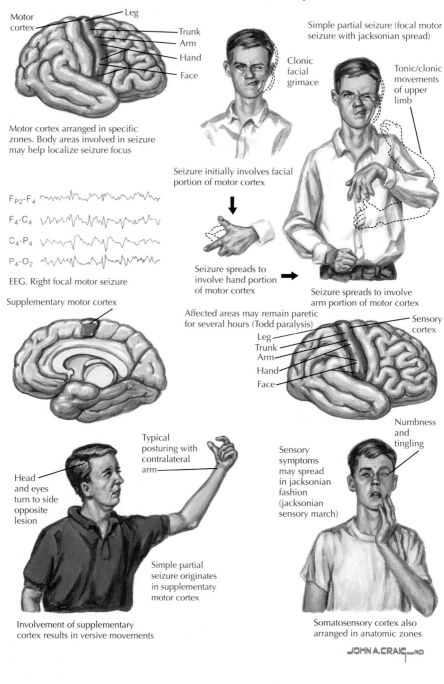

Motor cortex

Leg
Trunk
Arm
Hand
Face

Motor cortex arranged in specific zones. Body areas involved in seizure may help localize seizure focus

Simple partial seizure (focal motor seizure with jacksonian spread)

Clonic facial grimace

Tonic/clonic movements of upper limb

Seizure initially involves facial portion of motor cortex

F_{P2}-F_4

F_4-C_4

C_4-P_4

P_4-O_2

EEG. Right focal motor seizure

Supplementary motor cortex

Seizure spreads to involve hand portion of motor cortex

Seizure spreads to involve arm portion of motor cortex

Affected areas may remain paretic for several hours (Todd paralysis)

Leg
Trunk
Arm
Hand
Face

Sensory cortex

Typical posturing with contralateral arm

Head and eyes turn to side opposite lesion

Simple partial seizure originates in supplementary motor cortex

Involvement of supplementary cortex results in versive movements

Sensory symptoms may spread in jacksonian fashion (jacksonian sensory march)

Numbness and tingling

Somatosensory cortex also arranged in anatomic zones

JOHN A. CRAIG—AD

COMPLEX PARTIAL SEIZURES (CPS)	
Description	• A focal seizure that results in disturbance of consciousness • Complex symptomatology refers to the cognitive changes.
Pathophysiology	• Foci usually are structural lesions in the temporal or frontal lobes. Mesial temporal sclerosis, vascular malformations, tumors, and regions of encephalomalacia due to previous trauma or infarction, or neuronal migration abnormalities are some of the potential causes. • No pathological abnormality is seen in the foci after resection in some patients.
Clinical findings	• Aura prior to the seizure is common with CPS. • CPS is characterized by disturbance of responsiveness without major motor findings. • Automatisms are common. • There is often post-ictal confusion, which helps differentiation from absence seizures.
Laboratory studies	• Routine labs are normal. • Imaging with MRI and CT may show structural lesions in the area of the foci, as listed in the section above. • EEG often shows inter-ictal abnormalities when electrodes record from the region of the focus. However, the foci may be deep to the scalp, so that routine EEG is not able to detect the discharge. Because the discharge is not generalized, a seizure may not be associated with a discharge on routine scalp EEG.
Diagnosis	• CPS is suspected when a patient presents with episodes of alteration of consciousness but without the major motor activity of GTC seizures. • Inter-ictal abnormalities on EEG support the diagnosis. Ictal EEG abnormalities can confirm the diagnosis, but require long-term EEG monitoring. • Imaging is performed to look for a structural lesion.
Differential diagnosis	• *Absence seizures.* Episodic loss of consciousness without loss of posture is typical of absence seizures. Absence is differentiated from CPS by the very different EEG pattern, absence of aura, and absence of post-ictal confusion. • *Pseudoseizures.* Patients may have disturbance of consciousness without major motor activity as a manifestation of pseudoseizures.
Management	• Multiple anticonvulsants have been used for patients with CPS. In fact, most of the newly approved drugs have been studied predominantly in patients with CPS. • Vagal nerve stimulation is used for selected patients with frequent medically refractory CPS. • Seizure surgery, such as temporal lobectomy and focus resection, particularly is used for patients with CPS who are medically refractory.
Clinical course	Many patients have control with the first or second drug that is prescribed. If the seizures are not controlled with two drugs, the chance of control with additional drugs alone or as adjunctive therapy is low.

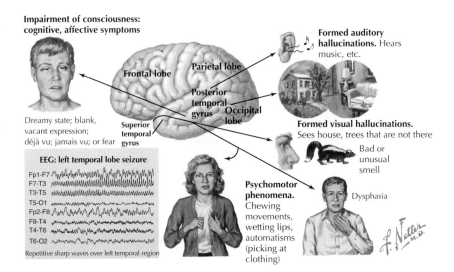

Impairment of consciousness: cognitive, affective symptoms

Frontal lobe

Parietal lobe

Posterior temporal gyrus

Occipital lobe

Superior temporal gyrus

Dreamy state; blank, vacant expression; déjà vu; jamais vu; or fear

Formed auditory hallucinations. Hears music, etc.

Formed visual hallucinations. Sees house, trees that are not there

Bad or unusual smell

Dysphasia

Psychomotor phenomena. Chewing movements, wetting lips, automatisms (picking at clothing)

EEG: left temporal lobe seizure

Fp1-F7
F7-T3
T3-T5
T5-O1
Fp2-F8
F8-T4
T4-T6
T6-O2

Repetitive sharp waves over left temporal region

ECLAMPSIA	
Description	• Characterized by hypertension during or shortly after pregnancy and associated with neurologic complications, including seizures and neurologic deficits • *Pre-eclampsia* is hypertension and proteinuria with pregnancy. • *Eclampsia* is defined as when seizures have developed in this setting.
Pathophysiology	• Pregnancy-induced hypertension likely is related to the effects of the placenta on vascular tone. • Vasospasm produces increased blood pressure, which can progress to the point of multisystem dysfunction.
Clinical findings	• Cardinal clinical findings indicating eclampsia are hypertension, proteinuria, and seizures. • Neurologic symptoms can include headache, visual disturbance, focal neurologic findings, confusion, and even coma. • Seizures can be partial but are more commonly generalized *tonic/clonic.* • Eclampsia may still occur anywhere from days to a couple of weeks following the birth.
Laboratory studies	• Imaging may be normal or show focal areas of T2-hyperintensity on MRI. Diffusion-weighted imaging (DWI) is normal, helping to differentiate the lesions from acute stroke. • EEG may show slowing and/or show discharges associated with the seizures. • Routine labs show the proteinuria.
Diagnosis	• Clinical features of hypertension, proteinuria, and seizures make the diagnosis. • Protienuria is seen in urine analysis. • MRI shows the typical abnormalities on T_2-imaging; however, DWI shows no abnormalities.
Differential diagnosis	• *Stroke.* Stroke has an increased incidence during pregnancy because of hypercoagulable state, and there may be reactive hypertension. Proteinuria is not expected. MRI can usually differentiate stroke from eclampsia. • *Substance use.* Drug overdose can result in mental status changes and seizures, from which a pregnant patient is not immune. • *Epilepsy.* Seizures can occur during pregnancy, so a previous history of seizures should be considered in a patient with suspected eclampsia.
Management	• Magnesium commonly is given and may be all that is needed for control. • Phenytoin and/or diazepam and similar agents also are often used, especially when magnesium is ineffective at controlling the seizures.
Clinical course	• Most patients improve with effective treatment. • Coma and death can occur in some patients.

Eclampsia Clinical Triad

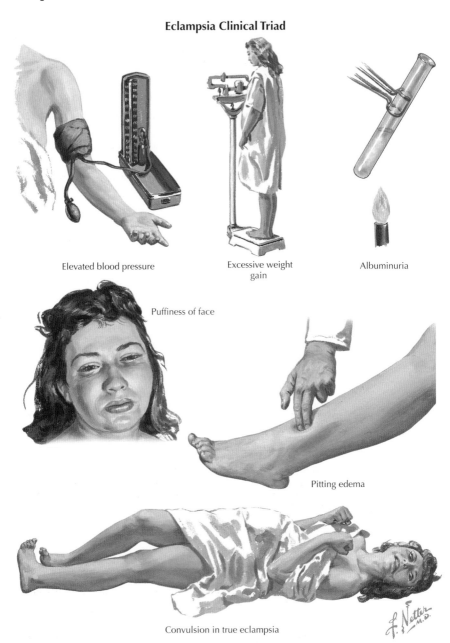

Elevated blood pressure

Excessive weight gain

Albuminuria

Puffiness of face

Pitting edema

Convulsion in true eclampsia

POST-TRAUMATIC SEIZURES	
Description	• Seizures occurring in association with head injury. The seizures may be acute, subacute, or delayed. • *Post-traumatic epilepsy* means recurrent unprovoked seizures, extending beyond the immediate recovery period.
Pathophysiology	• Acute trauma disturbs membrane function so that seizure activity can develop. • Acute and subacute seizures may be related to local tissue damage, edema, and hemorrhage. • Delayed seizures are likely due to the development of scar tissue in the region of damage. • Seizures are more common with penetrating trauma than with closed head injury.
Clinical findings	• Seizures may occur acutely, at the time of the head injury; subacutely with the first weeks after the injury; or delayed, months to more than a year following the injury. • Seizures can be partial or generalized. Without treatment, secondary generalized seizures are typically from a focal origin. • Exam results depend on the severity of the head injury. Seizures may develop in patients who have little or no deficit or have total incapacitation.
Laboratory studies	• Routine labs are normal. • Imaging with MRI or CT also may be normal, but with penetrating head injury, structural disruption is common. Encephalomalacia also seen in some patients long after the injury. • EEG can be normal in patients with little neurologic deficit. Slowing of the background can be seen especially if there is neurologic deficit. Focal slowing is also seen in patients with local hematomas or penetrating trauma.
Diagnosis	• Clinical seizure activity is seen after head injury. Acute and subacute seizures are easy to diagnose, but delayed seizures may or may not have an association with the previous injury. Seizures that occur for the first time years after an injury are less likely to be directly related to the insult. • Imaging always is performed in patients with head injury. Imaging with MRI also should be performed for patients with suspected delayed post-traumatic seizures to look for other pathology. • EEG is helpful for localizing the focus, but the diagnosis of seizures is seldom in doubt. Rare patients may have pseudoseizures after a head injury.
Differential diagnosis	• *Pseudoseizures.* Patients with head injury rarely may experience pseudoseizures. These patients also may have epileptic seizures, and, therefore, decisions regarding medication have to be carefully considered. • *Posturing.* Patients with severe head injury and neurologic deficits may have posturing that can look like seizure activity. This may be associated with autonomic symptoms, extensor posturing, and some clonus. Unlike seizures, posturing usually is of longer duration and is stimulus sensitive.

POST-TRAUMATIC SEIZURES—cont'd	
Management	• Anticonvulsants are given for seizures when they occur acutely. Often loading doses are needed; therefore, the intravenous options are phenytoin (or the intravenous prodrug fosphenytoin) or valproate. Maintenance after loading for acute seizures is done with the oral versions of these drugs. Other anticonvulsants are also effective, but cannot be used as loading doses. • Prophylaxis has not been shown to reduce the incidence of post-traumatic epilepsy.
Clinical course	• Most patients with acute and subacute seizures will not have recurrent seizures, and, therefore, long-term prevention is not needed. • Delayed seizures have a predisposition to recurrence, although not all will recur. Therefore, decision as whether to treat has to be individualized.

SURGICAL TREATMENTS FOR EPILEPSY	

Description	• Anticonvulsants do not fully control seizures in all patients. Therefore, surgical treatments have been tried with great success.
	• The most commonly used surgical treatments are:
	  • Temporal lobectomy
	  • Surgical resection of the focus
	  • Corpus callosum section
	  • Vagal nerve stimulation

Physiology	• Destruction or removal of the focus can result in control of the epilepsy where medications were not effective. • Recurrence of seizures can occur due to other foci not previously seen or due to scarring in the region of the surgery.
Patient selection	• Patients who should be considered for these procedures include those in whom the diagnosis of epilepsy is certain, and in whom there has not been control with medications. • Evaluation and treatment with one of these or other procedures should be left to physicians who are educated and experienced in evaluation and management of refractory seizures. The techniques should only be used by epilepsy programs—merely having the technical skill to perform the technique does not mean they should be done.
Technique	**Features**
Temporal lobectomy	• Patients with mesial temporal sclerosis and other pathologies of the anterior temporal lobe can have control of seizures with resection of the anterior temporal lobe. • Photon knife destruction of the same region can be performed, without an open surgery.
Surgical resection of the focus	• A defined focus can be identified through mapping, which begins with scalp EEG, then involves a subdural strip and/or depth electrodes. When the focus is identified, directed surgery can improve seizure control.
Corpus callosum section	• Certain patients with intractable seizures who are not candidates of cortical resection may have improvement in the seizures by section of the corpus callosum. • This mainly is done in children and adults with poor function of the hemisphere, which is the origin of the seizures. Also, the seizures may originate in a distribution not confined to a defined resectable focus.
Vagal nerve stimulator	• Performed for patients with refractory seizures, typically partial. Patients selected for VNS usually have frequent seizures or seizures in clusters, are insufficiently controlled with medications, and are not a candidate for surgery. • Improves seizure frequency, but is not expected to completely control the seizures.

Resective Surgery

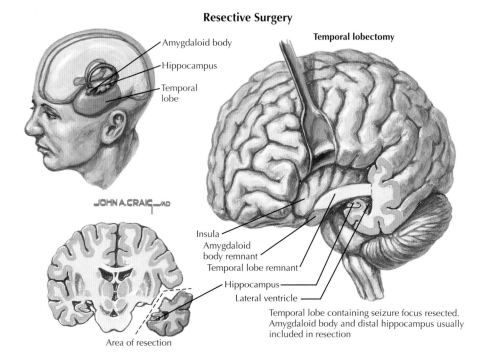

Amygdaloid body

Hippocampus

Temporal lobe

Temporal lobectomy

JOHN A.CRAIG—MD

Insula

Amygdaloid body remnant

Temporal lobe remnant

Hippocampus

Lateral ventricle

Area of resection

Temporal lobe containing seizure focus resected. Amygdaloid body and distal hippocampus usually included in resection

STATUS EPILEPTICUS (SE)	
Description	• Persistent or recurrent seizures of long duration. Although time is arbitrary, anything more than 30 minutes is long duration, but the definition depends on the neurologic and cardiorespiratory manifestations of the episode. • Can be one continuous seizure, or multiple seizures, where the patient has not recovered from the post-ictal period before the next seizure starts
Pathophysiology	• Seizures are common, and most seizures stop due to a combination of factors involving neuronal circuits and cellular mechanisms. In SE, the body has lost the ability to promptly stop a seizure, and the repetitive synchronous neuronal discharge is persistent. • SE can develop from almost any seizure type, from complex and simple partial seizures—to generalized *tonic/clonic* and absence seizures.

Clinical findings	• SE presents with a variety of symptoms. These include:
	
	  • Persistent generalized *tonic/clonic* seizure activity
	
	  • Persistent focal tonic and/or clonic activity
	
	  • Loss of awareness due to absence or complex partial status

Laboratory studies	• Routine labs are normal unless the SE is due to toxic/metabolic abnormality. • Imaging usually is normal unless the seizures are due to structural abnormality. • EEG is abnormal during SE, with a pattern that depends on the seizure type. Simple partial and complex partial seizures will have focal discharges from the scalp near the focus. *Absence status* shows the persistent 3/sec spike-wave pattern. *Generalized tonic/clonic* status is characterized by a generalized spike-wave pattern, which can be of varying frequency, although the EEG may be obscured by movement and muscle artifact.
Diagnosis	• SE is diagnosed by the observation of prolonged apparent seizures. Confirmation by EEG is good, but because of the adverse effects of SE, treatment should not await the performance of the EEG. • Labs including CMP, Ca^{2+}, Mg^{2+} are performed immediately. Drug screen, CBC, and other labs are performed as soon as possible. If there is doubt about whether the seizures are epileptic or psychogenic, prolactin level gives some sensitivity in this regard, being elevated in most patients with seizures. • Imaging is performed when able, although this usually has to wait until after the seizures have been controlled.

STATUS EPILEPTICUS (SE)—cont'd	

Management	• Emergency management protocols are in place in most emergency departments and intensive care units. In the absence of this, the key steps are as follows:
	
	  • ABCs—ensure that the patient has adequate airway, breathing, and circulation.
	
	  • Short-term and long-term medications can be used. Most patients need a short-acting agent, such as a benzodiazepine, for immediate cessation of the seizure.
	
	  • Prolonged anticonvulsant therapy begins with a load of either phenytoin or valproate. Phenytoin loading is most commonly performed using the prodrug fosphenytoin.
	
	  • Maintenance treatment of the seizures initially is with the oral version of the first drug use, usually phenytoin or valproate. Doses are adjusted to therapeutic levels and seizure control. Change to another agent is performed if needed.
	
	  • Seizures that do not respond to treatment with benzodiazepines and anticonvulsant therapy often need general anesthesia for control. Paralysis without treating the electrocerebral discharge is not recommended. Propofol is a commonly used anesthetic that can be used by continuous infusion. This has largely replaced intravenous barbiturates for the treatment of SE. Patients treated with these agents are intubated and mechanically ventilated.

Clinical course	• The outcome of SE depends on the cause. SE has a poorer prognosis if it is due to severe head injury, encephalitis, or other infection, or massive stroke. • SE related to a generalized or partial epilepsy has a better prognosis for neurologic recovery, providing that the patient did not have anoxia at the time of the SE.

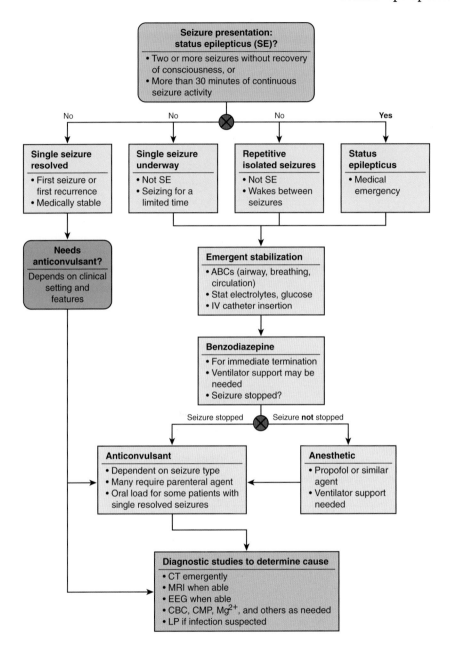

OVERVIEW OF STROKE	
Types of stroke	*Infarction*: • Thrombotic • Embolic • Lacunar • Venous *Hemorrhage*: • Subdural • Epidural • Subarachnoid • Intraparenchymal • Hemorrhagic transformation of ischemic stroke
Stroke Syndromes	**Likely Etiologies of the Syndrome**
Abrupt onset of focal deficit	• Embolic infarction, most likely, or • Thrombotic infarction
Awaken with focal deficit	• Thrombotic infarction, or • Lacunar infarction
Rapid but not abrupt onset of focal deficit	• Thrombotic infarction, or • Lacunar infarction, or • Venous infarction, or • Intraparenchymal hemorrhage
Acute onset of severe headache without deficit	• Subarachnoid hemorrhage (SAH) • Intraparenchymal hemorrhage (less likely)
Headache and focal deficit after injury	• Subdural hemorrhage • Epidural hemorrhage
Subacute onset of neurologic deficit	• Intraparencymal hemorrhage, or • Hemorrhagic transformation of ischemic stroke
Coma after head injury, with or without a lucid interval	Epidural hemorrhage (this is a classic history)

TYPES OF STROKE	
Description	Stroke is an acute neurologic event having foundation in pathology of the blood vessels supplying the brain.

Pathophysiology	• Vessel pathology can be congenital or acquired.
	• Strokes are ischemic or hemorrhagic.
	• Causes of ischemic stroke include:
	  • Thrombotic occlusion of arteries or veins,
	  • Embolic disease from the great vessels or heart, or
	  • Occlusion of the small penetrating blood vessels.
	Causes of hemorrhage can be breakage of the blood vessel due to hypertension or aneurysm, trauma, penetrating injury, shearing injury of the brain, or due to fragile vessels from infarction.

Clinical findings	Details of the clinical presentations are presented on subsequent pages, but in general, stroke presents with acute onset of focal deficit, including weakness, sensory loss, ataxia, speech deficit, or visual loss. Although there are other symptoms and signs, these are the most common.

Types of Infarction	Important Features
Embolic	• Embolic disease arises from the heart, aorta, or the carotid or vertebral arteries. • Cardiac emboli can be from valvular disease, akinetic myocardium with thrombus formation, or from the venous system via a right-to-left shunt from septal defect.
Thrombotic	• Thrombotic disease is occlusion of the vessel by propagation of thrombus. • The occlusion occurs over time, and the extent of the symptoms depends not only on the size and location of the vessel, but on collateral flow. These collaterals have more time to expand if the occlusion occurs over time.
Venous	• Venous infarction is much less common than arterial infarction. Pregnancy and other hypercoagulable states predispose to venous infarction. • Patients present any combination of focal weakness, headache, cognitive difficulty, and seizures.

Hemorrhage	Important Features
Subdural hematoma	• Subdural hemorrhage (SDH) can be spontaneous or due to trauma. In elderly patients, the trauma may be so mild as to be forgotten. • SDH can be acute, subacute, or chronic. Many patients present with layered blood in the subdural hematoma, suggesting various ages of hemorrhage.
Subarachnoid hemorrhage	• Subarachnoid hemorrhage is usually due to rupture of an intracranial aneurysm. • There is acute onset of headache and sometimes neurologic deficit. • SAH may be missed on CT, and, therefore, LP is indicated if this is considered despite the results of a CT.

Hemorrhage	Important Features
Epidural hematoma	• Epidural hemorrhage usually is due to trauma. The bleeding usually is arterial, from the middle meningeal artery. • Patients present with rapid deterioration in mental status after initially appearing to survive the injury alert and well. This rapid deterioration should trigger urgent CT for epidural hematoma.
Intraparanchymal hematoma	• Intraparenchymal hemorrhages usually are due to hypertension, although amyloid angiopathy and trauma can both cause intraparenchymal hemorrhage. Hemorrhagic infarction is another important cause of intraparenchymal bleeding. • Patients present with weakness, and may have seizures and decreased level of consciousness.

Diagnosis of Stroke

Ischemic ◀━━━ **Stroke** ━━▶ Hemorrhagic

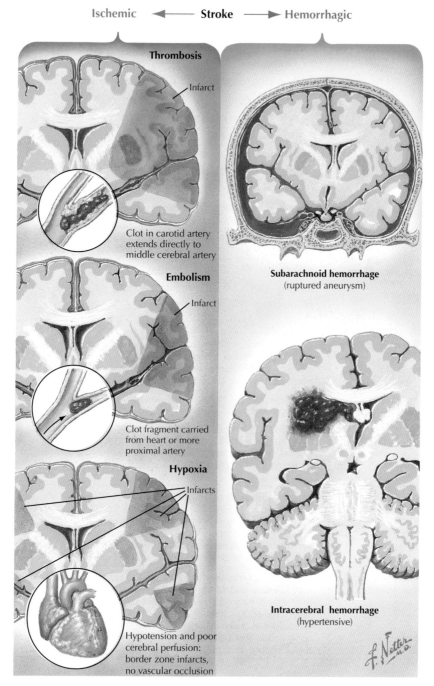

Thrombosis

Infarct

Clot in carotid artery
extends directly to
middle cerebral artery

Embolism

Infarct

Clot fragment carried
from heart or more
proximal artery

Hypoxia

Infarcts

Hypotension and poor
cerebral perfusion:
border zone infarcts,
no vascular occlusion

Subarachnoid hemorrhage
(ruptured aneurysm)

Intracerebral hemorrhage
(hypertensive)

EMERGENCY MANAGEMENT	
Steps in emergency management	• ABCs—**a**irway, **b**reathing, and **c**irculation, as with all emergencies. • Obtain vital signs. • Attach ECG leads, insert IV, and attach blood pressure (BP) monitoring device. • Perform initial medical and neurologic assessment. This includes: ◦ Level of consciousness ◦ Pupil response and eye movements ◦ Movement of arms and legs ◦ Cardiac and pulmonary ascultation ◦ Vascular survey. Look for pulses, cyanosis. • Obtain history from patient and others with the patient. • Perform detailed neurologic and medical exam to determine the diagnosis. • Determine candidacy for immediate stroke intervention, especially surgery or tissue-type plasminogen activator (t-PA).
Tests performed in the emergency department	• Blood—CMP, CBC, PT, PTT • Imaging—CXR, CT head without contrast • Urine—UA • Physiologic—ECG
Consideration of t-PA	• A patient who presents to the emergency department with suspected infarction should be considered for t-PA. If the patient arrives less than three hours since they were last seen to be normal, then they are considered a candidate for t-PA. • There are defined inclusion and exclusion criteria as shown on the management page. • Note that t-PA should not be given outside of the 3-hour window. Also, the clock starts from when the patient was last seen to be normal. A patient who awakens with a deficit may have had the stroke soon after going to sleep, and, therefore, the time of onset is not certain.
Consideration of surgery	• Patients with signs and symptoms of acute CNS bleed should have the CT performed as soon as possible. If the CT confirms bleed, then neurosurgery should be emergently consulted. The only exception to this would be a patient who would clearly not be a candidate for surgery, e.g., patient unstable for any procedure or a patient who refuses consideration of any procedure.
Consideration of neurointervention	• Interventional treatment of acute stroke is under development, and may become part of routine practice in the future. Meanwhile, it only should be performed on selected patients and at institutions where the staff is trained and experienced in the intervention. Specialists at those institutions will determine when these are appropriate. Just because a procedure can be done does not mean that it should be done.

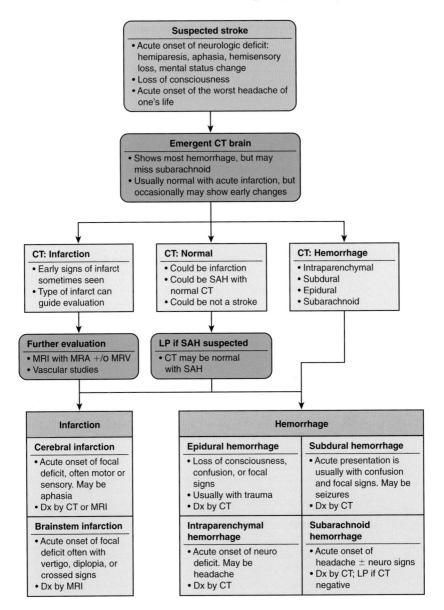

TRANSIENT ISCHEMIC ATTACK (TIA)	
Description	Temporary interruption of focal brain circulation, which results in neurologic deficit
Pathophysiology	• The most common cause of transient ischemic attack (TIA) is embolic disease from the heart or cerebral arteries. • The emboli temporarily block the vessels resulting in loss of function. The embolus can then break up and go downstream, resulting in return of flow to the region.

Clinical findings	• Temporary neurologic deficit lasts less than 24 hours, by definition. Commonly, the deficit lasts less than 1 hour, with a typical time of 15 minutes.
	• Almost any deficit can develop, but some of the most common are:
	  • Hemiparesis
	  • Hemisensory loss
	  • Aphasia
	  • Confusion
	  • Hemianopia
	  • Ataxia
	  • Vertigo
	• The onset of the deficit is abrupt, which helps differentiation from the neurologic deficit of migraine, and which has a progressive onset and migration of symptoms.
	• The recovery is gradual.

Laboratory studies	• Routine labs usually are normal. • Extended labs may show hyperlipidemia, hypercoagulable state, elevated C-reactive protein (CRP), elevated homocysteine, abnormal antinuclear antibody (ANA), and/or erythrocyte sedimentation rate (ESR). • Imaging usually is normal, although CT and MRI may show signs of previous infarction. Up to 40% of patients with TIA have signs of acute ischemic change on MRI diffusion-weighted imaging (DWI). This means that some TIAs are small strokes from which the patient clinically recovered. • Vascular imaging may show clot in the heart, valvular disease, right-to-left shunt, prominent aortic atheroma, carotid stenosis, or ulcerated plaque. • UA may show blood if there are multiple emboli throughout the body.
Diagnosis	• TIA is a clinical diagnosis. Abrupt onset of deficit, with recovery usually lasting less than an hour. • Imaging shows no abnormality or signs of previous strokes.

TRANSIENT ISCHEMIC ATTACK (TIA)—cont'd	
Differential diagnosis	• *Migraine.* Focal weakness or sensory loss can occur as a part of migraine, either during the aura or during the migraine. The neurologic deficit with migraine has a gradual march, rather than an abrupt onset. Headache with or after the deficit suggests migraine. • *Seizure.* Focal seizure activity usually produces focal shaking or stiffening, but transient paralysis can occur. The duration usually is shorter than TIA, lasting seconds to a few minutes. Also, focal seizures usually are recurrent whereas TIAs are single, although they can recur.

Management	• When the diagnostic tests have been performed, appropriateness of certain procedures can be performed:
	
	   • Carotid endarterectomy—for patients with high-grade carotid stenosis or ulcerated plaque in a vascular distribution appropriate to the deficit.
	
	   • Cardiac septal defect closure—for patients with patent foramen ovale (PFO) or other defect with a right-to-left shunt.
	
	   • Neurointervention—for selected patients with extra- or intracranial stenosis.
	
	 • Antithrombotic therapy is recommended for almost all patients. Some general guidelines are:
	
	   • Antiplatelets for most patients
	
	   • Warfarin for most patients with cardiac emboli and patients with antiphospholipid antibody syndrome
	
	   • Risk reduction includes smoking cessation, management of hypetension, diabetes, and hyperlipidemia, plus lifestyle changes such as a better diet and exercise program.
	
	 • All decisions regarding procedures and medications are individualized. A number of patient-specific factors would affect appropriateness for certain treatments, e.g., avoid warfarin in a noncompliant alcoholic, avoid surgery for a patient with end-stage cancer.

Clinical course	• Having a TIA places the patient at a markedly increased risk for subsequent TIA and stroke. The relative risk may be as high as 10 times. With antithrombotic therapy, procedures as indicated, and lifestyle changes, the belief is that a patient can reduce the incidence of stroke by half. • Patients with TIA have an increased incidence of MI, and, therefore, evaluation for cardiac and peripheral vascular disease is appropriate.

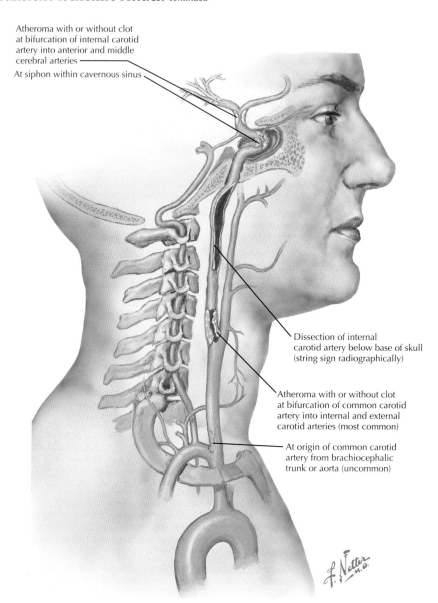

Atheroma with or without clot at bifurcation of internal carotid artery into anterior and middle cerebral arteries

At siphon within cavernous sinus

Dissection of internal carotid artery below base of skull (string sign radiographically)

Atheroma with or without clot at bifurcation of common carotid artery into internal and external carotid arteries (most common)

At origin of common carotid artery from brachiocephalic trunk or aorta (uncommon)

GENERAL FEATURES OF INFARCTION	
Symptoms	• Acute onset of neurologic deficit suggests infarction. • Differentiation from TIA is the persistence of the symptoms.

Signs	• Almost any deficit can occur.
	• Some common signs that should be looked for are:
	  • Hemiparesis
	  • Hemisensory loss
	  • Hemianopia
	  • Gait ataxia
	  • Limb ataxia
	  • Aphasia
	  • Neglect
	  • Ocular motor abnormality

Common affected vessels	• Middle cerebral artery (MCA) • Anterior cerebral artery (ACA) • Posterior cerebral artery (PCA) • Vertebrobasilar system • Penetrating arteries producing lacunar strokes • Veins and venous sinuses

Vascular Distributions	Overview of Clinical Features
Middle cerebral artery	• Contralateral hemiparesis and hemisensory loss, affecting arms more than legs • With left hemisphere CVA—aphasia • With right hemisphere CVA—neglect and constructional difficulty • Contralateral hemianopia is common, although not invariable.
Anterior cerebral artery	• Contralateral hemiparesis mainly affecting the leg. If the arm is affected, proximal arm is most prominent. • Bilateral infarction may produce bilateral leg weakness, which can be mistaken for myelopathy. • Frontal lobe signs can develop especially with bilateral infarction—apathy, disinhibition.
Posterior cerebral artery	• Contralateral hemianopia, which may spare the macula • Confusion with memory loss can occur acutely.
Vertebrobasilar	• Vertigo and ataxia are common. Ataxia can be of gait and/or limbs. • Ocular abnormalities can include diplopia, nystagmus, and anisocoria. • Dysarthria and dysphagia with medullary involvement. • Hemiparesis or quadriparesis with corticospinal tract involvement at any level.

Vascular Distributions	Overview of Clinical Features
Penetrating arteries	• Internal capsule or basal ganglia—contralateral hemiparesis and/or incoordination • Brain stem—contralateral hemiparesis. May have ipsilateral appendicular ataxia, depending on the location of the lesion. Ocular signs also are common. • Pure motor or pure sensory symptoms suggest penetrating vessel occlusion.
Veins and venous sinuses	• Focal deficit, often with headache and/or seizures, can suggest venous infarction. • Occurrence in postpartum women, or in young people generally at lower risk of arterial infarctions, suggests venous infarction.

Ischemia in Internal Carotid Artery Territory: Clinical Manifestations

A. Ocular

Internal carotid a.

Ophthalmic a.

Transient blindness in one eye from temporary occlusion by platelet-fibrin or cholesterol emboli (on side of involved artery)

Central retinal a.

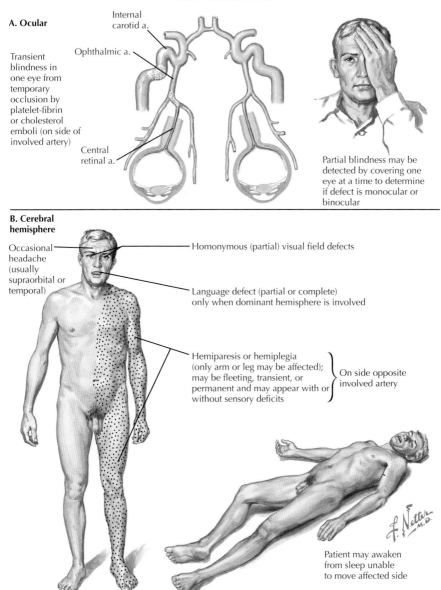

Partial blindness may be detected by covering one eye at a time to determine if defect is monocular or binocular

B. Cerebral hemisphere

Occasional headache (usually supraorbital or temporal)

Homonymous (partial) visual field defects

Language defect (partial or complete) only when dominant hemisphere is involved

Hemiparesis or hemiplegia (only arm or leg may be affected); may be fleeting, transient, or permanent and may appear with or without sensory deficits

} On side opposite involved artery

Patient may awaken from sleep unable to move affected side

DIAGNOSTIC TESTS FOR INFARCTION	
Diagnostic tests	• CT brain • CT angiography (CTA) • MRI brain • MR angiography (MRA) • MR venography (MRV) • LP • Echo • CDS • TCD • Catheter angiography
Test	**Features**
CT brain	• Performed in the emergency department for acute evaluation • Sensitive for hemorrhage and edema. Insensitive for acute infarction, with up to 3 days for signs of acute stroke to develop.
CT angiography	• High-resolution rapid CT performed after intravenous infusion of contrast • Performed for identification of intracranial or extracranial arterial or venous pathology • CTA has largely replaced conventional catheter angiography for many patients, although special equipment is required, not available at all institutions.
MRI brain	• Performed for definitive localization of the stroke • Diffusion-weighted imaging (DWI) is most sensitive for differentiating acute ischemia from chronic changes. • Usually not performed on patients with implanted devices and some prosthetic valves
MR angiography	• MRI technique for visualization of intracranial and extracranial arteries • Less resolution than angiography or CTA, but does not require iodinated contrast
MR venography	• MRI technique for visualization of the venous structures • Performed for patients with suspected venous infarction
Lumbar puncture	• Performed for patients with suspected subarachnoid hemorrhage if no blood is seen on CT. A small proportion of patients with SAH will not have sufficient blood in the CSF to be seen on CT.
Echocardiogram	• Routine transthoracic echocardiogram (TTE) is performed for most patients with stroke to assess cardiac function and look for source of emboli. • Transesophageal echo (TEE) is performed if the TTE suggests stroke etiology, and also is recommended for young people who are at risk for cardiac defect.

Test	Features
Carotid duplex study (CDS)	• Ultrasound evaluation of the extracranial arteries • Can identify carotid stenosis or ulcerated plaque • Most surgeons will not operate on the basis of CDS alone, and, therefore, confirmation of a lesion with catheter angiography or CTA usually is performed.
Transcranial doppler	• An ultrasound evaluation of intracranial arteries, but not of widespread use • Can be used to follow vasospasm with SAH
Catheter angiography	• Still performed but less so since the advent of MRA and CTA • Continues to be the gold standard for evaluation of intracranial and extracranial arteries

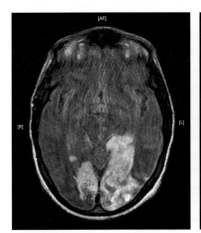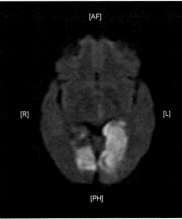

Cerebral infarction: Posterior cerebral artery infarction produces changes in both occipital lobes. Left side shows the FLAIR image, which is most sensitive for pathology. Right side shows the diffusion weighted imaging (DWI) which is sensitive for acute or subacute infarction.

MANAGEMENT OF INFARCTION	
Overview of management	• There are two phases of management—acute management and long-term maintenance therapy.
	• Acute management begins with emergency department admission.
	• Long-term maintenance issues should be addressed before hospital discharge.
Acute Management	
Thrombolytic agents	• Patients with acute infarction should be considered for thrombolytic therapy, as discussed in emergency management page.
	• Strict adherence to the criteria is recommended, and the package insert should be reviewed for details of the criteria for use.
	• *Inclusion criteria include:*
	• Acute ischemic stroke, with treatment within 3 hours from onset
	• No signs of hemorrhage
	• Does not meet any of the contraindications listed below or in the package insert.
	• Patient is felt to be a good candidate for treatment on the basis of age and medical condition.
	• *Contraindications include:*
	• Evidence of intracranial hemorrhage, including SAH
	• Stroke, brain or spine surgery, serious head injury within three months
	• History of intracranial hemorrhage
	• Uncontrolled hypertension at time of treatment
	• Active internal bleeding
	• Seizure at onset of the stroke
	• Intracranial neoplasm, arteriovenous malformation (AVM), or aneurysm
	• Known bleeding disorder, whether disease- or medication-induced
	• Thrombocytopenia
	• Refer to standard guidelines for use, dosages, and details of administration. Most emergency departments have written protocols with a checklist.
Anticoagulants	• Use is controversial. Some physicians place most patients with ischemic stroke on heparin infusion, aiming for therapeutic PTT. Others feel that the benefit is unproven and is overshadowed by the risk.
	• Low-molecular-weight heparins commonly are used when intravenous heparin is not, although the benefit on stroke recurrence is unproven. Because many patients with stroke are on bed rest, these agents do reduce the risk for deep vein thrombosis (DVT) and subsequent pulmonary embolism (PE).

Acute Management	
Blood pressure	• Commonly elevated immediately after a stroke, and this can be either a cause of or reaction to the infarction. • Emergent lowering of BP can adversely affect perfusion of a region of infarction, extending the region of damage. Therefore, most physicians recommend not treating BPs less than 210/110 mm Hg in patients with infarction unless there are compelling reasons to do so.
Cardiac monitoring	• Cardiac arrhythmia and ischemia is of increased incidence in patients with cerebrovascular accident (CVA), and, therefore, routine telemetry and ECG usually are performed. If there are signs of ischemia on the ECG, or if the patient develops symptoms or signs of myocardial infarction, an ROMI panel is performed, and cardiology consultation should be considered.
General medical management	• There are numerous aspects of medical management that are of importance in patients with infarction. General medical management is essential. • *Diabetes.* Hyper- and hypoglycemia have adverse effects on CVA, and, therefore, careful monitoring in patients with diabetes is suggested. • *Fever.* Fever from any cause has been shown to worsen the outcome of patients with CVA; therefore, the recommended course is observation for sources of fever, treat infections, keep adequate nutrition and fluid balance, and manage fever with antipyretics. • *Pulmonary status.* Aspiration is common in patients with CVA, especially with large CVAs, and in those with brainstem ischemia. Surveillance for aspiration and swallowing evaluation is performed for many patients. Tube feeding may be needed. • *Fluids and nutrition.* Patients with CVA may be dehydrated, which makes fever and vascular complications more likely; maintenance of adequate fluid balance and nutrition are considered important.
Long-Term Treatment	
Rehabilitation	• *Physical therapy.* Needed for most patients with stroke to improve physical functioning. The range of treatment can be from range-of-motion exercise of plegic limbs to gait and coordination assistance. • *Occupational therapy.* Helpful for working with patients on life care issues, activities of daily living (ADLs). OT does not necessarily mean returning to a job. • *Speech therapy.* Performed for patients with aphasia, dysarthria, and dysphagia. The speech therapists often help with swallowing evaluations.
Antithrombotic therapy	• Offered to most patients with TIA and ischemic stroke. The only patients not a candidate are those with bleeding disorders or known bleeding. • *Antiplatelets.* Aspirin, dipyridamole, clopidogrel, and ticlopidine are used, either individually or in combination, for prevention of subsequent stroke. The specific agent used depends on the clinical situation. Aspirin is used for primary prevention—when there has been no vascular event. Clopidogrel or the combination of dipyridamole plus aspirin is used for secondary prevention—when there has been a vascular event. Ticlopidine seldom is used because of adverse effects.

Long-Term Treatment	
	• *Warfarin.* Used less now as a result of recent studies. Currently, warfarin mainly is used for patients with cardioembolic disease and antiphospholipid antibody syndrome. Monitoring of PT is needed, and patients should adhere to dietary and activity recommendations, which is standard with warfarin therapy. Very elderly or noncompliant patients are not good candidates for warfarin therapy. • *Low-molecular-weight heparins.* Seldom used for long-term therapy. They have to be given by subcutaneous injection. • *Subcutaneous heparin.* Not routinely used for chronic anticoagulation.
Blood pressure control	• Allowed to autoregulate within limits acutely, but in the long-term, BP should be adequately controlled. Even moderate hypertension increases the risk of recurrent infarction or other vascular event. • Control of BP is thought to be among the best opportunities for reduction of subsequent vascular event.
Hyperlipidemia control	• Usually is diagnosed by the primary care physicians, but should be looked for during hospitalization for stroke • Statins reduce stroke risk dramatically. This reduction appears to be present even in patients without hypercholesterolemia. • Although there are certain risks with the use of these agents, for most patients, the risk overshadowed by the benefits.
Risk reduction	Self-care issues can significantly impact the risk for recurrent vascular event. Some of the important modifiable risks are: • *Smoking.* Cessation of smoking produces a marked reduction in the incidence of a secondary vascular event. The improvement does not occur immediately. • *Diet.* Appropriate diet can improve lipids, BP, and diabetes control and is an important adjunct to medical management of these problems. Without dietary change, the effectiveness of medical treatments is blunted. • *Alcohol.* Mild alcohol intake may reduce the incidence of stroke, although interpretation of the data is controversial. Heavy alcohol intake increases the risk for stroke and should be controlled. • *Vitamin supplementation.* Vitamin supplements are taken by many, and most do not have an effect on stroke risk. Patients with hyperhomocysteinemia may have homocysteine levels reduced by administration of B_6, B_{12}, and folate. Whether or not this produces a reduction in stroke risk is controversial, but it is still recommended.

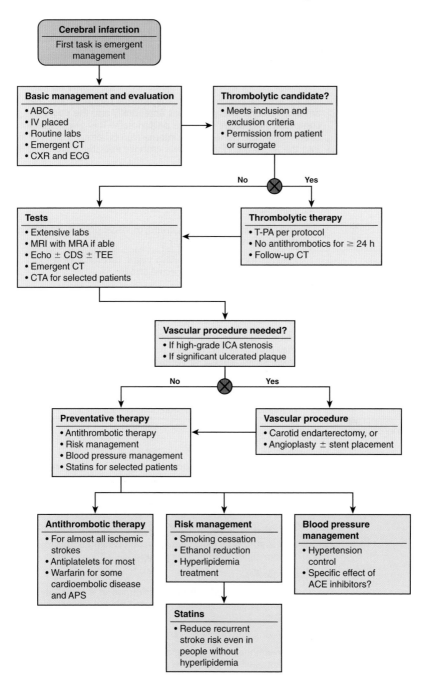

Cerebral infarction

First task is emergent management

Basic management and evaluation
- ABCs
- IV placed
- Routine labs
- Emergent CT
- CXR and ECG

Thrombolytic candidate?
- Meets inclusion and exclusion criteria
- Permission from patient or surrogate

No — ⊗ — Yes

Tests
- Extensive labs
- MRI with MRA if able
- Echo ± CDS ± TEE
- Emergent CT
- CTA for selected patients

Thrombolytic therapy
- T-PA per protocol
- No antithrombotics for ≥ 24 h
- Follow-up CT

Vascular procedure needed?
- If high-grade ICA stenosis
- If significant ulcerated plaque

No — ⊗ — Yes

Preventative therapy
- Antithrombotic therapy
- Risk management
- Blood pressure management
- Statins for selected patients

Vascular procedure
- Carotid endarterectomy, or
- Angioplasty ± stent placement

Antithrombotic therapy
- For almost all ischemic strokes
- Antiplatelets for most
- Warfarin for some cardioembolic disease and APS

Risk management
- Smoking cessation
- Ethanol reduction
- Hyperlipidemia treatment

Blood pressure management
- Hypertension control
- Specific effect of ACE inhibitors?

Statins
- Reduce recurrent stroke risk even in people without hyperlipidemia

Middle Cerebral Artery Infarction

MIDDLE CEREBRAL ARTERY INFARCTION (MCA)	
Description	Infarction in the distribution of the MCA produces contralateral hemiparesis and hemisensory loss, with additional features depending on the side and exact geometry of the lesion.
Pathophysiology	The MCA is the continuation of the internal carotid artery. The anterior cerebral artery branches anteriorly and the posterior communicating artery branches posteriorly. This gives emboli streaming in the center of the internal carotid artery a straight avenue into the MCA. Therefore, cerebral embolic infarctions are most likely to involve the MCA.
Clinical findings	*Symptoms:* • Patients have abrupt onset of contralateral weakness and numbness. • They may also have speech and/or visual deficits, depending on the location of the lesion. • Patients may additionally have vague dizziness, which is common in patients with acute stroke. *Signs:* • Neurologic exam shows contralateral hemiparesis, usually with some sensory loss as well. • Left hemisphere lesions result in language deficits. Mild lesions may only have anomia, but more commonly, we see Broca's (expressive) aphasia or Wernicke's (receptive) aphasia. • Right hemisphere lesions produce neglect. • Lesions affecting either side can produce contralateral hemianopia, if the optic radiations are affected.
Laboratory studies	*Blood:* • Routine labs are normal. • Risk factors for stroke should be looked for, including hyperlipidemia, diabetes, and vasculitis. *Imaging:* • CT is initially normal or only shows old findings. After 2–3 days, lucency in the region of the infarction commonly is seen. • MRI is abnormal early, with diffusion-weighted imaging showing abnormalities early in the course. *Vascular studies:* • Carotid ultrasound is usually performed as a first study, and may show high-grade stenosis, ulcerated plaque, or merely intimal plaque. • MRA or CT-angiography can show better detail. • Conventional catheter angiography is performed if the noninvasive techniques do not give adequate visualization.
Diagnosis	• Clinical features of acute onset of hemiparesis and cortical signs—aphasia or neglect—indicates the diagnosis, even in the absence of early imaging abnormalities. • CT is the initial study of choice to look for bleeding or mass lesion. Also, the CT is more readily available in the emergency department.

MIDDLE CEREBRAL ARTERY INFARCTION (MCA)—cont'd	
Differential diagnosis	• *Lacunar stroke.* Produces hemiparesis, which can resemble MCA infarction. However, there are no cortical signs, including aphasia or neglect. MRI is able to make the differentiation. • *Multiple sclerosis.* Can produce hemiparesis, but cortical findings are not expected. The onset of an MS attack is gradual, although it may be noticed overnight. MRI is able to differentiate these, since MS will show multiple lesions on T_2- and FLAIR imaging without abnormalities on DWI.
Management	Management of MCA infarction does not differ from that of other cerebral infarctions.
Clinical course	• Most patients with submaximal MCA infarctions improve with time. However, persistence of deficit is expected if the zone of infarction is extensive, and if there has not been reperfusion to the site. • Edema in the region of the infarction carries a poorer prognosis for recovery.

Occlusion of Middle and Anterior Cerebral Arteries

Lesion		Artery occluded	Infarct, surface	Infarct, coronal section	Clinical manifestations
Middle cerebral artery	Entire territory	Anterior cerebral — Superior division, Lenticulostriate Medial Lateral, Internal carotid — Middle cerebral, Inferior division			Contralateral gaze palsy, hemiplegia, hemisensory loss, spatial neglect, hemianopsia Global aphasia (if on left side) May lead to coma secondary to edema
	Deep				Contralateral hemiplegia, hemisensory loss Transcortical motor and/or sensory aphasia (if on left side)
	Parasylvian				Contralateral weakness and sensory loss of face and hand Conduction aphasia, apraxia, and Gerstmann's syndrome (if on left side) Constructional dyspraxia (if on right side)
	Superior division				Contralateral hemiplegia, hemisensory loss, gaze palsy, spatial neglect Broca's aphasia (if on left side)
	Inferior division				Contralateral hemianopsia or upper quadrant anopsia Wernicke's aphasia (if on left side) Constructional dyspraxia (if on right side)
Anterior cerebral artery	Entire territory				Incontinence Contralateral hemiplegia Abulia Transcortical motor aphasia or motor and sensory aphasia Left limb dyspraxia
	Distal				Contralateral weakness of leg, hip, foot, and shoulder Sensory loss in foot Transcortical motor aphasia or motor and sensory Left limb dyspraxia

ANTERIOR CEREBRAL ARTERY INFARCTION (ACA)	
Description	Infarction in the distribution of the anterior cerebral artery produces leg weakness, with relative sparing of arm strength.
Pathophysiology	• Whereas MCA infarcts often are embolic, ACA infarcts commonly are thrombotic. Patients with sustained hypertension and diabetes have atherosclerotic changes in the anterior cerebral arteries. • Infarction produces dysfunction, especially of the medial frontal lobe. Depending on the site of the occlusion and the vascular anatomy of the patient, the zone of damage can be more or less extensive.
Clinical findings	*Symptoms.* Patients complain of leg weakness or gait difficulty. They seldom complain of frontal lobe dysfunction, although that is often noticed by the family. Apathy and disinhibition can be seen. *Signs.* Contralateral leg weakness is the most common sign. If both ACAs arise from the same trunk—a common variant—the patient may have bilateral leg weakness. This can be mistaken for myelopathy. Frontal lobe signs including disinhibition or apathy, and the absence of back pain argue against a spinal site of the lesion.
Laboratory studies	*Blood.* No special abnormalities on routine blood are typical of ACA infarction. In general, ACA infarction is more likely to be due to uncontrolled hypertension and diabetes than MCA infarction. *Imaging.* CT initially shows no abnormalities in most patients. After 2–3 days, there is usually decreased density in the medial frontal lobe. Bilateral infarctions produce bilateral medial frontal lobe abnormalities. *Vascular studies.* CTA and MRA can show the occlusion and variant anatomy, if present of a common trunk of the ACAs.
Diagnosis	ACA infarction is suspected: • When a patient presents with unilateral leg weakness. Spinal causes are considered, but this is uncommon if one leg is affected and the weakness spans neural and dermatomal distributions. • In patients with bilateral leg weakness associated with clinical signs of frontal lobe dysfunction. Also, this is considered when a patient with bilateral leg weakness has no visible spinal cause. MRI shows the lesion almost immediately. CT can miss the lesion initially
Differential diagnosis	• *Lumbar spine disease.* Spondylotic change in the lumbar spine can produce leg weakness. Generally, the weakness is bilateral, although radicular distribution of weakness can occur. • *Peroneal neuropathy.* Foot drop can occur from peroneal neuropathy. Involvement of only distal peroneal-innervated muscles argues strongly against a central cause of this pattern of weakness. • *Myelopathy.* Spinal cord damage, above the lumbar spine, can produce leg weakness with Babinski signs and hyperactive tendon reflexes. This can be difficult to distinguish from ACA infarction, but with myelopathy there is often back pain and there are no frontal lobe signs.

ANTERIOR CEREBRAL ARTERY INFARCTION (ACA)—cont'd	
Management	• Management is detailed above. • Note that ACA infarction is less likely to be embolic than MCA infarction, and, therefore, optimal control of risk factors, including diabetes and hypertension, is important.
Clinical course	• Most patients have improvement, however, residual gait difficulty is common. • Bowel and bladder dysfunction can persist, being a management issue. • Frontal lobe symptoms may be less likely to improve than the motor findings.

POSTERIOR CEREBRAL ARTERY INFARCTION (PCA)	
Description	• Infarction in the distribution of the posterior cerebral artery • Typical presentation is hemianopia and confusion.
Pathophysiology	PCA infarction is usually due to embolization from the vertebrobasilar system. The PCAs are the terminal branches of the basilar artery. Therefore, embolization can affect one or both PCAs.

Clinical findings	*Symptoms:*
	  • PCA infarction most commonly produces vague complaints of visual difficulty; hemianopia may not be noted by the patient.
	  • Confusion may also be present.
	  • Patients are not able to read but are able to write (alexia without agraphia).
	Signs:
	  • Careful exam shows hemianopia.
	  • Memory deficit is common with medial temporal lobe involvement.
	Bilateral PCA infarction:
	  • Top of the basilar syndrome is infarction at the distal aspect of the basilar artery producing bilateral PCA infarctions.
	  • Bilateral PCA infarctions produces cortical blindness and prominent memory difficulty, often with confabulation (Anton's syndrome).

Laboratory studies	*Blood and urine.* No special abnormalities are seen with PCA infarction. Signs of coagulopathy may be present. Lab testing looks particularly for diabetes and hyperlipidemia. *Imaging.* CT usually does not show abnormalities for 2–3 days, then shows lucency in the medial occipital region. MRI shows abnormalities earlier than CT. *Vascular imaging.* MRA and CTA can show the disordered vascular supply with occlusion of one or more PCAs. These noninvasive procedures may also be able to determine whether there is basilar or vertebral pathology to correlate with the PCA infarction.
Diagnosis	• Clinical features of hemianopia and memory loss suggest PCA infarction. Note that hemianopia often is missed on casual exam, and, therefore, it must be routinely tested for. • Top of the basilar syndrome produces a characteristic presentation, with cortical blindness and confabulation.
Differential diagnosis	• *MCA infarction.* Hemianopia can develop from MCA infarction when the stroke affects the optic radiations. Weakness is not expected with PCA infarction, and is expected in MCA infarction unless the lesion is more posterior parietal with sparing of the central strips. • *Perichiasmal lesion.* Lesions posterior to the optic chiasm can produce hemianopia, but these are seldom acute, as a stroke. A gradual evolution of deficit is expected.

POSTERIOR CEREBRAL ARTERY INFARCTION (PCA)—cont'd	
Management	• Management is described above. • The management of PCA infarction typically does not differ from that of other stroke distributions, except that if there is the finding of significant basilar or vertebral disease, many clinicians are more likely to use warfarin than antiplatelets, although without good supporting clinical evidence.
Clinical course	• Hemianopia often does not improve. • Confusion due to unilateral infarction usually does improve; however, the prominent difficulty seen with bilateral infarction often results in persistent deficit.

Occlusion of "Top of Basilar" and Posterior Cerebral Arteries

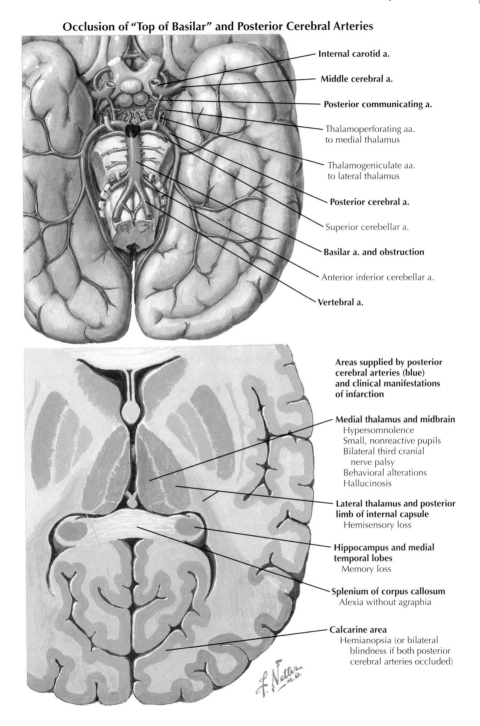

Internal carotid a.

Middle cerebral a.

Posterior communicating a.

Thalamoperforating aa.
to medial thalamus

Thalamogeniculate aa.
to lateral thalamus

Posterior cerebral a.

Superior cerebellar a.

Basilar a. and obstruction

Anterior inferior cerebellar a.

Vertebral a.

Areas supplied by posterior
cerebral arteries (blue)
and clinical manifestations
of infarction

Medial thalamus and midbrain
Hypersomnolence
Small, nonreactive pupils
Bilateral third cranial
    nerve palsy
Behavioral alterations
Hallucinosis

Lateral thalamus and posterior
limb of internal capsule
Hemisensory loss

Hippocampus and medial
temporal lobes
Memory loss

Splenium of corpus callosum
Alexia without agraphia

Calcarine area
Hemianopsia (or bilateral
    blindness if both posterior
    cerebral arteries occluded)

VERTEBROBASILAR INFARCTION	
Description	• Infarction in the distribution of the vertebral or basilar arteries • Commonly presents as a devastating stroke, with common symptoms being dizziness, diplopia, ataxia, paralysis, and coma
Pathophysiology	The basilar artery is supplied by the two vertebral arteries, one of which may be dominant or even absent. Infarction can be due to proximal embolic disease or vessel embolization from a more proximal vertebrobasilar lesion. Thrombotic occlusion also can occur.
Clinical findings	General symptoms are discussed here. Specific symptoms with differing levels of lesion are presented in the following pages. *Symptoms*: • Common complaints are dizziness, coordination and gait difficulty, difficulty speaking and swallowing, weakness on one or both sides. • Numbness usually on one side; numbness on one side of the face accompanied by numbness on the opposite side of the body raises special concern over a brainstem lesion. • Diplopia is common, and can have a variety of characteristics. *Signs*: • Exam findings can be multiple, including various combinations of mental status changes or coma. • Ataxia may affect gait and/or limbs. • Ocular motor difficulty can include gaze palsies, skew deviation, isolated ocular cranial nerve palsies, and anisocoria. • Weakness can be one side or both sides. • Dysarthria and dysphagia are common.
Laboratory studies	• Labs do not differ from those discussed above. • MRI usually shows the lesion, whereas CT usually does not initially. • Ultrasound does not adequately evaluate the vertebrobasilar circulation, and, therefore, MRA or CTA is needed.
Diagnosis	• Vertebrobasilar infarction is considered when a patient presents with ataxia, dizziness, diplopia, dysarthria/dysphagia, or weakness in any combination. • Clinical features usually are quite effective at localizing the lesion. • MRI confirms the infarction.

VERTEBROBASILAR INFARCTION—cont'd	
Differential diagnosis	• *Myasthenia gravis*. Patients with MG can present subacutely, and dysphagia, dysarthria, and diplopia are common symptoms. However, there are no signs of corticospinal tract dysfunction. • *Guillain-Barre syndrome*. Patients with GBS may present with bulbar signs early in the course, but then progress to diffuse weakness and areflexia. The onset may be rapid, but usually not stroke-like. • *Brainstem encephalitis*. This is a rare condition that can present with the subacute onset of bulbar signs. This is often a paraneoplastic condition.
Management	• Management does not differ from that discussed above. • Some clinicians are more likely to use anticoagulants in patients with vertebrobasilar disease than anterior-circulation stroke, although this is controversial.
Clinical course	Brainstem lesions are less likely to show improvement than cerebral hemisphere lesions. Therefore, persistent deficit is common.

Posterolateral medullary infarction and clinical manifestations

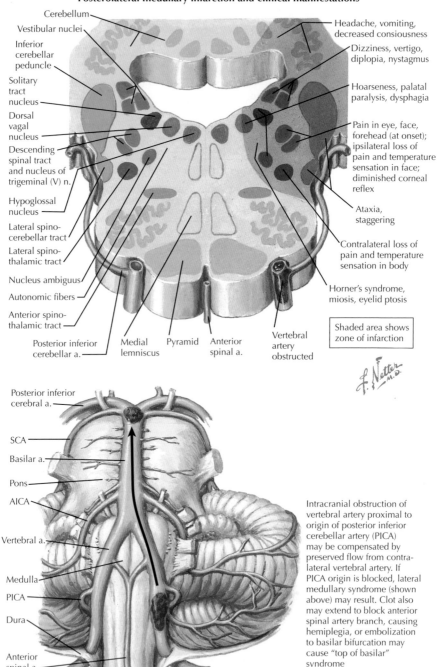

Cerebellum

Vestibular nuclei

Inferior cerebellar peduncle

Solitary tract nucleus

Dorsal vagal nucleus

Descending spinal tract and nucleus of trigeminal (V) n.

Hypoglossal nucleus

Lateral spino-cerebellar tract

Lateral spino-thalamic tract

Nucleus ambiguus

Autonomic fibers

Anterior spino-thalamic tract

Posterior inferior cerebellar a.

Medial lemniscus

Pyramid

Anterior spinal a.

Vertebral artery obstructed

Headache, vomiting, decreased consiousness

Dizziness, vertigo, diplopia, nystagmus

Hoarseness, palatal paralysis, dysphagia

Pain in eye, face, forehead (at onset); ipsilateral loss of pain and temperature sensation in face; diminished corneal reflex

Ataxia, staggering

Contralateral loss of pain and temperature sensation in body

Horner's syndrome, miosis, eyelid ptosis

Shaded area shows zone of infarction

Posterior inferior cerebral a.

SCA

Basilar a.

Pons

AICA

Vertebral a.

Medulla

PICA

Dura

Anterior spinal a.

Intracranial obstruction of vertebral artery proximal to origin of posterior inferior cerebellar artery (PICA) may be compensated by preserved flow from contralateral vertebral artery. If PICA origin is blocked, lateral medullary syndrome (shown above) may result. Clot also may extend to block anterior spinal artery branch, causing hemiplegia, or embolization to basilar bifurcation may cause "top of basilar" syndrome

VERTEBROBASILAR INFARCTION: BRAINSTEM SYNDROMES	
Pontine Infarction	**Features**
Superior cerebellar artery	• *Vessel.* The SCA supplies the superior and lateral aspect of the pons. • *Ipsilateral.* Gaze paresis to the side of the lesion. Limb and gait ataxia. • *Contralateral.* Sensory deficit to all modalities, arm and face are relatively spared for large-fiber sensations.
Anterior inferior cerebellar artery	• *Vessel.* The AICA supplies the lateral portion of the lower pons. • *Ipsilateral.* Facial paralysis, limb ataxia, gaze paralysis to the side of the lesion, sensation to the face • *Contralateral.* Impaired pain and temperature sensation to the body, sparing the face Note: This is one example of crossed sensory findings, where there is impaired sensation on the ipsilateral face and contralateral body.
Medial pons	• *Vessel.* Branches of the basilar artery supply the medial pons • *Ipsilateral.* Gaze paresis to the side of the lesion with lower lesions; internuclear ophthalmoplegia (INO) with higher lesions. Limb and gait ataxia. Diplopia with gaze to the side of the lesion. • *Contralateral.* Hemiparesis and hemisensory loss
Medullary Infarction	**Features**
Medial medullary syndrome	• *Vessel.* Usually the vertebral or a branch • *Ipsilateral.* Weakness of the tongue • *Contralateral.* Hemiparesis, sparing face. Sensory deficit over the body.
Lateral medullary syndrome	• *Vessels.* Can be vertebral, posterior inferior cerebellar, of medullary arteries • *Ipsilateral.* Sensory disturbance on the face and body, limb ataxia, Horner syndrome • *Contralateral.* Disordered pain and temperature sensation on the body • *Unsided.* Dysphagia, hoarse voice, diplopia, vertigo, nausea/vomiting
Basilar Infarction	**Features**
Locked-in syndrome	• *Vessel.* Basilar artery, including branches • Exam: Quadriplegia and facial weakness, with corticospinal tract signs— Babinski signs and hyperactive reflexes. Impaired horizontal eye movements with relative preservation of vertical eye movements. *Note:* These patients are commonly misdiagnosed as comatose because their only voluntary response may be vertical eye movement. When careful exam shows responsiveness, the level of the lesion is clear.
Basilar thrombosis	• *Vessel.* Basilar artery can be thrombosed with resultant infarction in the PCAs and smaller branches. Exam: Unresponsiveness with corticospinal tract signs

Occlusion of Basilar Artery and Branches

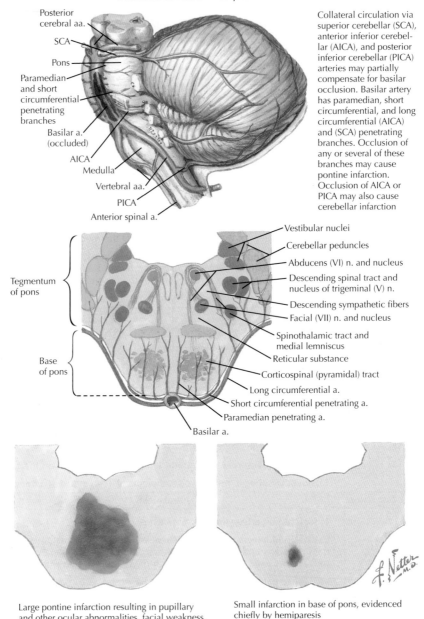

Posterior cerebral aa.

SCA

Pons

Paramedian and short circumferential penetrating branches

Basilar a. (occluded)

AICA

Medulla

Vestibular aa.

PICA

Anterior spinal a.

Collateral circulation via superior cerebellar (SCA), anterior inferior cerebellar (AICA), and posterior inferior cerebellar (PICA) arteries may partially compensate for basilar occlusion. Basilar artery has paramedian, short circumferential, and long circumferential (AICA) and (SCA) penetrating branches. Occlusion of any or several of these branches may cause pontine infarction. Occlusion of AICA or PICA may also cause cerebellar infarction

Vestibular nuclei

Cerebellar peduncles

Abducens (VI) n. and nucleus

Descending spinal tract and nucleus of trigeminal (V) n.

Descending sympathetic fibers

Facial (VII) n. and nucleus

Spinothalamic tract and medial lemniscus

Reticular substance

Corticospinal (pyramidal) tract

Long circumferential a.

Short circumferential penetrating a.

Paramedian penetrating a.

Basilar a.

Tegmentum of pons

Base of pons

Large pontine infarction resulting in pupillary and other ocular abnormalities, facial weakness, quadriplegia, and coma

Small infarction in base of pons, evidenced chiefly by hemiparesis

ARTERIAL DISSECTION	
Description	• An occasional cause of stroke is arterial dissection, rather than thrombotic or embolic occlusion. • Dissection is separation of the intima from the vessel wall, and extension of blood into this potential space. The intima can be pressed to the opposite wall to cause vessel occlusion.
Pathophysiology	• Many patients have a history of trauma to the neck resulting in separation of the intima of the carotid or vertebral arteries. • Arterial disease predisposes to dissection, including atherosclerotic disease, syphilis, some forms of arteritis.

Clinical findings	*Common symptoms and signs:*
	
	  • Symptoms are usually headache and neck pain. Weakness or ataxia is also common, with the symptoms depending on which artery is affected, as with infarction.
	
	  • Signs are typical of stroke, with deficits depending on the affected artery.
	
	  • The dissection may be induced by trauma to the neck, sudden twisting of the neck, or even coughing or sneezing.
	
	Carotid dissection:
	
	  • Carotid dissection produces pain in the head, face and/or upper neck.
	
	  • An ipsilateral Horner's syndrome may be present.
	
	  • Focal findings can develop from infarction distally in the internal carotid artery distribution, such as hemiparesis, hemianopia, language difficulty, neglect.
	
	Vertebral dissection:
	
	  • Vertebral dissection usually produces pain at the craniocervical junction and neck.
	
	  • Neurologic findings may occur from basilar or posterior cerebral infarction.

Laboratory studies	*Blood.* Routine labs are normal. Hypercoagulable states are occasionally identified, and are commonly tested for in younger patients who are more likely to have dissection. *Imaging.* CT usually is normal initially. If there has been infarction, lucency is seen after 2–3 days. MRI shows abnormalities earlier than CT. *Vascular imaging.* MRA, CTA, and CDS can often show the dissection. The appearance can be different than thrombotic or embolic occlusive disease.
Diagnosis	• Diagnosis is suspected in patients who have stroke symptoms at a young age with few risk factors. A history of neck trauma suggests the diagnosis. • Confirmation is by vascular imaging with CDS, CTA, or MRA.

ARTERIAL DISSECTION—cont'd	
Differential diagnosis	• *Thrombotic occlusion.* Thombotic occlusion of the carotid or vertebral arteries can produce pain and focal signs. Focal signs are more likely with acute occlusion than gradual occlusion.
	• *Embolic occlusion.* Embolic occlusion of the internal carotid or vertebral arteries produces acute onset of focal signs and may have associated headache. Differentiation is dependent on vascular imaging.
	• *Temporal arteritis.* Giant cell arteritis can present with headache with prominence in the temporal region. ESR is increased and vascular imaging shows no occlusion.
Management	• Initial treatment is with heparin to lower the risk for distal embolization.
	• Patients typically are changed to warfarin for at least 3 months; some for 6 months.
	• After warfarin has been discontinued, patients are maintained on antiplatelet therapy with aspirin or other agents.
Clinical course	• Most patients improve, with resolution of the pain and improvement in neurologic deficit.
	• Warfarin typically is discontinued after about 6 months, followed by institution of antiplatelet therapy.

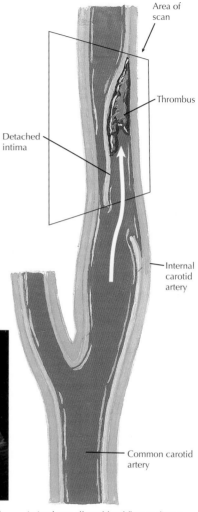

Area of scan

Thrombus

Detached intima

Internal carotid artery

Common carotid artery

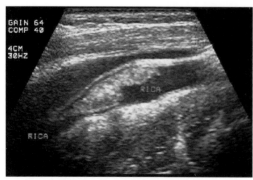

Carotid dissection: Left side is an ultrasound of the carotid arterty with clot formed between layers of the artery (near the upper RICA label). Right side shows a diagram of this dissection with separation of the layers of the artery and formation of clot in the potential space.

Intimal tear allows blood flow to dissect beneath intimal layer, detaching it from arterial wall. Large dissection may occlude vessel lumen

JOHN A. CRAIG—AD

VENOUS INFARCTION	
Description	• Occlusion of the venous system is less common than arterial occlusion. • Patients can have some hemorrhage associated with the infarction.

Pathophysiology	Most venous infarctions are due to hypercoagulable state, which can have a number of causes including:
	  • Pregnancy or recently postpartum
	  • Genetic disorder or other family predisposition
	  • Oral contraceptive use
	  • Smoking
	  • Cancer
	  • Autoimmune coagulopathy

Clinical findings	*Symptoms:*
	  • Weakness of one or both sides develops in a stepwise fashion, in keeping with the multifocal cortical infarctions seen in this condition.
	  • Seizures are much more common than with arterial infarction.
	  • Infarction of the sagittal sinus can produce prominent increased intracranial pressure with headache, decreased level of consciousness, nausea, vomiting.
	Signs:
	  • Multifocal infarction can produce weakness, sensory deficit, language deficit, and other symptoms that suggest more than one localized infarction.

Laboratory studies	*Blood.* Routine labs are normal. Labs should be done which look for hypercoagulable state. Among the labs that may be revealing are:
	  • Antiphospholipid antibody
	  • Factor V Leiden
	  • Prothrombin gene mutation
	  • Protein C or protein S deficiency
	  • Antithrombin III deficiency
	  • Sickle cell disease
	  • Pregnancy test
	Imaging. CT may be normal or show multifocal infarctions. Some bleeding in the affected parenchyma is common. MRI shows these changes, as well.
	Vascular imaging. Magnetic resonance venography (MRV) and CTA venous phase study can show the venous occlusive disease.
	Lumbar puncture. Performed when patients have symptoms and signs of increased intracranial pressure without a structural lesion seen on imaging. CSF pressure is increased, which should raise concern over this diagnosis. LP is usually not needed, unless infection is considered in the etiology.

VENOUS INFARCTION—cont'd	
Diagnosis	• Diagnosis is suspected particularly when a young patient presents with focal neurologic findings. • MRI can show the infarctions that can suggest venous disease. MRV can show the venous occlusive disease.
Differential diagnosis	*Arterial infarction.* Infarction affecting the arteries is more common than venous infarction.
Management	• Anticoagulation with heparin usually is used initially. • Warfarin therapy eventually is used in most patients.
Clinical course	• Most patients improve, but some residual deficit is common. • Cerebral edema from extension of the venous thrombosis can be fatal.

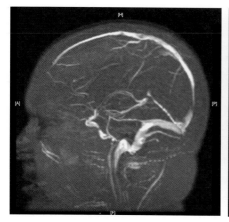

Normal MRV

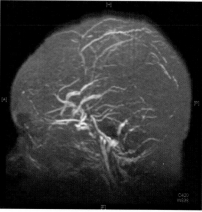

Venous thrombosis

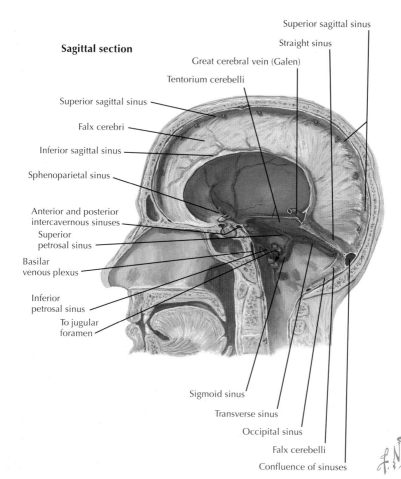

Sagittal section

Superior sagittal sinus

Straight sinus

Great cerebral vein (Galen)

Tentorium cerebelli

Superior sagittal sinus

Falx cerebri

Inferior sagittal sinus

Sphenoparietal sinus

Anterior and posterior intercavernous sinuses

Superior petrosal sinus

Basilar venous plexus

Inferior petrosal sinus

To jugular foramen

Sigmoid sinus

Transverse sinus

Occipital sinus

Falx cerebelli

Confluence of sinuses

PREVENTION OF INFARCTION	
Goals of prevention	Patients considered for preventive therapy of stroke fall into two treatment categories—primary prevention and secondary prevention. *Primary prevention* means that the patient has not had an event, but they often have risk factors. *Secondary prevention* means that the patient has had a vascular event, which places that patient at increased risk for stroke. Some of these risk factors include: • Previous TIA or CVA • MI or other CAD • PAD
Options for primary prevention	*Antiplatelets.* Aspirin mainly is used for primary prevention. Stronger antiplatelets and anticoagulants are not used for primary prevention. *Risk factor reduction.* Treatment of hypertension, diabetes, and hyperlipidemia reduces the incidence of stroke.
Options for secondary prevention	*Antiplatelets.* Used for almost all patients with cerebral infarction, but are not used when the patient has high risk of bleeding, i.e., a patient who has already bled or in whom full anticoagulation is given. *Anticoagulants.* Warfarin is used for patients with cardioembolic stroke and for some hypercoagulable states, including antiphospholipid antibody syndrome. *Risk factor reduction.* Essential for patients needing secondary stroke prevention.
Interventions	
Antiplatelets	Antiplatelets form the cornerstone of antithrombotic treatment for patients with TIA, cerebral infarction, and other vascular events. Options include: • Aspirin • Dipyrimadole • Clopidogrel • Ticlopidine *Primary prevention* for patients with risk factors for stroke usually is with aspirin. *Secondary prevention* for patients with previous stroke, TIA, MI, or PAD is with clopidogrel or the combination of aspirin and sustained-released dipyrimadole. *Antiplatelet failures.* Patients who have vascular events despite antiplatelet therapy should be considered for statin therapy a well as aggressive medical management and self-help guideline adherence. Warfarin does not appear to be helpful for most of these patients.
Anticoagulants	• Warfarin is used mainly for patients with cardiac emboli and antiphospholipid antibody syndrome. Some other hypercoagulable states also are treated with warfarin, including postpartum stroke. • Warfarin as not been shown to be better than ASA for treatment of patients with stroke or TIA, not due to the above clinical situations.

Interventions—cont'd	
Antihypertensives	Control of hypertension with medications and diet reduces the risk for both ischemic and hemorrhagic stroke. Uncontrolled hypertension predisposes patients to advancing atherosclerosis, as well as acute small-vessel infarction.
Lipid-lowering agents	• Statins have been shown to reduce the incidence of stroke. The effect is not only due to reduction in cholesterol, but also due to biochemical effects not related to cholesterol.
	• The American Heart Association Stroke Council has concluded that it is reasonable to use statins on patients with stroke and TIA, regardless of their lipid profiles.
Hypoglycemic agents	Improved glucose control reduces the risk of diabetic complications, including stroke. Diabetic ketoacidosis and hypoglycemia also predispose to or exacerbate stroke.
Self-help guidelines	*Diet.* Low-fat, low-salt diet improves control of hypertension and hyperlipidemia. A diabetic diet improves glucose control.
	Exercise. Frequent aerobic exercise is believed to improve insulin resistance, and is a helpful adjunct to diet in weight control.
	Compliance with treatment. Compliance is essential; management of hypertension, diabetes, and hyperlipidemia is markedly impaired in the absence of patient compliance with diet and medications.

Platelet Inhibitors

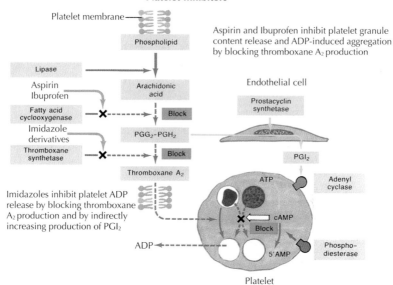

Platelet membrane

Phospholipid

Lipase

Aspirin
Ibuprofen

Fatty acid
cyclooxygenase

Imidazole
derivatives

Thromboxane
synthetase

Arachidonic
acid

Block

PGG$_2$-PGH$_2$

Block

Thromboxane A$_2$

Aspirin and Ibuprofen inhibit platelet granule
content release and ADP-induced aggregation
by blocking thromboxane A$_2$ production

Endothelial cell

Prostacyclin
synthetase

PGI$_2$

ATP

Adenyl
cyclase

cAMP

Block

5'AMP

Phospho-
diesterase

Imidazoles inhibit platelet ADP
release by blocking thromboxane
A$_2$ production and by indirectly
increasing production of PGI$_2$

ADP

Platelet

Dipyridamole impairs platelet ADP release by blocking phosphodiesterase
conversion of cAMP to inacive 5' AMP and by blocking uptake of adenosine,
which potentiates PGI$_2$ stimulation of cAMP production via adenyl cyclase

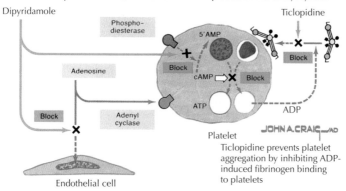

Dipyridamole

Ticlopidine

Phospho-
diesterase

5'AMP

Block

Adenosine

Block

cAMP

Block

Block

Adenyl
cyclase

ATP

ADP

JOHN A. CRAIG—AD

Platelet

Endothelial cell

Ticlopidine prevents platelet
aggregation by inhibiting ADP-
induced fibrinogen binding
to platelets

GENERAL FEATURES OF HEMORRHAGE	
Description	Hemorrhage is bleeding in the skull. The bleeding can be intraparenchymal, subarachnoid, subdural, or epidural.

Pathophysiology	• Hemorrhage is due to an acquired defect in an artery or, less likely, vein.
	• Factors which predispose to hemorrhage include:
	  • Hypertension—uncontrolled hypertension is the major risk factor for hemorrhage
	  • Risk factors for ischemic stroke—diabetes, hyperlipidemia, age
	  • Family predisposition to aneurysms and other vascular anomalies
	  • Aneurysm
	  • Vascular malformation
	  • Head injury
	  • Use of anticoagulants

Clinical findings	• Most patients with hemorrhage have the acute onset of headache, often with a neurologic deficit. Intraparenchymal hematomas are more likely to be associated with initial focal findings than extracerebral hematomas. • Increased intracranial pressure from the mass effect of hemorrhage can produce decreased level of consciousness, progressing to coma.

Laboratory studies	*Blood:*
	  • Routine labs are usually normal.
	  • Patients should be screened for coagulopathy, such as therapeutic anticoagulation or hepatic failure.
	Imaging:
	  • CT usually shows blood within, around, or overlying the brain.
	  • Occasional patient with subarachnoid hemorrhage will have negative CT scans, because the amount of blood in the CSF may be small.
	  • MRI is sensitive for intraparenchymal, subdural, and epidural blood, but may miss subarachnoid blood.
	Lumbar Puncture:
	  • LP is performed on patients with the clinical presentation of subarachnoid hemorrhage in whom the CT is negative.

Diagnosis	• Hemorrhage is suspected when a patient has the acute onset of headache with or without neurologic deficit. Decreased level of consciousness in this setting strongly suggests hemorrhage. • Diagnosis is confirmed when CT shows intracranial bleeding, or when a patient with suspected subarachnoid bleeding and a negative CT has blood on LP that is not due to a traumatic tap.

GENERAL FEATURES OF HEMORRHAGE—cont'd	
Differential diagnosis	• *Infarction.* Cerebral or brainstem infarction can be associated with headache, and the latter can produce fulminant neurologic deterioration, which may suggest hemorrhage. • *Meningitis and encephalitis.* Meningitis can be fulminant, and can give headache and neurologic findings that may suggest subarachnoid hemorrhage. • *Calcification of the basal ganglia.* Calcification of the basal ganglia can give an appearance on CT that might suggest basal ganglia hemorrhage. However, the calcification typically is bilateral and there are no neurologic findings that would correspond to the lesions. Careful evaluation of the CT with proper windowing of the image can make the diagnosis.
Management	• Management of hemorrhage depends greatly on the specific type and features (See pages on the specific types of hemorrhage.) • Common management of patients with hemorrhage includes control of blood pressure and reversal of coagulopathy.
Clinical course	• Intracranial hemorrhage can be fatal. Patients with decreased level of consciousness at presentation have a worse prognosis, and comatose patients have a poor prognosis for good neurologic recovery. • If the patient survives and the blood is metabolized, significant improvement can occur.

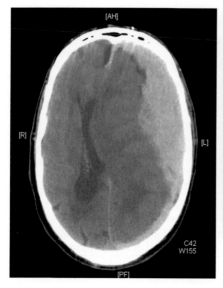

CT showing subdural hematoma

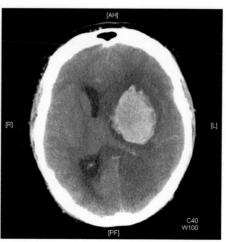

CT showing intrapenchymal hematoma

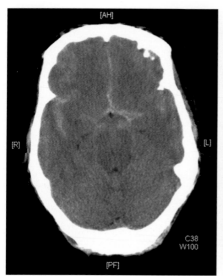

CT shows blood in the subarachnoid space consistent with subarchnoid hemorrhage

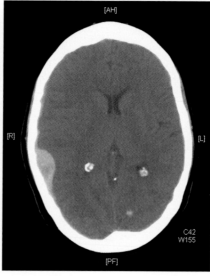

CT showing small epidural hematoma

SUBARACHNOID HEMORRHAGE (SAH)	
Description	Hemorrhage into the subarachnoid space, usually due to leak or rupture of an aneurysm.
Pathophysiology	• SAH is most commonly due to aneurysm. The aneurysm may leak or rupture. With a leak, the aneurysm may heal sufficiently, then rupture at a later date. With a rupture, the vessel may heal resulting in obliteration of the aneurysm. • Subarachnoid blood can cause vessel spasms in or near the circle of Willis, producing ischemic stroke superimposed on the signs of the hemorrhage. • Thrombus can form inside the aneurysm, which can break off, and become another potential cause of ischemia.
Clinical findings	*Symptoms:* • Classic presentation is a "thunderclap" headache, often with exertion. • Common precipitating activities are heavy athletic or occupational exertion or sexual intercourse. • The headache often is "the worst the patient has ever had." *Signs:* • Patients may have no abnormalities on examination or have focal findings, commonly diplopia or other cranial nerve palsy. • Meningeal signs are seen on examination. • If a patient has progressed to coma, the meningeal signs disappear. *Grading system:* • 1—Asymptomatic • 2—Headache with or without cranial nerve palsy • 3—Drowsy and mild deficit • 4—Stupor, moderate-severe hemiparesis, with or without rigidity • 5—Deep coma, decerebrate rigidity
Laboratory studies	*Blood.* Routine labs are usually normal. *Imaging.* CT usually shows subarachnoid blood. Some patients with small SAH may have a normal scan, although this is unusual. MRI may show the subarachnoid blood, but is less sensitive than the CT for this condition. *Lumbar puncture.* Performed on patients with suspected SAH who have a normal CT scan. Indicators for performing the LP include the worse headache of one's life, especially if the onset was abrupt. *Vascular imaging.* MRA and CTA may show the site of bleeding. However, the aneurysm cannot always be seen, and therefore repeat study often is needed after some of the subarachnoid blood has been reabsorbed. *Angiography.* Conventional catheter angiography is still the gold-standard for identifying aneurysms. As with noninvasive vascular imaging, re-study may be needed after the initial phase of hemorrhage and spasm, because aneurysms may not acutely be seen.

SUBARACHNOID HEMORRHAGE (SAH)—cont'd	
Diagnosis	• SAH is suspected when a patient presents with the abrupt onset of "the worst headache of their life." If CT is normal, LP is performed to look for blood. If the LP shows blood that is not due to a traumatic tap, then the diagnosis is confirmed. If the LP is normal, then the patient did not have SAH. • Vascular imaging with CTA or MRA or catheter angiography is performed to look for signs of aneurysm. The selection of study should follow consultation with neurology or neurosurgery.
Differential diagnosis	• *Migraine.* Most patients with acute onset of "the worst headache of their lives" do not have SAH, but rather migraine. When the headache occurs during sex or some other exertion, the concern is even further raised; therefore, many negative CTs and LPs are performed in emergency departments. • *Intraparenchymal hemorrhage.* Bleeding within the substance of the brain can have similar clinical features to SAH. Focal weakness or ataxia is more common with intraparenchymal bleeding, however.
Management	• Close monitoring is required for patients with SAH. Some are placed in the ICU, whereas others can be monitored in a telemetric bed. Frequent neurologic assessments and vital sign checks are important. • Blood pressure is monitored and controlled to avoid persistent hypertension or hypotension. • Vasospasm is a common occurrence in subarachnoid hemorrhage, and can be minimized by: • Cautious hydration • Plasma expanders • Nimodipine • Seizures can occur in patients with SAH, and, therefore, some clinicians routinely use phenytoin or other anticonvulsant prophylactically. • Dexamethasone or another corticosteroid often is used. • Timing of surgery for aneurysm is at the surgeon's discretion, and depends on the site and form of the aneurysm and the condition of the patient. In general, a patient with good functional status and accessible aneurysm is a good candidate for early surgery.
Clinical course	Although most patients with SAH survive, the mortality rate is higher than for ischemic stroke. Also, patients may be left with persistent deficit, especially due to vasospasm.

Common Locations of Aneurysms

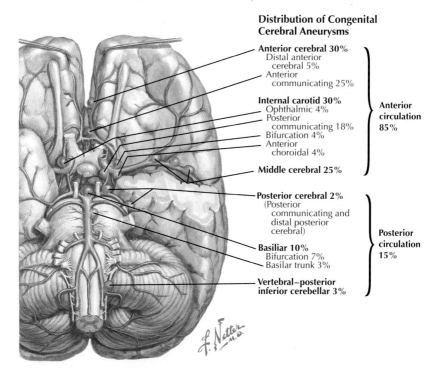

Distribution of Congenital Cerebral Aneurysms

Anterior cerebral 30%
Distal anterior
cerebral 5%
Anterior
communicating 25%

Internal carotid 30%
Ophthalmic 4%
Posterior
communicating 18%
Bifurcation 4%
Anterior
choroidal 4%

Middle cerebral 25%

} **Anterior circulation 85%**

Posterior cerebral 2%
(Posterior
communicating and
distal posterior
cerebral)

Basiliar 10%
Bifurcation 7%
Basilar trunk 3%

Vertebral–posterior inferior cerebellar 3%

} **Posterior circulation 15%**

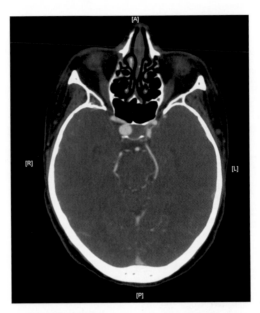

CT Angio source image showing an aneurysm

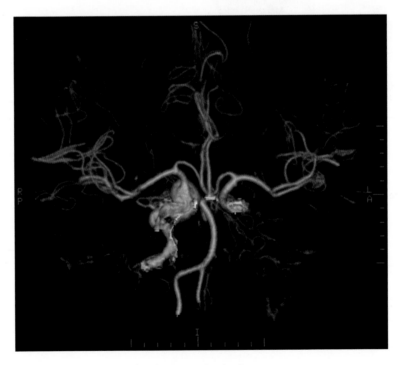

CTA 3-D reconstruction showing
detailed anatomy of the aneurysm

SUBDURAL HEMATOMA (SDH)	
Description	• Blood beneath the dura mater, but above the subarachnoid space. Blood is loculated so that it overlies one hemisphere, unless there are bilateral SDHs. • Can be acute, subacute, or chronic. Blood of differing ages may be seen in one hematoma.
Pathophysiology	• Bridging veins from the brain to the dura can break, resulting in blood into this potential space. • SDH is more common with trauma, which would damage these veins. • Elderly patients are more likely to have SDH because of cerebral atrophy stretching these bridging veins.

Clinical findings	*Symptoms:*
	  • Acute SDH can present with hemiparesis, decreased level of consciousness, ataxia, and headache.
	  • Chronic SDH can present with dementia, ataxia, and weakness.
	  • Seizures can occur.
	  • There may have been a head injury, although in susceptible patients the injury may have been mild and forgotten.
	Signs:
	  • Many patients have altered mental status; either decreased level of consciousness in patients with acute bleeding, or dementia without depressed consciousness in patients with chronic subdurals.
	  • A tendency to retropulsion commonly is seen in many patients with SDH of any chronicity.

Laboratory studies	*Blood.* Routine labs are normal unless there is a coagulopathy. *Imaging.* CT and MRI can show the subdural fluid collection. The appearance of acute, subacute, and chronic blood differs, and, therefore, the subdural can be timed not only by clinical presentation but also by radiological features. Often, there is a combination of old and new blood, especially in elderly patients on chronic anticoagulation.
Diagnosis	• SDH is suspected in a patient with a decreased level of consciousness, especially in patient groups at increased risk, e.g., elderly, anticoagulated, alcoholic. There may be a history of head injury, but this is not invariable. • Diagnosis is confirmed by CT or MRI, which shows fluid overlying one or both cerebral hemispheres and appears to be blood. The signal characteristics of the fluid differ, depending on whether the blood is new or old; a mixture of acute and chronic blood is common.

SUBDURAL HEMATOMA (SDH)—cont'd	
Differential diagnosis	• *Epidural hematoma.* Can present with somnolence after a head injury. The severity of the injury to produce this is usually greater than with SDH. Epidural hematoma is a much more acute problem than SDH. • *Intraparenchymal hematoma.* Can present in a fashion indistinguishable from SDH, with focal findings, seizures, and/or decreased level of consciousness. Focal findings are more common with intraparenchymal hemorrhage than with SDH. • *Normal pressure hydrocephalus (NPH).* Can give ataxia and confusion without focal findings. The mental status is disordered, but the patient is not typically somnolent.
Management	• Neurosurgical consultation is needed for most patients with SDH. Patients with small hematomas without critical brain compression can be followed. Patients with increased intracranial pressure, expanding hematomas, and decreased level of consciousness usually require surgery. • Anticonvulsants are needed if the patient has seizures, although prophylactic anticonvulsants are not routinely used.
Clinical course	• Most patients improve, but there is the possibility of persistent cognitive changes, weakness, and coordination difficulty after resolution of the hematoma. • Patients should be followed for the possibility of reaccumulation of subdural blood. Rescanning should be considered for patients who do not improve or who have any deterioration after initial improvement.

Natural History of Nonlethal Subdural Hematoma

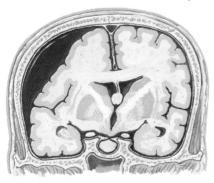

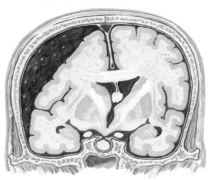

Stage 1: Dark blood spreads widely over brain surface beneath dura

Stage 2: (2 to 4 days) Blood congeals; becomes darker, thicker, and "jelly–like"

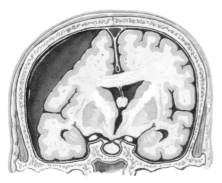

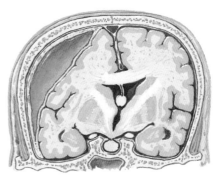

Stage 3: Clot breaks down and after about 2 weeks has color and consistency of crankcase oil

Stage 4: Organization begins with formation of encasing membranes; an outer thick, tough one derived from dura and thin inner one from arachnoid. The contained fluid becomes xanthochromic

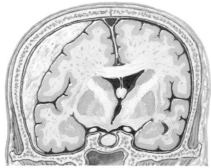

Stage 5: Organization is completed. Clot may become calcified or even ossified (or may resorb)

Intraparenchymal Hemorrhage

INTRAPARENCHYMAL HEMORRHAGE	
Description	**Hemorrhage within the Substance of the Brain**
Pathophysiology	• Hypertension is the most common cause. Marked elevations in BP can rupture small and medium-sized arteries. • Head injuries are a common cause of intracranial bleeding from mechanical damage to the blood vessels. • Vascular malformations predispose to bleeding. This is more common with arteriovenous malformations than with venous angiomas, which are generally under low pressure.
Clinical findings	*Symptoms:* • Usually begin with the acute onset of weakness, numbness, or incoordination, which has a distribution appropriate to the location of the blood. • Basal ganglia and thalamic hemorrhages affect the contralateral limbs. • Pontine bleeds can produce hemiparesis, quadriparesis, and even coma, depending on the location of the lesion. Headache is common. *Signs:* • Includes hemiparesis, hemisensory loss, ataxia, and decreased level of consciousness. Seizures can occur.
Laboratory studies	*Blood.* • Usually normal, unless there is coagulopathy due either to metabolic defect or warfarin. • Platelet studies may show impaired function especially in patients taking antiplatelet agents, and these predispose to intracranial hemorrhage. *Imaging.* CT or MRI shows the hemorrhage. Modern imaging techniques would not miss the diagnosis. *LP* is not performed for patients with confirmed or suspected intraparenchymal hemorrhage.
Diagnosis	• Intraparenchymal hemorrhage is suspected in a patient with acute onset of focal neurologic deficit and decreased level of consciousness in the setting of uncontrolled hypertension. Not all features will be present in all patients. Some patients with intraparenchymal hemorrhage can present in a fashion identical to infarction. • Diagnosis is confirmed with imaging.
Differential diagnosis	• *Infarction.* Can present with many of the same symptoms, although decreased level of consciousness is less common than with hemorrhage. • *Subdural or epidural hemorrhage.* Can present with focal deficit plus signs and symptoms of increased intracranial pressure. • *Calcification of the basal ganglia.* Can be mistaken for basal ganglia hemorrhage. Careful windowing of the CT scan usually can differentiate these possibilities. Also, basal ganglia calcifications are usually bilateral, which is not expected with most hemorrhages.

Description	Hemmorrhage within the Substance of the Brain
Management	• Blood pressure management is cautious. On the one hand, markedly elevated blood pressure should be lowered to reduce the risk for subsequent bleeding. However, overcorrection of the blood pressure can cause decreased cerebral perfusion pressure in the presence of increased intracranial pressure.
	• Surgical evacuation of the hematoma is rarely performed for intraparenchymal hemorrhages—the surgical procedure can be devastating. Retrospective analysis of the outcomes of patients who have had surgery for life-threatening intraparenchymal hemorrhages has generally indicated a poor outcome, with surgery making little impact in the results.
	• Ventricular drain occasionally is performed when the blood causes hydrocephalus, and can be an immediate life-saving maneuver.
Clinical course	• Patients who present comatose with intraparenchymal hemorrhage have a poor outcome, regardless of management. Although this is a controversial area in neurosurgery, there is little convincing evidence that emergency surgical evacuation of an intraparenchymal bleed has benefits that can be seen with an operation for subdural and epidural hemorrhage.
	• Patients who survive often have improvement in strength and coordination. Resolution of the interstitial blood can result in significant clinical improvement.

Intraparenchymal Hemorrhage *continued*

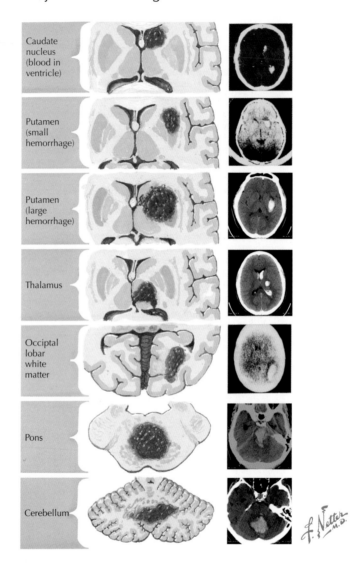

Caudate nucleus (blood in ventricle)

Putamen (small hemorrhage)

Putamen (large hemorrhage)

Thalamus

Occiptal lobar white matter

Pons

Cerebellum

EPIDURAL HEMATOMA (EDH)	
Description	Hemorrhage in the epidural space, usually due to trauma to the middle meningeal artery
Pathophysiology	• Trauma can cause a skull fracture, which can cross the middle meningeal artery. This may damage the artery without significantly displacing the bone. Arterial blood accumulates in the potential space, and compresses underlying brain. • Epidural hematomas occasionally are venous.
Clinical findings	• Classic presentation of an epidural hematoma is a patient with significant head injury having an initial phase of unresponsiveness followed by arousal—a.k.a., the lucid period. This is due to resolution of the initial neuronal shock from the injury. This phase is followed by decreased responsiveness as blood accumulates in the epidural space and presses on underlying brain with resulting increased intracranial pressure. • If the patient is hypotensive from other effects of the injury, the cerebral perfusion pressure (meaning arterial blood pressure minus intracranial pressure) may be compromised.
Laboratory studies	• Routine labs are usually normal. • Imaging shows the epidural hematoma in virtually all patients. • Skull radiographs usually show a fracture across the middle meningeal artery.

Diagnosis	Diagnosis is usually found in one of two ways:
	  • A patient with head injury is brought to the emergency department and scanned as part of routine protocol with significant head injury; or
	  • A patient initially appearing to have escaped unscathed from a head injury has deterioration in mental status minutes to hours after the injury.
	• Diagnosis is confirmed by imaging.

Differential diagnosis	• *Subdural hematoma.* Can present in a similar fashion, although the rapidity of deterioration is typically faster with epidural hematoma. • *Subarachnoid hemorrhage.* Can present with unresponsiveness and can occasionally be the result of injury. • *Shearing injury with head trauma.* Can present with neurologic deterioration without the extensive bleeding of epidural hematoma.
Management	• Surgical evacuation is needed for most patients with epidural hematoma. Because the blood is arterial, accumulation often does not stop without intervention. • Blood pressure is controlled but not overly lowered, because of concerns over decreases in perfusion pressure, as discussed above.
Clinical course	• Patients who have good functional status with epidural hematoma have a better prognosis than those who are neurologically devastated. • Surveillance for reaccumulation of blood is performed, because rebleeding can occur at the site.

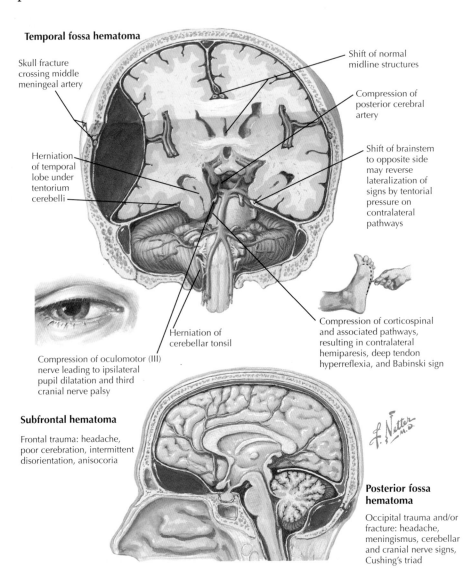

Temporal fossa hematoma

Skull fracture crossing middle meningeal artery

Shift of normal midline structures

Compression of posterior cerebral artery

Herniation of temporal lobe under tentorium cerebelli

Shift of brainstem to opposite side may reverse lateralization of signs by tentorial pressure on contralateral pathways

Herniation of cerebellar tonsil

Compression of oculomotor (III) nerve leading to ipsilateral pupil dilatation and third cranial nerve palsy

Compression of corticospinal and associated pathways, resulting in contralateral hemiparesis, deep tendon hyperreflexia, and Babinski sign

Subfrontal hematoma

Frontal trauma: headache, poor cerebration, intermittent disorientation, anisocoria

Posterior fossa hematoma

Occipital trauma and/or fracture: headache, meningismus, cerebellar and cranial nerve signs, Cushing's triad

HYPERCOAGULABLE STATES	
Description	• Some individuals have a predisposition to have their blood clot within the vessels, predisposing them to stroke and other ischemic events. • Can be genetic or acquired
Pathophysiology	• The clotting system is a delicate balance between freedom from clotting within the vessels, and ability to establish hemostasis in the event of internal or external bleeding. • Some individuals have a predisposition to clotting within the vessels, resulting in increased incidence of stroke, DVT, and other thrombotic events.
Clinical findings	• Patients with stroke due to hypercoagulable state do not have a different presentation than other strokes. Symptoms are focal motor or sensory deficit, language disturbance, or other abnormality in a vascular distribution. • Patients with stroke due to a hypercoagulable state are more likely to have multifocal infarctions, have a history of previous stroke, or have a history of other thromboembolic events.
Laboratory studies	Routine labs are often normal, although routine coagulation studies may be abnormal. Imaging studies and vascular studies do not differ between these patients and others with stroke. Evaluation of a patient with possible hypercoagulable state includes study for the following: • Antiphospholipid antibody syndrome (anticardiolipin antibody and lupus anticoagulant) • Antithrombin deficiency • Factor V Leiden • Prothrombin gene mutation • Activated protein C resistance • Protein C and protein S deficiency • Hyperhomocysteinemia • Malignancy
Diagnosis	• Hypercoagulable state is suspected when a patient presents with stroke and has few risk factors, is young, or has had thromboembolic events previously. • Diagnosis is confirmed by not only routine imaging studies, but by the aforementioned labs.
Differential diagnosis	• Differentiating between the causes of hypercoagulable states is by the aforementioned labs. • *Stroke.* The main differential diagnosis. Not due to coagulopathy, which can occur even in young patients and in patients without risk factors.

HYPERCOAGULABLE STATES—cont'd	

Management	• Initial treatment of a patient with stroke due to hypercoagulable state does not differ from that of other patients. However, low-molecular-weight heparins may be preferable to use of unfractionated heparin, initially.
	
	• Long-term anticoagulation with warfarin often is routinely given to patients with stroke and hypercoagulable state; however, it is likely needed only for patients with:
	
	  • Persistently elevated anticardiolipid antibody
	
	  • Persistent lupus anticoagulant
	
	  • Antithrombin deficiency
	
	  • Homozygous factor V Leiden
	
	  • Prothrombin gene mutation
	
	  • Cancer with hypercoagulability
	
	• Some patients may be treated with warfarin for 3–6 months, then changed to an antiplatelet agent.

Clinical course	Most patients improve, although there is persistent risk for repeated thromboembolic event.

SUBACUTE BACTERIAL ENDOCARDITIS (SBE)	
Description	A bacterial infection of the heart valves, which predisposes to the neurologic complications of brain abscess and stroke
Pathophysiology	• *Streptococcus viridans* and *Staphylococcus aureus* are responsible for most cases of infectious endocarditis. *Enterococcus*, *Haemophilus influenzae*, *Pseudomonas*, and fungi are also potential causes. • Involvement usually is of the mitral and/or the aortic valves. Mitral valve infection is most common. • Septic emboli can break off from the infected valves then lodge in vessels throughout the body, including the brain. The result is infarction or abscess.
Clinical findings	• The classic triad is fever, heart murmur, and hemiparesis, although this presentation is not universal. • Common symptoms are confusion, transient or persistent focal deficits, and spine pain. • Exam shows fever and often heart murmur, although these are not always present. Focal neurologic findings are common. • Osler nodes may be found on the fingers, as well as Janeway lesion on the palms. Roth spots in the eyes are harder to see.
Laboratory studies	• Routine labs show anemia with normal white blood cells in most patients. ESR and CRP are usually elevated, and can be used to follow disease activity during treatment. • Blood cultures usually are positive, but repeat samplings must be obtained. • UA often shows hematuria and/or proteinuria.
Diagnosis	• SBE is suspected in a patient with stroke who has a fever and heart murmur. However, elevation in ESR and/or CRP in the absence of fever and heart murmur should still raise the concern over SBE. • Confirmation is by blood culture and supportive data such as echocardiogram. • Echo often shows valvular changes, although transthoracic echo does not have the sensitivity of a transesophageal echocardiogram.
Differential diagnosis	• *Ischemic stroke.* Often presents with hemiparesis, and patients are at increased risk for fever and elevated inflammatory indicators suggestive of SBE. • *Cerebral hemorrhage.* Can present with focal signs and fever, although the possibility of SBE producing hemorrhage must be considered.
Management	• Antimicrobial therapy is given to all patients with infectious endocarditis. • Surgical repair or replacement of the valve is considered, but is high risk near the time of the stroke. • Anticoagulants often are used chronically in patients with prosthetic valves, but are contraindicated in patients with stroke with nonvalvular endocarditis.
Clinical course	Most patients improve after stroke, but there is risk for subsequent infarction. Also, patients need ongoing follow-up of their cardiac status.

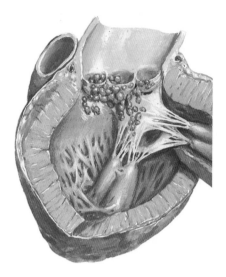

Subacute bacterial endocarditis vegetations

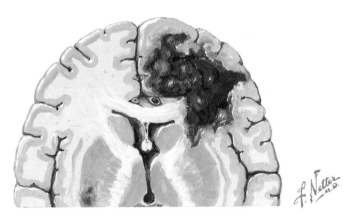

Infarct of brain with secondary hemorrhage from embolism to r. ant.
cerebral artery; also small infarct in l. basal gangila

CONGENITAL HEART DEFECTS (CHDs)	
Description	Some selected CHDs predispose to stroke. These mainly involve right-to-left shunts.
Pathophysiology	• Patients with certain congenital heart defects have an increased incidence of stroke. • Septal defects allow for right to left shunts, thereby increasing the incidence of clot from the venous circulation ending up on the arterial side without being trapped in the lungs.
Clinical findings	• Patients present with stroke that does not clinically differ from stroke due to other causes. However, patients with septal defects tend to be younger and have few other risk factors for stroke.
Laboratory studies	• Routine labs are normal. • Imaging with MRI and CT shows brain infarction, which does not differ from the appearance of infarction due to other causes. • Transthoracic echo may show the defect, but transesophageal echo is more likely to show the defect, and should be ordered in patients at risk, i.e., younger patients without many risk factors for stroke.
Diagnosis	• Stroke is diagnosed by the acute onset of neurologic deficit. • CT and MRI can show the stroke, but CT is less sensitive. CT is more likely to show the stroke after 2–3 days, whereas diffusion-weighted imaging is able to show an acute stroke on MRI almost immediately. • Heart defect is seen on echo. If there is reasonable suspicion, transesophageal echo is done, rather than transthoracic.
Differential diagnosis	• *Stroke from any cause.* Gives the same neurologic presentation as stroke from a septal defect. • *Mural thrombus.* Another cause of cardiac emboli.
Management	• Initial management of stroke possibly due to heart defect does not differ from stroke in general. • Options for treatment of a septal defect include long-term anticoagulation or use of a closure device. If the defect can be closed, then this is usually the preferred treatment.
Clinical course	The chance of repeat stroke with a defect is increased, but with treatment, the incidence of recurrent stroke is reduced.

Ostium secundum defect

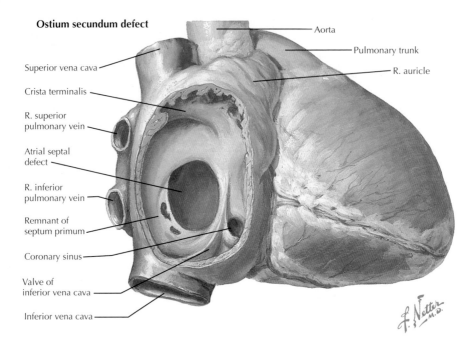

Aorta

Pulmonary trunk

Superior vena cava

R. auricle

Crista terminalis

R. superior
pulmonary vein

Atrial septal
defect

R. inferior
pulmonary vein

Remnant of
septum primum

Coronary sinus

Valve of
inferior vena cava

Inferior vena cava

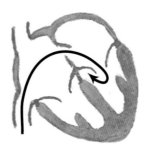

Probe-patent
foramen ovale
transmitting
venous clots

REHABILITATION	
Description	Combination of physical therapy, occupational therapy, and speech therapy is usually offered to patients with stroke who have a persistent neurologic deficit.
Physiology	• Improvement occurs in most patients after a stroke, although perhaps as many as 20% can show deterioration despite adequate treatment. • Therapy can aid the spontaneous improvement process. This not only involves helping to strengthen impaired muscles (physical therapy [PT]) but also to rework connections that can improve functional and self-care activities (occupational therapy [OT]).
Goals of therapy	• The principal purpose of therapy is to return the patient to the highest level of function possible. • Self-care can be improved with aggressive therapy, thereby reducing the cost of continuing care for the patient, whether at home or in a long-term care facility.
Types of Therapy	
Physical therapy	• Concentrates on muscle strength range of motion and ambulation. • The main goal of PT is to improve motor function and mobility.
Occupational therapy	• Concentrates on use of the body for self-care. Although the term "occupational" might suggest returning to work, this is not the main goal of OT.
Speech therapy	• Deals not only with speech, but also swallowing. • *Language therapy* is generally more effective for expressive aphasias than receptive aphasias, because the latter's patients have difficulty understanding commands and difficulty understanding their own errors. • *Therapy for swallowing* is needed for most patients with brainstem strokes and for some patients with hemispheric strokes. Aspiration is a major problem for stroke patients and can be improved with vigilance, limitation of oral intake for patients at risk, and changing manners of eating. Speech therapy evaluation is standard for many patients with stroke.
Other forms of therapy	There are other forms of therapy, including *recreation therapy*, *cognitive therapy*, and *music therapy*. These all have clear benefits for some patients. The rehabilitation specialist is in the best position to determine which forms of therapy are most appropriate.

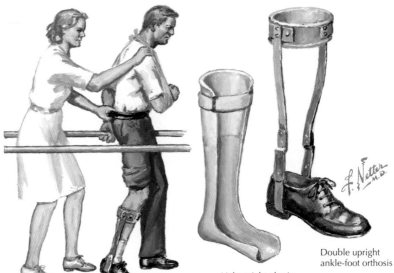

Patient relearns to walk between parallel bars wearing ankle-foot brace or orthosis. Support by attendant usually necessary at first

Lightweight plastic orthosis for weakness of ankle dorsiflexion fits easily into most shoes

Double upright ankle-foot orthosis

OVERVIEW OF PAIN DISORDERS	
Physiology of pain	• Pain is a protective sensation. Pain is evoked when tissues are either damaged or subjected to stresses that could cause damage. • Pain is not just a high-intensity sensation, rather, there are specific pain receptors and pathways that are responsible for transduction, transmission, and appreciation of pain.
Types of pain	Pain can be subdivided in a number of ways. Commonly discussed types include neuropathic, musculoskeletal, and visceral. • *Neuropathic pain* is due to damage directly to the nerve fibers. The membrane of the nerve is depolarized and unstable. Therefore, there are repetitive action potentials in the nerve. Although the pain is generated in the nerve, the pain is perceived in the part of the body innervated by the nerves. Neuropathic pain is stabbing, shooting, or burning. • *Musculoskeletal pain* is due to strain or inflammation of muscle fibers and surrounding tissues. Damage to bony structures results in distortion of nociceptors resulting in pain. Musculoskeletal pain usually is steady and is exacerbated by movement or weight bearing on the bone. • *Visceral pain* is due to stretching, twisting, or inflammation of tissues of the internal organs. This can be tumor, cyst, anatomic distortion, or other pathology. Ischemia of the tissues can achieve the same result. Pain is steady or crampy and is perceived as a deep pain.
Causes of pain	• *Neuropathic pain* can be due to numerous etiologies, including trauma, nutrition, toxins, metabolism, and vasculature. The most common cause is diabetic neuropathy. • *Musculoskeletal pain* is due to osteoarthritis, disc disease, damage to cartilage, or damage to tendons, ligaments, and/or muscles. Major or repeated minor trauma is the most common cause. • *Visceral pain* can be due to tumor, ischemia, twisting, or inflammation of the internal organs.
Treatment of pain	• All pain should be treated by removing the damage, if at all possible. Compression of nerve by osteophyte can be treated by removal of the compression. Pain from infiltrating tumor is particularly resistant to medical therapy, and, therefore, radiation therapy and/or chemotherapy is effective for most patients. • Neuropathic pain often is treated by anticonvulsants and/or antidepressants. The combination of an element from both groups often is needed.
Common Treatments	
Anticonvulsants	• Anticonvulsants treat mainly neuropathic pain, and are especially helpful for shooting and stabbing pains. They can also be helpful for burning pain. • Agents commonly used include carbamazepine, gabapentin, and pregabalin, although multiple agents in this class can be helpful.
Antidepressants	• Tricyclic antidepressants are used for headache and neuropathic pain. They mainly help the steady burning pain of peripheral neuropathy and can be especially helpful in diabetics. • Selective serotonin re-uptake inhibitors (SSRIs) also occasionally are used for headache and neuropathic pain, but less so than TCAs. • Serotonin-norepinephrine re-uptake inhibitors (SNRIs) are used for neuropathic pain.

Common Treatments—cont'd	
Analgesics	• Analgesics can be taken on an as needed basis or by regular administration. Use of sustained release opiates is not first line for most physicians. Other treatments should generally be used first with PRN analgesics.
	• Acetaminophen, tramadol, propoxyphene, and nonsteroidal anti-inflammatory drugs (NSAIDs) usually are used for milder pain. Opiates such as hydrocodone, oxycodone, morphine, and fentanyl are used for severe and refractory pain.
Miscellaneous agents	Baclofen used for some patients with neuropathic pain, especially trigeminal neuralgia.

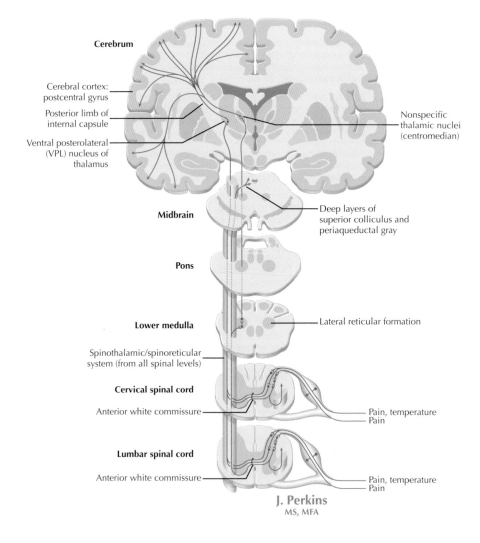

Cerebrum

Cerebral cortex: postcentral gyrus

Posterior limb of internal capsule

Ventral posterolateral (VPL) nucleus of thalamus

Nonspecific thalamic nuclei (centromedian)

Midbrain

Deep layers of superior colliculus and periaqueductal gray

Pons

Lower medulla

Lateral reticular formation

Spinothalamic/spinoreticular system (from all spinal levels)

Cervical spinal cord

Anterior white commissure

Pain, temperature
Pain

Lumbar spinal cord

Anterior white commissure

Pain, temperature
Pain

J. Perkins
MS, MFA

MIGRAINE HEADACHE	
Description	• Episodic headache due to neurovascular inflammation • Can be with or without aura
Pathophysiology	• Neurovascular inflammation affecting cerebral and scalp arteries • Neural trigger that is sensitive to internal host factors for triggering a migraine • Spreading electrical depression across the cortex results in the aura symptoms when present.
Clinical findings	• The headache is episodic with periods of no headache. Constant headache is not migraine. Features that suggest migraine include unilateral distribution, throbbing, nausea/vomiting, photophonia, phonophobia, and sensitivity to smell. Not all of these features will be present in all patients with all headaches. None of the features are invariable. • *Migraine with aura* is preceded by an aura, which typically is sensory. Visual aura is most common, although other sensory and motor symptoms can develop. Scintillating scotoma is a visual obscuration that is variably described as shifting jagged lines, whirling prisms, or other positive visual phenomenon. Vision is obscured in the area of the scotoma. • *Migraine without aura* is more common than migraine with aura, and the headache is similar but without the aura. • Neurologic and medical exams are normal between migraines. During the migraine, patient distress may make examination impossible.
Laboratory studies	• Labs are normal and may include CBC, CMP, ANA, ESR, TSH. Routine labs are not essential. Labs are performed if the patient has atypical features or fails to respond to medical treatment. • Imaging with magnetic resonance imaging (MRI) and computer tomography (CT) is normal. They are not needed unless the patient has atypical features or fails to respond to treatment.
Diagnosis	• Migraine is suspected with a clinical presentation of episodic headache with associated symptoms of nausea and sensory sensitivity in the setting of a normal examination. • Absence of abnormalities of labs and scans (if performed) supports the diagnosis.
Differential diagnosis	• *Subarachnoid hemorrhage.* Acute onset of severe headache can be due to migraine, but subarachnoid hemorrhage (SAH) has to be considered. • *Cluster headache.* Episodic unilateral periorbital and frontal pain is typical of cluster headache. Cluster is briefer than migraine—less than 1 hour. Also, cluster often begins in midlife. Cluster headaches occur as a series, over days to weeks, and often wakes the sleeping patient, all of which are unusual features for migraine. • *Stroke.* Hemorrhagic stroke can present with headache, but there usually is focal neurologic deficit or alteration of consciousness. The deficit may be ascribed to migraine, but the deficit persists, rather than being transient with migraine. Infarction also may present with headache, although this is less likely. The neurologic deficit is persistent.

MIGRAINE HEADACHE—cont'd	
	• *Temporal arteritis.* Temporal headache in a middle-aged to elderly patient raises concern over TA. The temporal artery is usually thickened and tender. Erythrocyte sedimentation rate (ESR) is elevated.
	• *Sinusitis.* Can give a headache that is similar to migraine. Migraines are often misdiagnosed as sinus-related; nausea and photophobia argue against sinus-related causes. Fever and drainage suggest sinusitis.
Management	*Acute treatment.* Triptans are the agents of choice for most patients. Response or adverse effects to one does not necessarily indicate intolerance to all in this group. ***Note:*** Triptans should not be used in patients with uncontrolled hypertension and with basilar migraine.
	Dihydroergotime (DHE) is effective for typical migraine, and can be given nasally or by intravenous, intramuscular, or subcutaneous injection. ***Note:*** Precautions with use of DHE are similar to those of triptans. DHE and triptans should not be used within 24 hours of each other.
	Preventative treatment. Use of preventive agents is indicated for patients with headaches that are frequent (e.g., at least 4 per month) or refractory to abortive therapy. The choices are multiple, including β-blockers, calcium channel blockers, tricyclic antidepressants, and many anticonvulsants. Young patients often are treated with β-blockers. Anticonvulsants are powerful and are effective for many people. Tricyclics often are used, but seldom first line, because of sedation and anticholinergic effects.
	Self-help. Patients can reduce the incidence of migraine by following some general guidelines:
	• *Sleep.* Too much or too little sleep makes headaches more likely.
	• *Diet.* Migraines are more likely with skipping meals, and with intake of certain substances, including monosodium glutamate (MSG), aspartame, nitrates, nitrites, caffeine, tyramine, ethanol, and sugar. The triggers differ between patients.
	• *Exercise.* Regular exercise reduces the incidence of headaches, including migraine. The occasional patient, however, will have exercise-induced headache.
Clinical course	• Most patients improve with treatment. With selective treatment, abortive therapy is effective for up to 75% of headaches. In the rest, the headache eventually abates.
	• Preventive therapy, plus self-help guidelines, can reduce the incidence of headache by at least 50%.
	• Patients should be cautioned that abortive therapy is not effective for 100% of headaches, and the first failure does not mean that medications have to be changed. Similarly, preventive therapy does not prevent all headaches, and, therefore, having headaches does not necessitate changing of medications.

Migraine

Attack

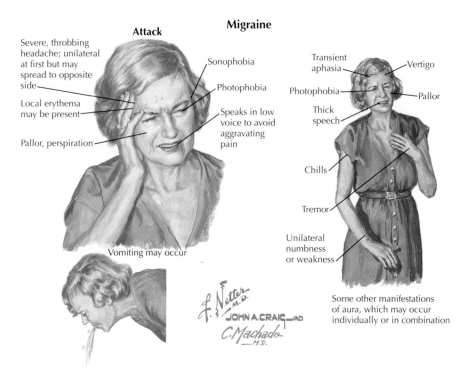

Severe, throbbing headache; unilateral at first but may spread to opposite side

Local erythema may be present

Pallor, perspiration

Sonophobia

Photophobia

Speaks in low voice to avoid aggravating pain

Vomiting may occur

Transient aphasia

Photophobia

Thick speech

Chills

Tremor

Unilateral numbness or weakness

Vertigo

Pallor

Some other manifestations of aura, which may occur individually or in combination

Scintillating Scotoma and Fortification Phenomena

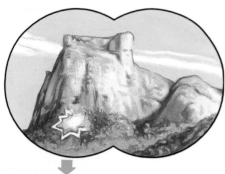

Early phase: isolated paracentral scintillating scotoma

Scintillating edge

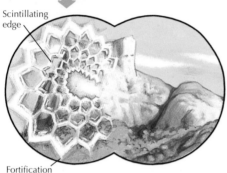

Spread of scotoma to involve entire unilateral visual field

Fortification pattern

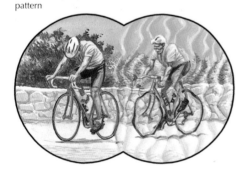

Wavy lines (heat shimmers)
Wavy line distortions in part of visual field similar to shimmers above hot pavement

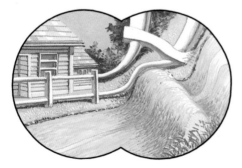

Metamorphopsia
Distortions of form, size, or position of objects or environment in part of visual field

CLUSTER HEADACHE	
Description	• Episodic headache centered over the eye and frontal region. Headache unilateral, brief (less than 1 hour).
	• Occurrence is in clusters, i.e., groups of headaches over days to weeks.
Pathophysiology	• Pathophysiology is thought to be neuropathic, although the details are not known. Although considered in association with migraine, many features differ.
Clinical findings	• Episodic, brief headaches centered around one eye. The pain may extend to the frontal region, but does not involve both sides, and does not extend to the posterior aspects of the head.
	• "Cluster" is so called because groups of headaches occur over days to weeks. There may be multiple episodes per day, and they may wake the patient from sleep. Duration of the headache is less than 1 hour, and more typically 20–30 minutes.
	• Cluster is most common in men, whereas migraine is more common in women. Nausea, vomiting, photophobia, and phonophobia are not typical of cluster, whereas they are seen with migraine.
Laboratory studies	• Routine labs are normal. With typical presentations, labs are not needed.
	• Imaging is normal. MRI and CT usually are not needed unless there are atypical features or the patient fails to respond to medication.
	• Lumbar puncture (LP) is performed if the patient is thought to have meningitis or subarachnoid hemorrhage; however, these are seldom in the differential diagnosis because of the longer duration of these headaches—when they begin, they do not stop.
Diagnosis	• Clinical features of brief, episodic, and periorbital headache suggests cluster. The absence of prominent autonomic symptoms is supportive.
	• Normal examination argues against many other diagnoses.
	• Normal imaging is supportive, but usually not needed for diagnosis.
Differential diagnosis	• *Migraine.* Episodic headaches are typical of migraine. Migraines are longer in duration and often bilateral. Associated symptoms also are suggestive of the diagnosis.
	• *Sinusitis.* Can cause headache in the same distribution as cluster; however, the headache is not episodic and recurrent.
Management	*Acute treatment.* Medications for migraine are commonly used, including triptans. Pure analgesics also are used, and some unfortunate patients require strong opiate analgesics. Inhalation of 100% O_2 is helpful for some patients. DHE can be very helpful, both as acute treatment and short-term prevention.
	Preventive treatment. Prevention can be with some of the meds used for migraine, including valproate and some calcium channel blockers. Anti-inflammatory agents are tried, and brief courses of corticosteroids are used for patients with refractory cluster.
Clinical course	• Most patients respond to triptans or one of the other abortive agents, although some patients become opiate-dependent.
	• Cluster persists into midlife for many patients.

Cluster Headache

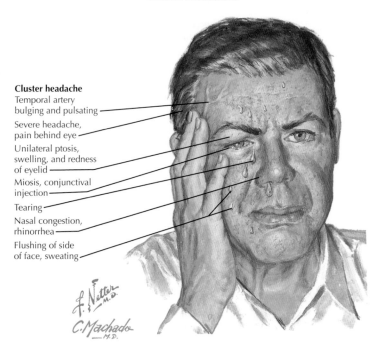

Cluster headache

Temporal artery bulging and pulsating

Severe headache, pain behind eye

Unilateral ptosis, swelling, and redness of eyelid

Miosis, conjunctival injection

Tearing

Nasal congestion, rhinorrhea

Flushing of side of face, sweating

TENSION (MUSCLE CONTRACTION) HEADACHE	
Description	• Most prominent in the craniocervical region and regions of the temporalis and frontalis muscles • Tension headache and muscle contraction headache are synonyms; they refer to the same pathophysiologic process.
Pathophysiology	• Muscle contraction/tension headaches are likely multifactorial, with the final path being contraction and irritation of the paraspinal and cranial muscles. • Factors that predispose to this muscle contraction include cervical spine disease, poor posture, anxiety, prolonged postures with limited movement (e.g., office worker staring at a computer screen), and upper body deconditioning.
Clinical findings	• Constant pain in the craniocervical and temporal regions is the most common symptom. The headache may be frequent, and in some patients be almost continuous. • Symptoms distinctly not present are photophobia, nausea, vomiting, and phonophobia. These symptoms suggest migraine or other meningeal inflammatory pathology. • Neurologic and medical exams are normal, although patients may have increased tone of the paraspinal muscles.
Laboratory studies	• Routine labs are normal. Patients who are middle-aged, with constant pain in this region, should have ESR checked, specifically looking for temporal arteritis and polymyalgia rheumatica—both treatable expressions of giant cell arteritis. • Imaging with MRI and CT are normal, and often are not needed. Imaging is indicated when the headache is continuous, or if the headaches do not respond to management. • LP is performed in some patients with constant headache accompanied by neck pain, but the diagnostic yield in the absence of fever, lab signs of infection, and/or meningeal signs on examination is quite low.
Diagnosis	• Clinical features make the diagnosis of muscle contraction headache. • Tests usually are not needed unless the patient does not respond to therapy.
Differential diagnosis	• *Migraine.* More episodic, with briefer and less frequent headaches. • *Chiari malformation.* Can present with craniocervical pain, but most symptomatic patients also have other neurologic symptoms of brainstem compression. • *Pseudotumor cerebri.* Benign intracranial hypertension, or pseudotumor cerebri, presents with constant headache associated with papilledema distinctly not present in tension headache. • *Brain tumor.* Can present with constant or fluctuating headache, which can resemble muscle contraction. Most patients have neurologic deficits, which argue against a benign diagnosis. Seizures also are common with tumor, and not expected with muscle contraction.

TENSION (MUSCLE CONTRACTION) HEADACHE—cont'd	
Management	*Acute treatment.* Analgesics can be used for occasional muscle contraction headache; however, they should be avoided for frequent or chronic use because of the risk for developing rebound headache. *Preventative treatments.* Physical methods are recommended, including short course of physical therapy followed by sustained upper-body conditioning routine. Biofeedback also is used, although this is not a long-term solution. Tricyclic antidepressants are the most commonly used meds. NSAIDs also are used, although their long-term safety has been questioned. Many patients can be managed without long-term preventive therapy.
Clinical course	• Most patients improve with treatment, but a chronic level of muscle contraction pain is common. Aggressive therapy and conditioning can lower the incidence of persistent muscle contraction headache. • Some patients with muscle contraction headache take daily analgesics, predisposing to rebound headache. These patients will not have resolution of the rebound headache until they have ceased the daily use of analgesics.

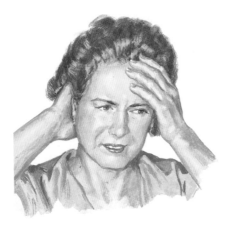

Intermittent, recurrent, or constant head pain, often in forehead, temples, or back of head and neck; commonly described as "bandlike," "tightness," or "viselike"

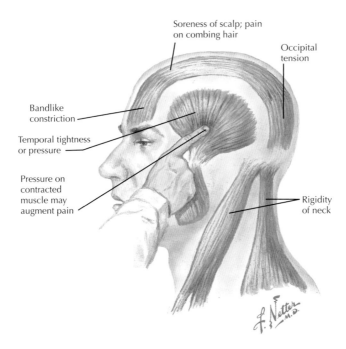

Soreness of scalp; pain on combing hair

Occipital tension

Bandlike constriction

Temporal tightness or pressure

Pressure on contracted muscle may augment pain

Rigidity of neck

REBOUND HEADACHE	
Description	• Persistent headache related to the overuse of some medications, usually analgesics. • This is the most common diagnosis of patients referred to headache clinics.
Pathophysiology	• Patients with rebound headaches typically have a history of migraine. The headaches are treated with the offending agent, which can be an analgesic or even a triptan. The details of the pathophysiology are unknown.
Clinical findings	• Chronic holocephalic headache is typical. The headache may even be present in the morning, when the patient has gone for several hours without analgesics. Treatment with analgesics produces attenuation, but seldom abolition, of the headache. • The history typically is of migraine treated with analgesics. The headache becomes increasingly frequent and eventually virtually daily. The occasional patient will have headaches on most, but not all, days. • Exam is normal. Detailed examination for neurologic deficit and papilledema is important.
Laboratory studies	• Routine labs are normal. • Imaging is normal. MRI often is performed to look for other causes of chronic craniocervical pain, including mass lesion, hydrocephalus, and Chiari malformation. • LP seldom is needed; patients present with headache that is of a duration long enough to make chronic meningitis extremely unlikely.
Diagnosis	• Clinical features of constant headache, frequent use of analgesic or tryptan, and a normal examination • Imaging often is needed to rule out serious causes of constant headache.
Differential diagnosis	• *Brain tumor.* Can present with constant headache, and patients may take analgesics. Neurologic deficit or papilledema usually is present. Imaging makes the diagnosis. • *Pseudotumor cerebri.* Benign intracranial hypertension, or pseudotumor cerebri, presents with constant headache and papilledema. • *Chiari malformation.* A malformation of the craniocervical junction that can present with pain in that region. Most patients have symptoms or signs of brainstem compression or hydrocephalus, although not all.

	REBOUND HEADACHE—cont'd
Management	*Acute treatment.* The key to treatment of rebound headaches is avoidance of PRN medications. This requires long discussions with the patient, and often his family as well. Some patients are able to abruptly stop analgesics, whereas others taper over days to weeks, similar to smoking cessation. Along with cessation of acute treatments, initiation of preventive therapy often is helpful, as mentioned below. *Preventive treatment.* Because many patients initially had migraines, initiation of therapy for prevention of migraine headaches can be effective. Tricyclic antidepressants in particular are helpful. Institution of a preventive treatment allows suppression of the episodic migraines, which commonly follow withdrawal of the analgesics. Also, patients psychologically appreciate having a medicine that is expected to reduce their headaches.
Clinical course	If patients are able to reduce their intake of analgesics, they usually are able to reduce their chronic headaches. Then, the episodic migraines can be treated with PRN triptan or another agent. Unfortunately, many patients are not successful.

TEMPORAL ARTERITIS (TA)	
Description	One manifestation of giant cell arteritis. This is a cause of temporal pain in middle-aged and elderly patients.
Pathophysiology	• Inflammation of the temporal arteries often is associated with inflammation of other tissues, including those in the shoulder girdle (polymyalgia rheumatica [PMR]). • Although the immune system is implicated, the root cause is unknown.

Clinical findings	*Symptoms*:
	  • Patients present with pain most prominent in the temporal regions.
	  • Some patients also have pain in the muscles of the neck and shoulders (PMR), and some will have more diffuse aches and pains.
	Signs:
	  • Exam shows temporal arteries that are thickened and tender.
	  • There are usually no other findings.
	  • Patients who are untreated can progress to blindness.

Laboratory studies	*Labs.* ESR is usually elevated, although occasionally normal. *Imaging.* MRI and CT are normal. *Pathology.* Temporal artery biopsy is diagnostic, although occasionally the biopsy may miss the pathology.
Diagnosis	• Clinical presentation of temporal area pain with thickened and tender temporal artery and elevated ESR suggests the diagnosis. • Temporal artery biopsy is diagnostic, and should be performed in most patients.
Differential diagnosis	• *Tumor.* Can produce focal pain in an older patient, which can be mistaken for temporal arteritis. Scan is needed to rule out brain mass. • *Subacute bacterial endocarditis.* Can present with neck pain, fever, malaise, and elevated ESR. The pain is more in cervical muscles, and focal pain in the temporal region is not expected. • *Migraine.* Unusual in the older age group, which is susceptible to temporal arteritis. The pain is episodic, however, and there is almost always a history of episodic, migraine-type headaches in the younger years.
Management	• Prednisone is the most commonly used corticosteroid. Treatment should begin when the diagnosis is suspected, even prior to obtaining the results of the temporal artery biopsy. • ESR and clinical symptoms are followed during maintenance and titration phase of the prednisone.

TEMPORAL ARTERITIS (TA)—cont'd	
Clinical course	• Most patients have prompt improvement in headache with administration of prednisone therapy. Because of the risk for blindness, the administration of prednisone should not await the biopsy results. • Systemic symptoms of PMR also improve in response to prednisone. • Ongoing monitoring of ESR and clinical presentation is required for the possibility of recurrence.

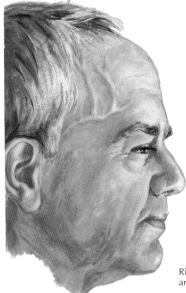

Rigid, tender, nonpulsating temporal arteries may be visible or palpable

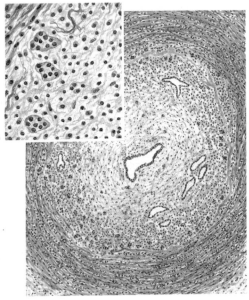

Biopsy of superficial temporal artery. Lumen almost completely obliterated, with some recanalization. High-power insert shows infiltration with lymphocytes, plasma cells, and giant cells; fragmentation of elastica

PSEUDOTUMOR CEREBRI	
Description	Also called *benign intracranial hypertension*. Patients have increased intracranial pressure not due to mass lesion or hydrocephalus.
Pathophysiology	• Etiology is unknown in most patients. • The occasional patient may have venous insufficiency.
Clinical findings	*Demographics.* Most patients are young women who are moderately to markedly overweight. *Symptoms.* Patients have headache that is constant, and may be positional, i.e., greater pain when recumbent. Visual obscuration is common. *Signs.* Papilledema is typical, and raises concern over the diagnosis. Neurologic and medical exams are otherwise normal.
Laboratory studies	*Blood.* Routine labs are normal. *Imaging.* CT and MRI are normal. The absence of mass lesion or increased ventricular size is essential. MRV is recommended for many patients and may show intracranial venous occlusive disease. *Lumbar puncture.* Cerebrospinal fluid (CSF) opening pressure is elevated, greater than 20 cm H_2O and usually greater than 30 cm H_2O. Fluid has normal CSF profile and chemistries.
Diagnosis	• Clinical features of headache and papilledema in the absence of structural lesion on MRI make the diagnosis of pseudotumor cerebri. • MRV may show venous outflow obstruction, which is consistent with the diagnosis.
Differential diagnosis	• *Tumor.* Symptoms of brain tumor can be indistinguishable from pseudotumor cerebri. Imaging is required for diagnosis. • *Cavernous sinus thrombosis.* Another form of venous sinus disease, which presents with orbital pain and typically cranial nerve palsies, with ocular motor and trigeminal being predominantly affected. • *Optic neuritis.* Bilateral optic neuritis may present with bilateral papilledema, which can be clinically indistinguishable in appearance from the papilledema of pseudotumor cerebri. Retrobulbar pain is common with ON, which is exacerbated by turning of the globes. However, prominent headache is unusual. • *Chiari malformation.* Can result in hydrocephalus, which may present with headache and papilledema. Many of these patients will have cognitive disturbance and/or other neurologic deficits, however.

PSEUDOTUMOR CEREBRI—cont'd	
Management	*Lumbar puncture.* Diagnosis and initial management is with LP. CSF opening pressure is measured, after scanning has shown no Chiari or other structural lesion. When the opening pressure is elevated, sufficient CSF is removed not only for analysis but also to reduce the CSF pressure to normal levels. When the closing pressure is normal, CSF draining stops. If the symptoms worsen, the LP can be redone, but repeated high-volume CSF drainage procedures are seldom performed nowadays.
	Medications. Some medications have been used to reduce CSF pressure, including, specifically, carbonic anhydrase inhibitors. Acetazolamide is the most commonly used medication. Topiramate and zonisamide have weaker carbonic anhydrase effects and additionally aid with weight loss for many patients, and are helpful for many patients.
	Surgery. Needed for a minority of patients with pseudotumor cerebri. The most commonly used techniques are optic nerve fenestration and lumboperitoneal shunt placement.
	Self-help. Weight loss greatly improves pseudotumor cerebri, to the point that a loss of 10% or more of total body weight is recommended. This can normalize the pressure so that further CSF drainage or medications are not needed.
Clinical course	• Few patients can lose the weight that is required to obviate the use of direct medical or surgical treatment. Maintenance therapy, with acetazolamide or one of the other medications listed, is common.
	• Surgery can give the definitive treatment that can protect the visual loss that can develop as a result of the increased intracranial pressure.

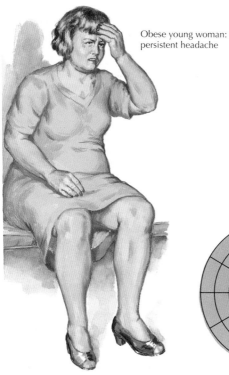

Obese young woman:
persistent headache

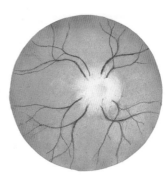

Papilledema: nasal blurring
of optic disc vessels

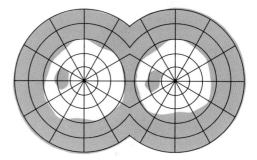

Concentrically contracted visual
fields, large blind spots

May be related to pregnancy; menstrual
disturbances; hypervitaminosis A; use
of steroids, tetracycline, or nalidixic acid;
chronic otitis media with dural sinus
occlusion; endocrinopathy (Addison's or
Cushing's disease, hypoparathyrodism)

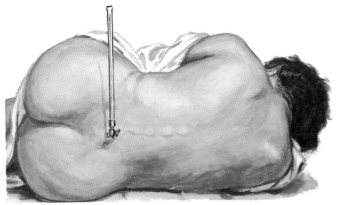

Cerebrospinal fluid
pressure elevated

NEUROPATHIC PAIN	
Description	Produced by repetitive neuronal discharge
Pathophysiology	• Peripheral nerve damage from any cause can bring about neuropathic pain. • Common causes are peripheral neuropathy from diabetes or other causes, entrapment neuropathy in the arm or leg, and nerve root compression. • The final common pathway for neuropathic pain is depolarization of the membrane and fluctuation in membrane potential. This causes episodic action potentials, which can be sustained and repetitive.
Clinical findings	• Pain can be stabbing, shooting, or burning. The distribution of the pain depends on the location. Mononeuropathies, such as carpal tunnel syndrome and radiculopathy, produce focal pain in the cutaneous distribution of the affected nerve. Peripheral neuropathy, such as diabetes, produce distal burning pain. • Diabetics can have a combination of pain from mononeuropathy and polyneuropathy.
Laboratory studies	• Routine labs are commonly normal, although diabetics will have signs of glucose intolerance on chemistries, and elevated glycosylated hemoglobin. • Imaging is needed if there are symptoms or signs of radiculopathy. • Electromyography (EMG) can document peripheral neuropathy or mononeuropathy.
Diagnosis	• Neuropathic pain is a clinical diagnosis. Laboratory studies, imaging, and EMG can help to show the cause, but they do not make the diagnosis.
Management	• Anticonvulsants are effective for multiple modalities of neuropathic pain, especially shooting and stabbing pain. • Antidepressants mainly help burning pain, but can help shooting and stabbing pain as well. TCAs and SSRIs are mainly used. • Light therapy can be of benefit to patients with distal polyneuropathy.
Clinical course	• Most patients have improvement with medications. • Eventually, patients improve with or without treatment. In general, dysfunctional neurons exhibit painful discharges, but when the neurons have degenerated, they do not exhibit such discharges.

Mechanisms of Neuropathic Pain

1. Sprouting of sympathetic postganglionic nerve fibers on 1° afferent endings and 1° sensory cell bodies
2. Lowered threshold for firing of C fibers (hyperesthesia) and Aδ fibers (allodynia)
3. Proliferation of α-adrenergic receptors on 1° sensory afferent endings and 1° sensory cell bodies
4. Possible ephaptic afferent activation
5. Permanent hyperactivation of wide dynamic range neurons
6. Glutamate excitotoxic cell death of inhibitory neurons (glutamate storms)
7. Inadequacy of central descending serotonin, norepinephrine, opioid peptide pathways to control nociception
8. Immobilization by pain decreases gating of nociceptive input, limiting physical therapy to initiate gating
9. Sprouting of C fibers in spinal cord
10. Extension of interneuron dendrites into additional spinal cord laminae

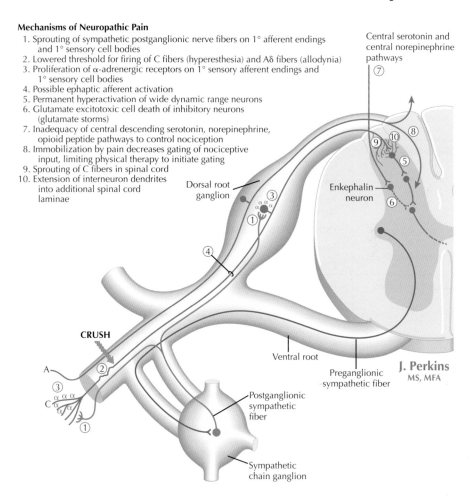

Central serotonin and central norepinephrine pathways

Dorsal root ganglion

Enkephalin neuron

CRUSH

Ventral root

A

C

Postganglionic sympathetic fiber

Sympathetic chain ganglion

Preganglionic sympathetic fiber

J. Perkins
MS, MFA

TRIGEMINAL NEURALGIA	
Description	Neuropathic pain in the distribution of one trigeminal nerve
Pathophysiology	• Microvascular compression is thought to be the cause in many cases. Compression of part of the trigeminal nerve causes repetitive action potentials in the nerve, thereby producing pain. • Tumors and other lesions at the cerebellopontine angle rarely are seen.
Clinical findings	• Severe lancinating pain, always confined to the distribution of the trigeminal nerve on one side. One division is commonly affected. • Pain is lancinating, shooting, or stabbing. • Pain occurs in attacks, which are often triggered by talking, eating, chewing, or brushing teeth. • Patients typically are late middle-aged to elderly. • Spontaneous remissions can occur. • Exam is normal, including facial motor and sensory function.
Laboratory studies	• Routine labs are normal. • Imaging also is usually normal. Cerebellopontine angle lesions can occasionally be seen; these are better seen on MRI than CT. • Although the cause commonly is microvascular, angiography seldom is revealing and not needed for most patients.
Diagnosis	• Diagnosis is suspected by the clinical features of lancinating pain in one trigeminal distribution. • Imaging is done to look for other causes of neuropathic pain.
Differential diagnosis	• *Hemifacial spasm.* Occasionally is misdiagnosed as trigeminal neuralgia. However, hemifacial spasm is an episodic facial muscle contraction, whereas trigeminal neuralgia is a sensory disorder. The confusion arises because some patients with trigeminal neuralgia grimace from the pain. • *Bell's palsy.* Should not be confused with trigeminal neuralgia, but because there is some periauricular pain in many patients with trigeminal neuralgia, the diagnoses can be confused.

TRIGEMINAL NEURALGIA—cont'd	
Management	• Anticonvulsants are considered first-line therapy for many patients. Although carbamazapine has traditionally been first line, newer agents also are used, including gabapentin, oxcarbazepine, and many of the other second generation agents.
	• Baclofen often is used alone or in combination with other agents.
	• Radiofrequency nerve lesion is one of the options available for medically refractory patients.
	• Stereotactic radiosurgery often is used, although there is incomplete information on the long-term efficacy of this treatment. Many surgeons use this technique prior to considering more aggressive surgery.
	• Microvascular decompression is used as a last resort when medical treatment has been ineffective, and other less invasive procedures have been ineffective or judged as inappropriate.
Clinical course	• Most patients have improvement with medical or surgical therapy.
	• Some unfortunate patients continue to have pain and require long-duration opiate analgesics; the duration of the paroxysms is too short to benefit from PRN dosing of analgesics.

Sensory distribution of trigeminal (V) nerve

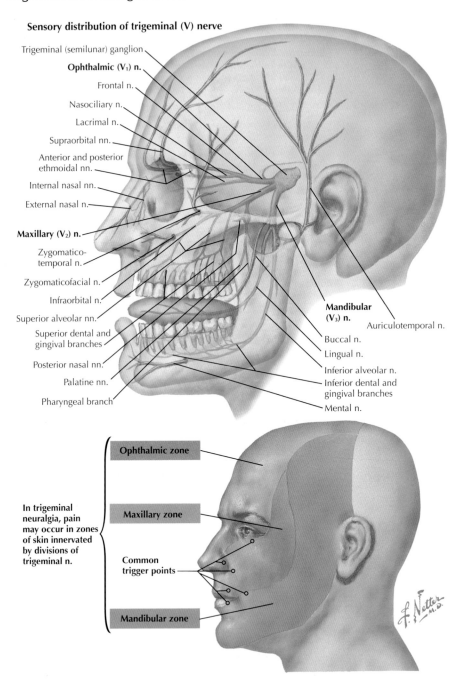

Trigeminal (semilunar) ganglion

Ophthalmic (V₁) n.

Frontal n.

Nasociliary n.

Lacrimal n.

Supraorbital nn.

Anterior and posterior ethmoidal nn.

Internal nasal nn.

External nasal n.

Maxillary (V₂) n.

Zygomatico-temporal n.

Zygomaticofacial n.

Infraorbital n.

Superior alveolar nn.

Superior dental and gingival branches

Posterior nasal nn.

Palatine nn.

Pharyngeal branch

Mandibular (V₃) n.

Auriculotemporal n.

Buccal n.

Lingual n.

Inferior alveolar n.

Inferior dental and gingival branches

Mental n.

Ophthalmic zone

Maxillary zone

In trigeminal neuralgia, pain may occur in zones of skin innervated by divisions of trigeminal n.

Common trigger points

Mandibular zone

FIBROMYALGIA	
Description	A syndrome of pain prominent in the muscles. It is a syndrome rather than a disease.
Pathophysiology	• There is no pathologic correlate to the reports of pain. • Multiple factors appear to predispose to fibromyalgia. In general, fibromyalgia is more common in females, with depression, sleep disturbance, connective tissue disease, and a family history.
Clinical findings	• Diffuse muscle and soft tissue pain is typical of fibromyalgia. The pain is in tissues bilaterally, and involves the upper and lower extremities and body. • Exam is normal except for tenderness in multiple focal regions.
Laboratory studies	• Routine labs are normal. Unless there is a coexisting connective tissue disease, additional labs for autoimmune diseases are normal. • EMG is normal. • Imaging is usually not necessary, but if performed is normal. • LP is usually not performed, but would be normal.
Diagnosis	• Fibromyalgia is suspected when a patient presents with multifocal pains without objective findings on examination. • Labs for connective tissue disease are performed to look for systemic lupus erythematosus and other disorders that can produce symptoms of fibromyalgia. • EMG is performed to look for neuropathy or myopathy. • Diagnosis is established by clinical features and the absence of another cause.
Differential diagnosis	• *Polyneuropathy.* Can produce diffuse pain, although the sensory loss is common and the symptoms are distal. NCS and EMG show neuropathic findings. • *Polymyalgia rheumatica.* Produces pain in the neck and upper shoulders. In general, the duration is more subacute than fibromyalgia. ESR is elevated. • *Systemic lupus erythematosus.* Can produce pains in tissues which can resemble fibromyalgia. Some investigators associate fibromyalgia with SLE, but most feel the diagnosis of SLE is a more specific disagnosis and separate from fibromyalgia.

Management	Treatment is symptomatic and supportive.
	A host of medications are used, including:
	  • Antidepressants—helpful for pain control and management of comorbid depression
	  • Analgesics—helpful for pain control
	  • Anti-inflammatories—helpful for pain control. There is no certainty that the anti-inflammatory effects are beneficial.
	  • Anticonvulsants—helpful for some patients as an adjunct to pain control
	Sleep disturbance should be considered in patients with fibromyalgia, and should be tested for and treated if found.

Clinical course	Patients may improve, but long-term treatment is needed.

Chronic Fatigue Syndrome
Signs and Symptoms

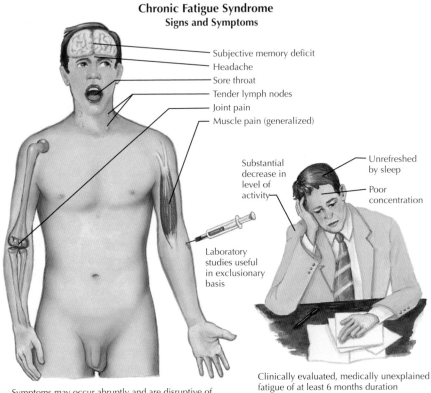

Subjective memory deficit

Headache

Sore throat

Tender lymph nodes

Joint pain

Muscle pain (generalized)

Substantial decrease in level of activity

Laboratory studies useful in exclusionary basis

Unrefreshed by sleep

Poor concentration

Clinically evaluated, medically unexplained fatigue of at least 6 months duration

Symptoms may occur abruptly and are disruptive of othewise productive life. Post-viral onset is often noted.

Underlying pathophysiology is uncertain

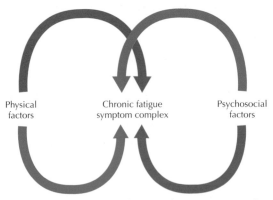

Physical factors

Chronic fatigue symptom complex

Psychosocial factors

Chronic fatigue syndrome is best viewed as a symptom complex resulting from interaction of physical and psychosocial factors

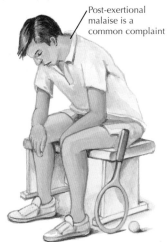

Post-exertional malaise is a common complaint

Malaise in excess of 24 hours

JOHN A. CRAIG—AD
with
E. Hatton

OVERVIEW OF IMMUNE DISORDERS	
Description	• Immune disorders may affect any part of the nervous system.
	• Some disorders are primary, in that they affect the nervous system predominantly, whereas others affect the nervous system in conjunction with other systems.
Pathophysiology	• The mechanisms of immune disease are not completely understood.
	• One possible mechanism is antigenic stimulation producing a persistent immune response, which targets the host tissues.
Clinical findings	• Immune disorders have myriad of central and peripheral manifestations.
	• Some important disorders are discussed here and in other sections.
Disorders	**Features**
NEUROLOGIC DISORDERS	
Myasthenia	• Weakness affecting ocular muscles or ocular, bulbar, and limb muscles due to antibodies to the acetylcholine receptor
	• Diagnosed by antibody testing
	• Treated by corticosteroids and pyridostigmine. Additional immune-modulating therapy with intravenous immunoglobulin (IVIG), plasma exchange, or certain chemotherapies sometimes are needed.
Acute inflammatory demyelinating polyneuropathy (AIDP)	• An acute-onset immune-mediated neuropathy
	• Treated with IVIG or plasma exchange
Chronic inflammatory demyelinating polyneuropathy (CIDP)	• A chronic immune-mediated neuropathy
	• Treated with IVIG or corticosteroids
Multiple sclerosis	• A multifocal demyelinating disease affecting the brain and spine
	• Treated with corticosteroids for acute attacks, and a variety of immune modulators for reduction in attacks
Optic neuritis	• Acute demyelination of one or both optic nerves
	• May be a component of MS or occur independently
	• Treated with corticosteroids, usually intravenously to start then orally with a taper
Acute disseminated encephalomyelitis (ADEM)	• A postinfectious condition, which is felt to have an immune basis
	• Multifocal demyelinating changes develop over hours to days.
	• Treatment with corticosteroids is commonly used, but is of uncertain benefit.
Transverse myelitis	• Demyelinating changes to the spinal cord, which can occur in association with MS or neuromyelitis optica or can be a single event
	• Treated with corticosteroids or plasma exchange, although the data supporting this is not as solid as with treatment of MS.

SYSTEMIC DISORDERS	
Systemic lupus erythematosus	• Multisystem immune disease, with involvement especially of the skin, blood vessels, kidneys, brain, and heart • Treated with corticosteroids and other immune suppressants
Sarcoidosis	• Immune condition, which may be precipitated by an infectious disease • Treated with corticosteroids and other immune suppressants
Polyarteritis nodosa (PAN)	• A vasculitis affecting the entire body. Patients can present with signs of transient and persistent cerebral ischemia, i.e., TIA and cerebrovascular accident (CVA). • Treated with immune suppressants, especially corticosteroids

SYSTEMIC LUPUS ERYTHEMATOSUS (SLE)	
Description	• A multisystem disease characterized by multiorgan damage • An immune attack results in systemic and neurologic symptoms.
Pathophysiology	• Affects the nervous system in a number of ways • Vasculitis is a common cause of encephalopathy. • Antiphospholipid antibodies predispose to cerebral thrombosis. • Peripheral neuropathy can be demyelinating, suggesting a direct immune attack or vasculitis. • Myopathy has the inflammatory appearance of polymyositis or dermatomyositis.
Clinical findings	The clinical presentation depends on the type of deficit. Specific presentations are as follows: • *Encephalopathy.* The most common manifestation of SLE, and can be acute or chronic. Acute encephalopathy can be associated with confusion and lethargy. Chronic changes can present as dementia. Lupus cerebritis presents with subacute mental status changes, and seizures can occur. • *Optic neuritis.* Can be a sign of SLE, although this is uncommon. Other cranial nerve disorders can occur as well. Optic neuropathy presents with visual loss. Other cranial nerve involvement may present with diplopia and ocular motor weakness. • *Stroke.* Can develop without encephalopathy, and may be associated with vasculitis, antiphospholipid antibody syndrome, or cardiac disease. • *Peripheral neuropathy.* Common, usually in association with other neurologic and systemic involvement. Patients present with sensory and motor symptoms that are mainly distal. Neuropathic pain, decreased sensation, and distal weakness are seen. • *Myopathy.* Can present with progressive proximal weakness without sensory findings. The myopathy can be painful, although arthralgias and myalgias may cause muscle-area pain even in the absence of myopathy.
Laboratory studies	• Routine labs usually are normal. • Antinuclear antibodies (ANA) are usually positive. Extractable nuclear antibody (ENA) and anti-DNA studies usually are performed to follow up on the positive ANA. • Antiphospholipid antibodies are found in some patients, and correlate with thrombotic events. Lupus anticoagulant often is positive. • MRI may show cerebritis or multiple infarctions.
Diagnosis	• SLE is suspected when a patients presents with neurologic and systemic symptoms. • Labs are supportive, including positive ANA. Follow-up lab testing with anti-DNA, ENA, complement studies, and antibody studies typically is tested. • Defined criteria for diagnosis of SLE exist.

SYSTEMIC LUPUS ERYTHEMATOSUS (SLE)—cont'd	
Differential diagnosis	• *Polyarteritis nodosa.* Produces multifocal neurologic deficits and can affect the central (CNS) and peripheral nervous systems (PNS). Criteria for SLE are not met. • *Multiple sclerosis.* Can produce multifocal CNS lesions, which may resemble SLE; however, none of the peripheral signs of immune disease are seen.
Management	• Treatment is with immune suppression. Corticosteroids often are used as first line, but there are multiple options for treatment, including plaquenil, cyclophosphamide, and methotrexate.
Clinical course	• Most patients improve with immune-modulating treatment; however, patients need long-term treatment and relapses are common.

Major Diagnostic Criteria of Systemic Lupus Erythematosus (SLE)*
(At least 4 should be present for diagnosis)

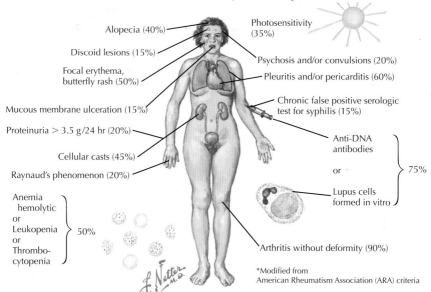

Alopecia (40%)

Discoid lesions (15%)

Focal erythema, butterfly rash (50%)

Mucous membrane ulceration (15%)

Proteinuria > 3.5 g/24 hr (20%)

Cellular casts (45%)

Raynaud's phenomenon (20%)

Anemia hemolytic or Leukopenia or Thrombo-cytopenia } 50%

Photosensitivity (35%)

Psychosis and/or convulsions (20%)

Pleuritis and/or pericarditis (60%)

Chronic false positive serologic test for syphilis (15%)

Anti-DNA antibodies

or } 75%

Lupus cells formed in vitro

Arthritis without deformity (90%)

*Modified from American Rheumatism Association (ARA) criteria

MULTIPLE SCLEROSIS (MS)	
Description	An immune disease characterized by multifocal regions of demyelination, with lesions of varying ages
Pathophysiology	Demyelination is seen in the CNS, with optic nerve involvement common. White matter changes can have a characteristic appearance with the orientation of the demyelination, producing the "Dawson's fingers" seen radiographically and pathologically.
Clinical findings	MS is considered when a young to middle-aged patient develops focal or multifocal neurologic deficits. In these patients, there are few risk factors for stroke, and vasculitis is uncommon, but still considered. Common findings are visual loss, hemiparesis, paraparesis, and ataxia.
Laboratory studies	• Routine labs are normal. • Magnetic resonance imaging (MRI) shows multiple regions of increased signal intensity on T_2 and FLAIR imaging. Although these findings are not definitive for MS, radiographic appearance can suggest MS over vascular changes. • CT is much less sensitive for the demyelinating changes than MRI. • Lumbar puncture (LP) shows normal CSF pressure and profile. However, immune studies often show elevated immunoglobulin (Ig)G index, especially at the time of an attack. Oligoclonal IgG banding is seen in many patients, with isolation from the cerebrospinal fluid (CSF) but not from the blood.
Diagnosis	• Diagnosis of MS is suspected when a patient presents with focal neurologic deficit, and they have low risk for vascular disease. Onset of the symptoms over hours to days also suggests demyelinating disease. A history of previous neurologic deficits supports the diagnosis of MS. • MRI shows multiple areas of increased signal intensity on T_2-weighted and FLAIR imaging. Although MRI is not definitive, there are differences that can favor MS versus infarctions. • EPs can support the diagnosis if they identify other lesions in the spine, brain, or optic nerves. • CSF can be supportive of the diagnosis with increased IgG-index in patients with an acute attack and oligoclonal IgG in many patients with MS. • There are defined criteria for MS, but these mainly have been used for research studies, where the diagnosis must be absolutely certain. In practice, the combination of history, examination, MRI, and CSF abnormalities differentiates between possible, probable, and definite MS.
Differential diagnosis	• *Vasculitis.* From any cause, can produce multiple CNS lesions. This can include SLE and PAN. • *ADEM.* A monophasic demyelinating disorder that is a post-infectious condition. MRI may look identical to MS. • *Small-vessel cerebrovascular disease.* Can cause multifocal neurologic deficits over time. MRI usually can differentiate between vascular and demyelinating changes.

MULTIPLE SCLEROSIS (MS)—cont'd	
Management	• Acute attacks are treated with corticosteroids. Classic treatment has been with intravenously administered methylprednisolone. Recently, oral methylprednisolone or dexamethasone have been used and may be as effective.
	• Relapses can be reduced by administration of interferons or glatiramer. If these agents are ineffective, chemotherapy and other immune modulators are sometimes used.
	• Spasticity and muscle spasms are treated with the usual agents, including baclofen, tizanidine, diazepam and other benzodiazepines, and gabapentin.
Clinical course	• Most patients improve with intermittent relapses. Remissions may result in improvement to baseline, but accumulation of fixed neurologic deficit is common.
	• Patients can transition from relapsing-remitting to secondary-progressive MS. This is characterized by progressive deficit, and is not thought to respond as well to immune-modulating therapy.

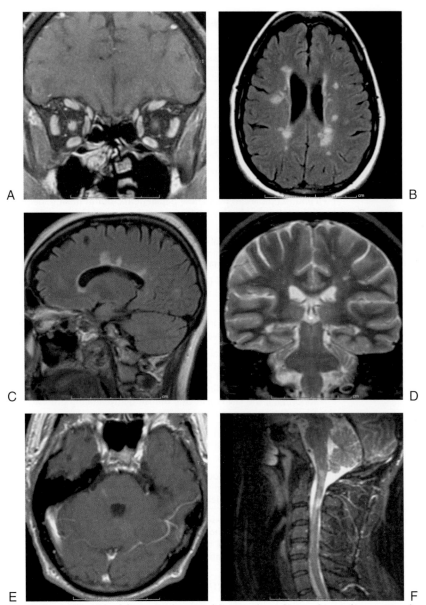

(**A**) Coronal T1-weighted, fat-saturated, post–gadolinium-enhanced image shows enhancement and enlargement of the right optic nerve (*arrow*). (**B** and **C**) Axial and sagittal FLAIR images with increased T2 signal within the corpus callosum and paraventricular white matter with extension into central white matter along vascular pathways, also illustrated in **D**, coronal T2, where the typical oval lesions are oriented along vascular pathways, typical of "Dawson fingers" (*arrowheads*). (**E**) Axial T1-weighted post–gadolinium-enhanced image shows enhancement of T2 bright lesion shown in other sequences in the right cerebellar peduncle. The enhancement suggests disease activity. (**F**) Sagittal T2-weighted image shows T2 bright lesion in posterior cord at C2-3.

OPTIC NEURITIS (ON)	
Description	Inflammatory demyelination of the optic nerve. May occur independently or as a component of another demyelinating disease.
Pathophysiology	• Demyelination can occur as an isolated entity or as a component of MS or neuromyelitis optica. • Inflammatory demyelination produces a disruption in vision.
Clinical findings	• Visual disturbance is the most common symptom. Loss of visual acuity, occasionally with loss of vision, and difficulty with differentiation of colors is prominent. • Pain with movement of the eye may develop with a retrobulbar location. • Funduscopic exam may show papilledema, but in most patients there is no visible abnormality, since the area of the involvement is behind the eye. • Can be bilateral or unilateral
Laboratory studies	• Routine labs are normal. • MRI often is normal if ON is an isolated entity. ON associated with MS shows regions of increased T2-intensity, suggestive of multifocal demyelination. • CSF shows a normal profile. Findings that would suggest MS are oligoclonal bands, elevated IgG index, and myelin basic protein. • Visual evoked potential (VEP) usually is abnormal, showing delay or loss of the normal response, consistent with unilateral or bilateral ON. Nonvisual evoked potentials (Somatosensory evoked potential [SSEP], Brainstem auditory evoked potential [BAEP]) may be abnormal if the ON is part of a diffuse demyelinating disease, but otherwise are normal.
Diagnosis	• ON is suspected when a patient presents with visual loss in one or both eyes. Pain with movement of the eye supports the diagnosis. Papilledema is seen in a minority of patients. • MRI is performed to look for structural and demyelinating lesions. Normal study favors idiopathic ON. MRI lesions suggest an increased change for later development of MS.
Differential diagnosis	• *Multiple sclerosis.* Considered in patients with ON, although most patients with ON do not go on to present with MS. Patients with ON who have the CSF markers mentioned above or white matter lesions on MRI have an increased risk for subsequent development of MS. • *Neuromyelitis optica (Devic's disease).* Presents with optic neuritis, plus transverse myelitis. • *Acute glaucoma.* Can present with visual changes and pain in the globe. The pain is in the eye itself rather than behind the eye. Differentiation is by eye exam.

OPTIC NEURITIS (ON)—cont'd	
Management	• Intravenous corticosteroid regimens, followed by a tapering dose of prednisone, are the most commonly used for treatment. Use of purely oral steroids is not favored on the basis of current information. • Long-term immunosuppressant treatment is not needed for ON, except if ON develops as a component of MS.
Clinical course	• Most patients show improvement in vision, although residual visual loss is common. • There is a risk for recurrent optic neuritis or development of other demyelinating lesions.

Multiple Sclerosis: Clinical Manifestations

Visual manifestations — Optic Neuritis

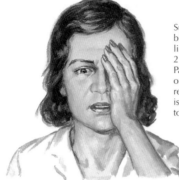

Subacute onset of unilateral or bilateral blindness, self-limited (usually 2 to 3 weeks). Patient covering one eye, suddenly realizes other eye is partially or totally blind

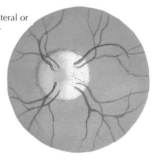

Temporal pallor in optic disc, caused by delayed recovery of temporal side of optic (II) nerve

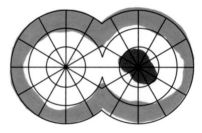

Visual fields reveal central scotoma due to acute retrobulbar neuritis.

Oculomotor defects — Internuclear Opthalmoplegia

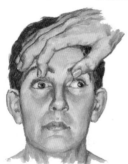

Eyes turned to left, right eye lags

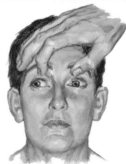

Eyes turned to right, left eye lags (to lesser degree)

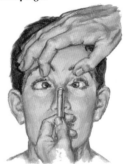

Convergence unimpaired

SARCOIDOSIS	
Description	Granulomatosis disease with systemic and neurologic involvement
Pathophysiology	Sarcoidosis is an immune disease of unknown cause, but may be related to infection.

Clinical findings	• Patients commonly present with multiple neurologic abnormalities. Among the common neurologic manifestations are:
	
	  • Peripheral polyneuropathy
	
	  • Facial palsy or other cranial neuropathy
	
	  • Visual loss and/or diplopia
	
	  • Vertigo and/or hearing loss
	
	  • Diabetes insipidus
	
	  • Cognitive deficits
	
	  • Ataxia—gait and/or appendicular
	
	  • Seizures
	
	• Patients commonly present with one or more deficits, but not all are present.

Laboratory studies	• Routine labs are normal. • Angiotensin-converting enzyme (ACE) levels are increased in most patients. • Imaging with MRI may show enhancing lesions in the subarachnoid space. Mass lesions also can be seen. • CSF usually shows mild lymphocytic pleocytosis, if there has been neurologic involvement with root or cranial nerve deficit. Oligoclonal bands may be present, and IgG index may be elevated.
Diagnosis	• Sarcoidosis is suspected when a patient presents with cranial neuropathy or other neurologic deficit and is found to have pulmonary granulomas. • MRI is performed for identification of focal structural lesions and to look for demyelinating disease. • Biopsy of nerve or muscle can confirm the diagnosis.
Differential diagnosis	• *Neoplastic meningitis.* Can produce multiple nerve root lesions and cranial neuropathies. MRI can show enhancement of the meningeal lesions. CSF cytology is confirmatory. • *Multiple sclerosis.* Can produce multiple neurologic lesions; however, meningeal abnormalities are not expected, and cranial neuropathies are uncommon.
Management	• Corticosteroids are the most commonly used agents. Cyclophosphamide and methotrexate occasionally are also used. • Long-term immune suppression often is needed.
Clinical course	Patients usually improve with treatment, although recurrent symptoms are common.

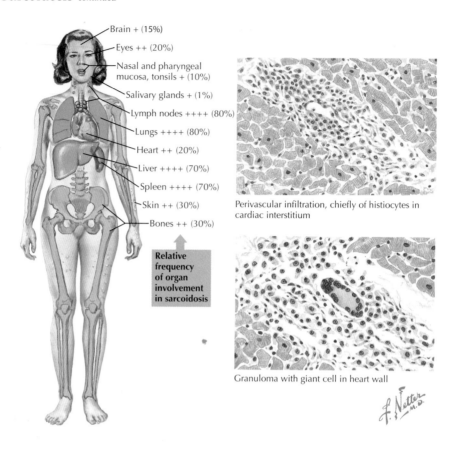

Brain + (15%)

Eyes ++ (20%)

Nasal and pharyngeal
mucosa, tonsils + (10%)

Salivary glands + (1%)

Lymph nodes ++++ (80%)

Lungs ++++ (80%)

Heart ++ (20%)

Liver ++++ (70%)

Spleen ++++ (70%)

Skin ++ (30%)

Bones ++ (30%)

Relative
frequency
of organ
involvement
in sarcoidosis

Perivascular infiltration, chiefly of histiocytes in
cardiac interstitium

Granuloma with giant cell in heart wall

OTHER IMMUNE DISORDERS	
Disorder	**Features**
Neuromyelitis optica	• An immune disease related to multiple sclerosis. There is demyelination in the optic nerves and spinal cord.
	• Apparent neuromyelitis optica that develops eventual demyelination elsewhere in the nervous system is really MS. Neuromyelitis optica that develops after a cold or other infection and does not progress to other neurologic involvement is considered a form of acute disseminated encephalomyelitis (ADEM).
	• Clinical features include visual loss from the optic neuritis, and spasticity, bladder control difficulty, and loss of sensation develops from the spinal cord involvement.
	• Treatment is supportive. Corticosteroids are often used, although their benefit is unproven.
Acute disseminated encephalomyelitis (ADEM)	• A postinfection acute demyelinating disorder of the CNS. It develops after cold or other illness. Can also develop after vaccination.
	• Clinical features can include headache, encephalopathy, seizures, and findings of optic neuritis and/or transvers myelitis.
	• Treated with corticosteroids
	• Some patients appear to totally recover, but many are left with residual neurologic deficit.
Transverse myelitis (TM)	• An inflammatory demyelinating lesion of the spinal cord, usually in the thoracic region
	• Patients develop paraparesis and sphincter control deficits. Spasticity develops after the onset of the paraparesis. Neurologic deficits related to the brain are not present. Back pain is common at onset.
	• Treated with corticosteroids initially, and further immune treatment may be needed.
	• Patients often are left with residual deficit.
Polyarteritis nodosa (PAN)	• An immune disease that can affect the CNS or PNS
	• Stroke and seizures can develop from brain involvement. PNS involvement can produce sensory deficit and/or neuropathic pain, or motor deficit with weakness.
	• Treated with immunosuppressants. Corticosteroids often are used as first-line therapy.
Wegener's granulomatosis	• A vasculitis with multiorgan involvement
	• Non-neurologic involvement includes findings of sinus inflammation, often with bacterial superinfection. Cough and other signs of pulmonary involvement also are common. Joint swelling and pain is common and present in the majority of patients.
	• Neurologic involvement includes polyneuropathy or mononeuropathy multiplex. Cranial neuropathies are much less frequent. The occasional patient may develop stroke or cerebritis, resulting in mental status changes, focal neurologic signs, or seizures.
	• Immunosuppression with cyclophosphamide is the most common initial treatment.

Acute Disseminated Encephalomyelitis (ADEM)

CT scan without contrast medium (left) shows several areas of low density in frontal and parietal lobes, primarily involving periventricular white matter. CT scan with contrast medium (right) shows gyral enhancement.

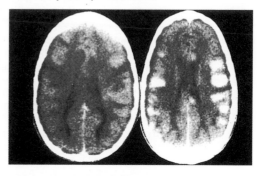

Multiple Sclerosis: Central Nervous System Pathology

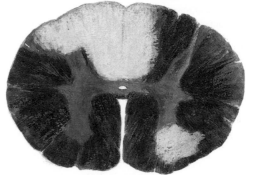

In thoracic spinal cord

OVERVIEW OF NEUROMUSCULAR DISEASES	

Introduction	• Neuromuscular disorders comprise a huge variety of disease states and conditions, producing an often confusing plethora of signs and symptoms.
	• A thorough history and neurologic examination is the best approach to initial diagnosis, which then can be supplemented by appropriate neurophysiologic testing.
	• Specific laboratory investigations are available for confirmatory diagnosis of some disorders in this group. Neuroimaging and muscle/nerve biopsy also can be useful in certain settings.
	• Disorders are categorized into four groups:
	  • Motor neuron diseases
	  • Peripheral neuropathies
	  • Neuromuscular transmission abnormalities
	  • Myopathies

Category	**Representative Disorders**
Motor neuron diseases	• Amyotrophic lateral sclerosis • Primary lateral sclerosis • Spinal muscular atrophy
Peripheral neuropathies	• AIDP (Guillain-Barre syndrome) • CIDP • Sensorimotor neuropathy (e.g., diabetic neuropathy) • Mononeuropathies (e.g., carpal tunnel syndrome) • Multifocal motor neuropathy
Neuromuscular transmission disorders	• Myasthenia gravis and ocular myasthenia • Myasthenic syndrome (Eaton-Lambert syndrome) • Botulism
Myopathies	• Muscular dystrophies • Inflammatory myopathies • Metabolic myopathies • Toxic myopathies

Peripheral Nervous System

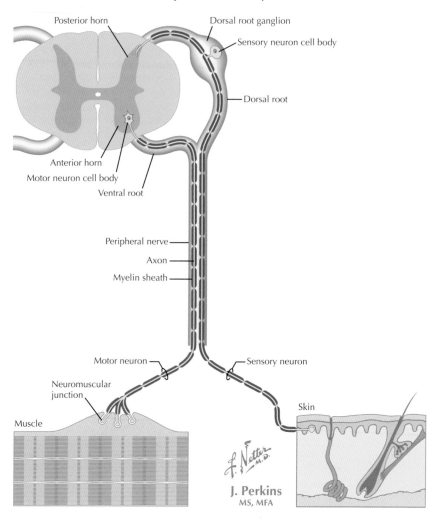

Posterior horn

Dorsal root ganglion

Sensory neuron cell body

Dorsal root

Anterior horn

Motor neuron cell body

Ventral root

Peripheral nerve

Axon

Myelin sheath

Motor neuron

Sensory neuron

Neuromuscular junction

Skin

Muscle

J. Perkins
MS, MFA

OVERVIEW OF NEUROPATHY	
Description	• Neuropathy is extremely common in clinical practice, and presents with varying degrees of sensory and/or motor loss. The distribution and character of the symptoms depends on the type of neuropathy. • The clinical presentation often provides the most valuable information regarding diagnosis. When history and clinical examination are indicative of peripheral neuropathy, a standard diagnostic approach will include neurophysiologic studies, laboratory investigations, and rarely—cerebrospinal fluid (CSF) analysis.
Pathophysiology	The causes of neuropathy are multiple, including metabolic, traumatic, genetic, toxic, paraneoplastic, immune-mediated, and idiopathic.
Clinical findings	Neuropathy is usually worse distally than proximally and typically presents with some combination of sensory loss, paresthesias, weakness, and/or pain of varying intensity and quality.
Laboratory studies	Common laboratory tests for neuropathy include: • ANA, ENA, pANCA, cANCA, ESR, CRP • Serum immunoelectrophoresis (SIEP) • Hemoglobin A1C • B_{12}, folate • Heavy-metal screen • Hepatitis or HIV Screening when indicated *EMG* (electromyogram) is performed to determine the location and character of the neuropathy. *Nerve biopsy* can be performed to look for specific disorders such as inflammatory neuropathies. *Imaging* is of limited value for neuropathy, unless a mononeuropathy is thought to be due to a mass lesion, such as neuroma.
Diagnosis	Neuropathy is considered when a patient presents with sensory and/or motor complaints that suggest a peripheral nerve distribution rather than a central origin. Some of the suggestive presentations include: • Distal bilateral numbness and/or pain of the legs with or without involvement of the arms • Numbness and/or weakness in the distribution of a single nerve or nerve root distribution • Diagnosis confirmed by EMG • Imaging usually is not needed, except to rule out other causes of the symptoms.
Differential diagnosis	• *Spinal lesions.* Can produce peripheral symptoms, although back pain is common. Compression of the distal spinal cord and nerve roots can reproduce some of the symptoms of distal neuropathy. • *Neoplastic meningitis.* Can present with symptoms and signs of single or multiple radiculopathies.

OVERVIEW OF NEUROPATHY—cont'd	
Subsets of neuropathy	• Polyneuropathy • Mononeuropathy • Mononeuropathy multiplex
Subset	**Basic Features**
Polyneuropathy	• A variety of conditions can produce axonal or demyelinating changes in the peripheral nerves. • These conditions present with any combination of sensory loss, pain, and motor loss most prominent distally.
Mononeuropathy	• Single nerve lesions can be due to trauma, focal entrapment, ischemia, tumors, infections, or other focal structural lesions. • Symptoms are confined to the distribution of a single nerve or nerve root distribution. • Mononeuropathy can be superimposed on a polyneuropathy.
Mononeuropathy multiplex	• The most common cause of multiple mononeuropathies is diabetes, with other causes including polyarteritis nodosa and leprosy. • Multiple mononeuropathies can appear to be superimposed on polyneuropathy.

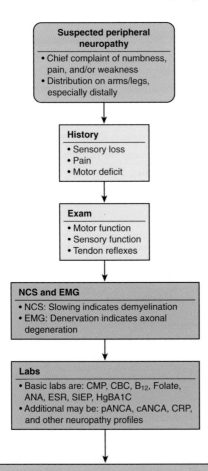

Suspected peripheral neuropathy
- Chief complaint of numbness, pain, and/or weakness
- Distribution on arms/legs, especially distally

History
- Sensory loss
- Pain
- Motor deficit

Exam
- Motor function
- Sensory function
- Tendon reflexes

NCS and EMG
- NCS: Slowing indicates demyelination
- EMG: Denervation indicates axonal degeneration

Labs
- Basic labs are: CMP, CBC, B_{12}, Folate, ANA, ESR, SIEP, HgBA1C
- Additional may be: pANCA, cANCA, CRP, and other neuropathy profiles

Classification of neuropathy

Demyelinating neuropathy	Mixed neuropathy	Axonal neuropathy
• Motor and/or sensory deficit • Decreased or absent reflexes • NCS shows slowed conduction with block • Types include AIDP, CIDP, and MMN	• Sensory ± motor deficit • Reflexes usually decreased but not absent • NCS shows slowed conduction • EMG shows chronic denervation, occasionally some active denervation, also	• Motor and/or sensory deficit • Reflexes are usually normal or only reduced distally • NCS normal except for low amplitude • EMG shows chronic denervation, occasionally some active, also

NEUROPATHY EVALUATION	
Classification of neuropathy	Classification of the neuropathy into the following categories can be of tremendous help in diagnosing a neuropathy: • Polyneuropathy vs. mononeuropathy vs. mononeuropathy multiplex • Axonal vs. demyelinating • Motor vs. sensory vs. sensory-motor • Acute vs. subacute vs. chronic These differentiations are made on the basis of history, exam, and EMG. Additional information from labs and biopsy can help to nail down the diagnosis.
Classification	**Features**
Polyneuropathy vs. mononeuropathy vs. Mononeuropathy multiplex	• *Polyneuropathy* is suggested by symmetric symptoms and signs. Decreased distal reflexes are common, and sensory and motor loss is distal. Legs are affected earlier than the arms. These usually are metabolic, toxic, genetic, and idiopathic in origin. • *Mononeuropathy* is suggested by symptoms and signs in the distribution of one nerve, such as median or peroneal. The location along the nerve can be suggested by which muscles and skin areas are affected, e.g., proximal vs. distal median neuropathy. These usually are compressive or ischemic in origin. • *Mononeuropathy multiplex* is the presentation of symptoms and signs of multiple mononeuropathies. These usually are metabolic, immune-mediated, or infectious in origin.
Axonal vs. demyelinating	• This differentiation applies mainly to polyneuropathy. • *Axonal neuropathy* is suggested by relative preservation of reflexes. EMG is confirmatory. This is the most common type, and includes most metabolic, toxic, genetic, and nutritional neuropathies. • *Demyelinating neuropathy* is suggested by marked suppression or absence of reflexes. Nerve conduction study (NCS) and EMG are confirmatory. These neuropathies are more likely to be immune-mediated but can be genetic.
Motor vs. sensory vs. sensory-motor	• *Motor neuropathies* are uncommon, and present with weakness in the absence of pain and sensory loss. The most important motor neuropathies in adults are ALS and multifocal motor neuropathy. In children, the most important are the spinal muscular atrophies (SMA). • *Sensory neuropathies* present with sensory symptoms without motor deficit. Important causes are diabetes and AIDS. • *Sensory-motor neuropathies* are the most common and represent most genetic and acquired neuropathies.
Acute vs. subacute vs. chronic	• *AIDP (Guillain-Barre syndrome)* is the prototypic acute to subacute neuropathy. Most other neuropathies are chronic. • *Acute to subacute neuropathies* are more likely to be immmune-mediated and toxic, whereas *chronic neuropathies* are more likely to be metabolic, genetic, and idiopathic. • History and EMG help to make the differentiation within this scheme.

Individual Tests	
Nerve conduction study (NCS) and electromyogram (EMG)	• NCS is a nerve conduction study, which is performed by stimulating peripheral nerves and recording from other nerves or muscles. Motor nerve conduction is assessed by recording from muscles. Sensory nerve conduction is performed by recording from parts of the nerve that do not contain motor fibers, e.g., fingers. • NCS and EMG can differentiate axonal from demyelinating changes. Also, the chronicity of changes can be determined from the EMG component.
Blood and urine	• Multiple lab tests can be performed, as listed above. These are done predominantly to look for acquired disorders of the peripheral nerves. • Genetic tests can be performed to look for inherited disorders. • Urine can be analyzed for heavy metals, an uncommon but important cause of neuropathy.
Nerve biopsy	• Nerve biopsy is performed on a small proportion of patients with neuropathy, and mainly is done when there is concern over immune-mediated neuropathy or metabolic disorder, e.g., amyloidosis. • A portion of nerve is biopsied that is pure sensory, so that there is no motor loss.

Electrodiagnostic Studies in Compression Neuropathy

Electromyography (EMG)

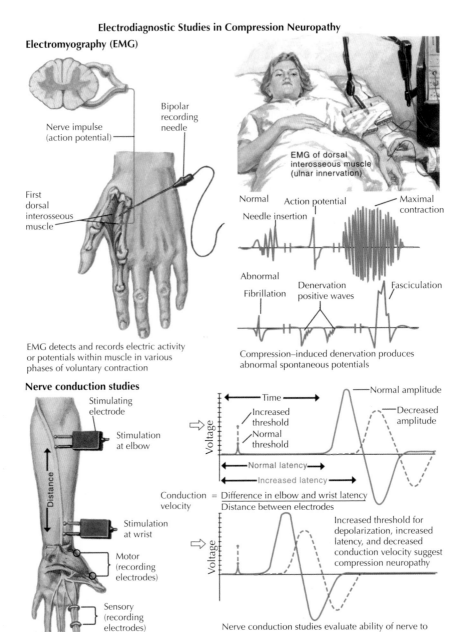

Nerve impulse
(action potential)

Bipolar
recording
needle

First
dorsal
interosseous
muscle

EMG of dorsal
interosseous muscle
(ulnar innervation)

Normal   Action potential   Maximal
contraction

Needle insertion

Abnormal

Fibrillation   Denervation   Fasciculation
positive waves

EMG detects and records electric activity
or potentials within muscle in various
phases of voluntary contraction

Compression–induced denervation produces
abnormal spontaneous potentials

Nerve conduction studies

Stimulating
electrode

Stimulation
at elbow

Distance

Stimulation
at wrist

Motor
(recording
electrodes)

Sensory
(recording
electrodes)

Time

Increased
threshold

Normal
threshold

Voltage

Normal amplitude

Decreased
amplitude

Normal latency

Increased latency

$$\text{Conduction velocity} = \frac{\text{Difference in elbow and wrist latency}}{\text{Distance between electrodes}}$$

Voltage

Increased threshold for
depolarization, increased
latency, and decreased
conduction velocity suggest
compression neuropathy

Nerve conduction studies evaluate ability of nerve to
conduct electrically evoked action potentials. Sensory
and motor conduction stimulated and recorded

F. Netter M.D.
JOHN A. CRAIG—MD

MEDIAN NEUROPATHY CARPAL TUNNEL SYNDROME (CTS)	
Description	• CTS is the most common mononeuropathy.
	• Patients have numbness and commonly pain on the palms.
Pathophysiology	• CTS is caused by entrapment of the median nerve at the wrist. This causes damage to the motor nerves supplying some of the intrinsic muscles of the hand and sensory loss over the palm from near the thumb to the border of digit 4.
	• Several medical conditions predispose to CTS, including diabetes, rheumatoid arthritis, and obesity.
	• The role of occupational exposure is debatable. Strenuous activity involving palm and wrist pressure and twisting likely plays a role, whereas routine computer and mouse use may not.
Clinical findings	*Symptoms:*
	• Sensory loss, usually with pain on the palm. The distribution is on the radial side of the palm, extending from the thumb to the margin of digit 4.
	• Pain can be aching or shooting, with exacerbation by movement, pressure, or other activity. Patients often awaken with pain at night and have to move the hand.
	• Weakness is usually a late symptom but when present causes difficulty with jar opening and other hand tasks.
	Signs:
	• Sensory loss in the distal median nerve distribution is typical.
	• Weakness may be present, and the abductor pollicis brevis is easy to test. The palm is held upright and the thumb forcibly lifted off of the table. Weakness indicates median nerve motor deficit. This should be paired with normal function of more proximal median-innervated muscles, including the flexor digitorum profundus, which allows for contraction of the deep flexors of digits 2 and 3 (index and middle).
	• Signs of peripheral neuropathy may be seen. Peripheral neuropathy predisposes to CTS—distal sensory loss and decreased ankle reflexes, perhaps with distal weakness.
Laboratory studies	• Routine labs may be normal, but the following studies should be considered: B_{12} level, RA latex, TSH, T4, and glycosylated hemoglobin.
	• Imaging is normal, and usually is not needed. The occasional patient with hand pain may be considered for cervical radiculopathy, and have MRI done. MRI of the wrist can show the region of nerve compression, but usually is not needed.
	• EMG shows slowing of conduction of the sensory and/or motor nerves through the wrist. This may be superimposed on generalized abnormalities if the CTS is in the setting of polyneuropathy. Denervation is usually not seen except in severe CTS or with polyneuropathy.

MEDIAN NEUROPATHY CARPAL TUNNEL SYNDROME (CTS)—cont'd	
Diagnosis	• CTS is suspected when a patient presents with pain and numbness of the palm. Careful examination reveals the anatomic distribution of the median neuropathy. • EMG confirms the median neuropathy. • Labs are performed to look for treatable causes.
Differential diagnosis	• Cervical radiculopathy can present with pain and numbness of the hand, but symptoms in the arms are expected; both the palmar and dorsal surfaces would be affected; and EMG would differentiate the two. • Ulnar neuropathy produces sensory symptoms similar to CTS, but overlying digits 4 and 5.
Management	• Splints often are helpful in stabilizing the carpal tunnel. • Nonsteroidal anti-inflammatory drugs (NSAIDs) commonly are used for pain control. • Injection of steroids into the carpal tunnel can be helpful. • Surgical decompression of the carpal tunnel often is helpful, and is considered especially when patients are refractory to conservative care or when there is weakness.
Clinical course	Most patients improve, although even surgery does not guarantee a good clinical response.

Median Nerve

Anterior view

Note: Only muscles innervated by median nerve shown

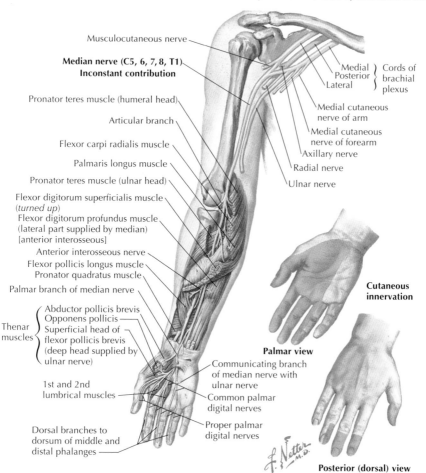

Musculocutaneous nerve

Median nerve (C5, 6, 7, 8, T1)
Inconstant contribution

Pronator teres muscle (humeral head)

Articular branch

Flexor carpi radialis muscle

Palmaris longus muscle

Pronator teres muscle (ulnar head)

Flexor digitorum superficialis muscle
(*turned up*)
Flexor digitorum profundus muscle
(lateral part supplied by median)
[anterior interosseous]

Anterior interosseous nerve
Flexor pollicis longus muscle
Pronator quadratus muscle

Palmar branch of median nerve

Thenar
muscles
{
Abductor pollicis brevis
Opponens pollicis
Superficial head of
flexor pollicis brevis
(deep head supplied by
ulnar nerve)
}

1st and 2nd
lumbrical muscles

Dorsal branches to
dorsum of middle and
distal phalanges

Medial) Cords of
Posterior } brachial
Lateral) plexus

Medial cutaneous
nerve of arm
Medial cutaneous
nerve of forearm
Axillary nerve
Radial nerve

Ulnar nerve

Cutaneous
innervation

Palmar view

Communicating branch
of median nerve with
ulnar nerve
Common palmar
digital nerves
Proper palmar
digital nerves

Posterior (dorsal) view

ULNAR NEUROPATHY	
Description	Dysfunction of the ulnar nerve, supplying sensation to the ulnar aspect of the hand and motor to many of the intrinsic muscles of the hand
Pathophysiology	• The ulnar nerve is susceptible to compression in the ulnar grove at the elbow, distal to the elbow and at the wrist as it enters the hand. • Any cause of polyneuropathy predisposes to ulnar nerve compression. This includes diabetes, which is the most common predisposing disorder.
Clinical findings	*Symptoms:* • Numbness and/or pain in the distal ulnar nerve distribution, affecting both the palmar and dorsal sides of the hand's ulnar aspect. Digit 5 and the ulnar half of digit 4 are affected. • Patients may complain of weakness of hand motion with severe ulnar neuropathy. *Signs:* • Sensory loss in an ulnar nerve distribution is common. • Weakness of ulnar-innervated muscles is sometimes seen. This is easiest to determine in the interossei—weakness of the spreading of fingers. Long finger flexors weakness affecting digits 4 and 5 also can be demonstrated.
Laboratory studies	• Routine labs are normal. • Imaging is normal; magnetic resonance imaging (MRI) and computed tomography (CT) show no consistent abnormalities. • EMG shows slowed conduction of the sensory and/or motor nerves through the affected region.
Diagnosis	• Ulnar neuropathy is suspected when a patient has sensory loss and pain, especially with weakness in a distal ulnar nerve distribution. • Confirmation is with EMG, showing the focal slowing and/or denervation isolated to ulnar-innervated muscles.
Differential diagnosis	• *Carpal tunnel syndrome.* Can be mistaken for ulnar neuropathy; however, the distribution of the deficit is very different, and the EMG would be definitive. • *C8 radiculopathy.* Can produce sensory disturbance and weakness that can resemble ulnar neuropathy. Usually, EMG is able to differentiate these. In C8 radiculopathy, the C8-innervated, median-innervated muscles are also affected, such as the abductor pollicis brevis. • *Brachial plexopathy.* Can produce a pattern of weakness similar to ulnar neuropathy, but median-innervated muscles also are affected.

ULNAR NEUROPATHY—cont'd	
Management	• Wrist splints are of little benefit for ulnar neuropathy. Padding the elbow and having the patient avoid trauma to the ulnar nerve near the elbow can also help.
	• Surgical transposition of the ulnar nerve at the elbow or decompression distally, depending on the site of the lesion, can be done but is usually reserved for patients with refractory symptoms or in whom weakness is prominent.
Clinical course	Improvement in the ulnar neuropathy is expected; however, it is not uncommon for there to be persistent numbness in an ulnar nerve distribution. Some persistent weakness is also not uncommon.

Ulnar Nerve

Anterior view

Note: Only muscles innervated by ulnar nerve shown

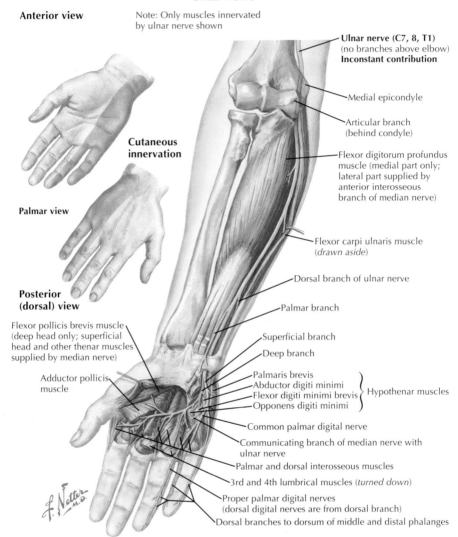

Ulnar nerve (C7, 8, T1)
(no branches above elbow)
Inconstant contribution

Medial epicondyle

Articular branch
(behind condyle)

Flexor digitorum profundus
muscle (medial part only;
lateral part supplied by
anterior interosseous
branch of median nerve)

Cutaneous innervation

Palmar view

Flexor carpi ulnaris muscle
(*drawn aside*)

Dorsal branch of ulnar nerve

Palmar branch

Posterior (dorsal) view

Superficial branch

Deep branch

Flexor pollicis brevis muscle
(deep head only; superficial
head and other thenar muscles
supplied by median nerve)

Palmaris brevis
Abductor digiti minimi
Flexor digiti minimi brevis
Opponens digiti minimi
} Hypothenar muscles

Adductor pollicis
muscle

Common palmar digital nerve

Communicating branch of median nerve with
ulnar nerve

Palmar and dorsal interosseous muscles

3rd and 4th lumbrical muscles (*turned down*)

Proper palmar digital nerves
(dorsal digital nerves are from dorsal branch)

Dorsal branches to dorsum of middle and distal phalanges

RADIAL NEUROPATHY	
Description	Dysfunction of the radial nerve, with the main finding being wrist drop
Pathophysiology	• Compression of the radial nerve in the spiral groove of the humerus is the most common cause. This is most common in alcoholics who fall asleep on the arm and do not shift position. Therefore, they have pressure on the nerve and resultant conduction block. • The nerve may function immediately upon relief of pressure, or it may have persistent axonal damage requiring months of recovery. Any cause of polyneuropathy can predispose to radial neuropathy.
Clinical findings	• Wrist drop is the most common symptom, especially on awakening. Pain and numbness in a radial nerve distribution can occur. • Weakness is in the wrist and finger extensors. The triceps may also be weak, depending on the level of the lesion. • Tendon reflexes are usually normal, but the triceps reflex may be reduced if that muscle is affected.
Laboratory studies	• Routine labs usually are normal. If the radial neuropathy is superimposed on a polyneuropathy, then there may be some abnormalities on testing such as diabetes, B_{12} deficiency, and hypothyroidism. If the patient is an alcoholic, then metabolic abnormalities associated with that may be seen, such as hyponatremia, hypomagnesemia, or abnormal liver function tests. • Imaging is normal and usually not needed. Occasionally, central lesions such as stroke can produce wrist drop, but other muscles are affected as well; if there is still doubt, cerebral and/or spine imaging with MRI can be performed. • EMG may show slowing of the conduction of the radial nerve if there has been continued impairment in radial nerve function. It is more difficult to see radial nerve dysfunction on nerve conductions than it is with other mononeuropathies. Denervation can be seen in radial innervated muscles, which include not only the wrist and finger extensors, but also the triceps, if this muscle is affected. Abnormalities of the radial-innervated muscles paired with normalcy of median and ulnar-innervated muscles are important for this diagnosis.
Diagnosis	• Radial neuropathy is suspected when a patient presents with weakness of wrist and finger extension, especially upon awakening. • EMG is helpful for confirmation of the diagnosis but is not positive in all patients, since it may be difficult to test conduction across the lesion. Also partial denervation may not be seen for weeks. • Imaging is usually not needed.
Differential diagnosis	• *Stroke.* Can cause weakness of wrist extension; however, other muscles also are affected. Tendon reflexes in the arm usually will be brisk with stroke and most other central causes. • *Brachial plexopathy.* Can cause weakness of radial-innervated muscles, but the deficit includes median and ulnar-innervated muscles.

RADIAL NEUROPATHY—cont'd	
Management	• Treatment includes avoidance of further injury and detection of predisposing factors, such as polyneuropathy and alcoholism. • Physical therapy and occupational therapy are helpful. As part of this, splinting of the wrist and fingers sometimes is needed with severe lesions. • Pain can be severe, but is uncommon. When present, can be treated by anticonvulsants and/or selected antidepressants, just as with other causes of neuropathic pain.
Clinical course	Weakness usually improves. The rate of improvement varies, from within weeks for some to many months for others with severe axonal lesions. Avoidance of further damage is the key to preventing second injuries.

Radial Nerve in Forearm

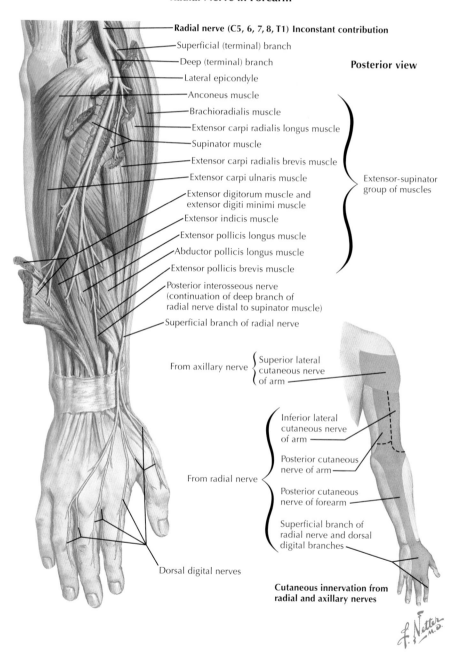

Radial nerve (C5, 6, 7, 8, T1) Inconstant contribution

Superficial (terminal) branch

Deep (terminal) branch

Lateral epicondyle

Posterior view

Anconeus muscle

Brachioradialis muscle

Extensor carpi radialis longus muscle

Supinator muscle

Extensor carpi radialis brevis muscle

Extensor carpi ulnaris muscle

Extensor digitorum muscle and extensor digiti minimi muscle

Extensor-supinator group of muscles

Extensor indicis muscle

Extensor pollicis longus muscle

Abductor pollicis longus muscle

Extensor pollicis brevis muscle

Posterior interosseous nerve (continuation of deep branch of radial nerve distal to supinator muscle)

Superficial branch of radial nerve

From axillary nerve

Superior lateral cutaneous nerve of arm

Inferior lateral cutaneous nerve of arm

Posterior cutaneous nerve of arm

From radial nerve

Posterior cutaneous nerve of forearm

Superficial branch of radial nerve and dorsal digital branches

Dorsal digital nerves

Cutaneous innervation from radial and axillary nerves

PERONEAL NEUROPATHY	
Description	Lesion of the peroneal nerve most commonly produces foot drop.
Pathophysiology	• Compression of the peroneal nerve is most common at the fibular neck, where the nerve is most exposed. Prolonged bedrest, especially in hospitalized patients, can result in peroneal compressive neuropathy. • Improper intramuscular injection can result in damage to the sciatic nerve in the buttocks. This usually results in dysfunction of both the peroneal and tibial divisions, but the peroneal can be affected predominantly. Also, compressive and traumatic lesions of the sciatic nerve can affect the peroneal division, predominantly.
Clinical findings	• Foot drop from weakness of foot extensors is the most common symptom. Specific examination of the tibialis anterior shows weakness. The peroneii muscles also may be affected, giving impaired lateral stabilization. • There are no reflex abnormalities. • Sensation may be altered or diminished on the dorsum of the foot. • Function of tibial-innervated muscles, especially the plantar flexors and inverters, are normal.
Laboratory studies	• Routine labs are normal, unless malnutrition, alcoholism, or another cause of polyneuropathy is identified. • Imaging of the back and leg usually are normal, and seldom is needed. • EMG may show slowing of conduction of the peroneal nerve across the fibular neck, but this is not invariable. EMG can show denervation in the peroneal-innervated muscles, but it may take 4 weeks for EMG abnormalities to develop.
Diagnosis	• Peroneal neuropathy is suspected when a patient presents with foot drop. The history of prolonged bed rest supports the diagnosis. • EMG can confirm the diagnosis, but careful clinical exam usually is able to make the diagnosis.
Differential diagnosis	• *Lumbar-5 (L5) radiculopathy.* Can present with foot drop and is the main item in the differential diagnosis. Back pain is common, and radicular pain radiating down the leg is expected. MRI of the spine supports this diagnosis. • *Sciatic neuropathy.* Sciatic neuropathy from any cause can give the presentation of peroneal neuropathy, because the peroneal division of the sciatic is more sensitive to injury than the tibial. The diagnosis can be confirmed by exam and EMG. • *Critical illness polyneuropathy (CIP).* Can present with leg weakness, a component of which is foot drop. However, weakness spans more than just the peroneal nerve distribution, and is usually bilateral. • *Critical illness myopathy.* Can produce foot drop, but diffuse weakness is expected. EMG and muscle biopsy help with the differentiation.

PERONEAL NEUROPATHY—cont'd	
Management	• Foot splint (ankle-foot orthosis [AFO]) is commonly used to aid walking, to help prevent the drop that impairs the swing-through of gait. • Physical therapy can help strength. • Surgical decompression of the peroneal nerve is seldom needed. • Avoidance of peroneal nerve compression, and movement of the limbs in bed-bound patients, can be a tremendous help.
Clinical course	Most patients improve, although some residual weakness is common, such that patients may drag a toe or occasionally stumble.

Common Peroneal (Fibular) Nerve

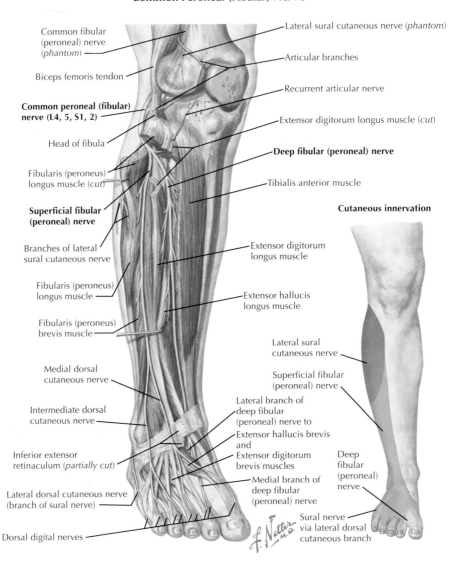

Common fibular (peroneal) nerve (*phantom*)

Biceps femoris tendon

Common peroneal (fibular) nerve (L4, 5, S1, 2)

Head of fibula

Fibularis (peroneus) longus muscle (*cut*)

Superficial fibular (peroneal) nerve

Branches of lateral sural cutaneous nerve

Fibularis (peroneus) longus muscle

Fibularis (peroneus) brevis muscle

Medial dorsal cutaneous nerve

Intermediate dorsal cutaneous nerve

Inferior extensor retinaculum (*partially cut*)

Lateral dorsal cutaneous nerve (branch of sural nerve)

Dorsal digital nerves

Lateral sural cutaneous nerve (*phantom*)

Articular branches

Recurrent articular nerve

Extensor digitorum longus muscle (*cut*)

Deep fibular (peroneal) nerve

Tibialis anterior muscle

Extensor digitorum longus muscle

Extensor hallucis longus muscle

Lateral branch of deep fibular (peroneal) nerve to Extensor hallucis brevis and Extensor digitorum brevis muscles

Medial branch of deep fibular (peroneal) nerve

Cutaneous innervation

Lateral sural cutaneous nerve

Superficial fibular (peroneal) nerve

Deep fibular (peroneal) nerve

Sural nerve via lateral dorsal cutaneous branch

SCIATIC NEUROPATHY	
Description	Damage to the sciatic nerve, usually due to injury in the buttocks
Pathophysiology	• Damage to the sciatic nerve usually is traumatic. Direct pelvic injury, positioning of the hip during a medical procedure, and needle stick intended for intramuscular injection are among the possible causes. • Tumor infiltration is an uncommon cause. • Piriformis syndrome can be sciatic compression at the piriformis muscle.
Clinical findings	• Pain in one leg is expected that is associated with sensory disturbance, with loss of sensation, and/or dysesthesias. • Weakness spans dermatomal distributions, with involvement of ankle flexors and extensors, inverters, and knee flexors. The quadriceps (femoral nerve) are normal, and, therefore, knee extension is preserved. • Ankle reflex typically is reduced, and knee reflex is normal.
Laboratory studies	• Routine labs are normal. • Imaging usually is normal, unless there is a tumor, fracture, or some other prominent structural lesion. • EMG shows denervation in sciatic nerve innervated muscles, although the denervation may not appear for 4 weeks.
Diagnosis	• Sciatic neuropathy is suspected when a patient presents with weakness and/or sensory change in one leg, especially if an injury to the pelvis or buttock has occurred. • Abnormal sciatic function on exam and EMG, combined with normal functioning of the knee extensors (femoral) and leg adductors (obturator), supports the diagnosis.
Differential diagnosis	• *Lumbosacral radiculopathy.* Can produce back pain that radiates down the leg, similar to sciatic neuropathy. However, there typically is involvement of only one nerve root, which can be distinguished from motor or sensory exam, and on EMG. Also, imaging of the spine should show the source of the root damage. • *Lumbosacral plexopathy.* Can result in unilateral leg pain and weakness. Most patients will also have some difficulty with non-sciatic nerve-innervated muscles, including the adductors and knee and hip flexors. • *Peroneal neuropathy.* Presents with foot drop, but can be mistaken for sciatic neuropathy. The peroneal division of the sciatic nerve is more sensitive to injury than the tibial division, but sciatic neuropathy should have at least some clinical findings in a tibial nerve distribution.
Management	• No medications have been found to be helpful to encourage reinnervation, but typical meds for neuropathic pain can be used if needed, including anticonvulsants, select antidepressants, and analgesics. • Physical therapy can help restoration of muscle function and gait. • Surgery seldom is warranted for sciatic neuropathy.
Clinical course	Most patients improve over time, although the time to reinnervation with such a proximal lesion is long, and the recovery often is incomplete.

Sciatic Nerve and Posterior Cutaneous Nerve of Thigh

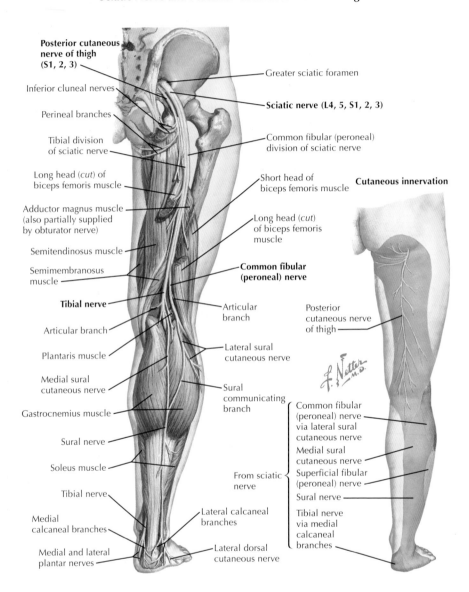

Posterior cutaneous nerve of thigh (S1, 2, 3)

Inferior cluneal nerves

Perineal branches

Tibial division of sciatic nerve

Long head (*cut*) of biceps femoris muscle

Adductor magnus muscle (also partially supplied by obturator nerve)

Semitendinosus muscle

Semimembranosus muscle

Tibial nerve

Articular branch

Plantaris muscle

Medial sural cutaneous nerve

Gastrocnemius muscle

Sural nerve

Soleus muscle

Tibial nerve

Medial calcaneal branches

Medial and lateral plantar nerves

Greater sciatic foramen

Sciatic nerve (L4, 5, S1, 2, 3)

Common fibular (peroneal) division of sciatic nerve

Short head of biceps femoris muscle

Long head (*cut*) of biceps femoris muscle

Common fibular (peroneal) nerve

Articular branch

Lateral sural cutaneous nerve

Sural communicating branch

Lateral calcaneal branches

Lateral dorsal cutaneous nerve

Cutaneous innervation

Posterior cutaneous nerve of thigh

Common fibular (peroneal) nerve via lateral sural cutaneous nerve

Medial sural cutaneous nerve

Superficial fibular (peroneal) nerve

Sural nerve

Tibial nerve via medial calcaneal branches

From sciatic nerve

DIABETIC NEUROPATHY	
Description	Diabetes mellitus remains the most common cause of peripheral neuropathy in the United States, and produces a variety of clinical presentations.
Pathophysiology	• The precise pathophysiology has not been determined, but is thought to be a combination of metabolic, vascular, and immune-mediated factors. • Axons degenerate, resulting in dysfunction of sensory neurons, with motor axons usually, but not invariably, being affected.
Clinical findings	• A number of clinical neuropathic syndromes are associated with diabetes. • *Distal small-fiber axonal neuropathy* usually presents with burning feet and toes and over several months or years can progress to involve more proximal portions of the feet and lower legs. Eventually the hands may become involved. There usually is very little weakness, although reflexes may be diminished. • *Diabetic polyradiculopathy* presents with pain most prominent in the thighs, followed by weakness that persists after the pain has abated. • *Symmetrical sensory-motor polyneuropathy* has axonal and demyelinating features. More rapid development of weakness and demyelination is suggestive of an inflammatory component, and investigation for this is warranted. • *Mononeuritis* and *mononeuritis multiplex* commonly are seen in the setting of diabetes and are suggestive of microvasculitis or, at least, microvascular disease.
Laboratory studies	• Routine labs usually are normal; however, there may be evidence of diabetes. • Special testing for diabetes is warranted in most patients with neuropathy. • Imaging has little value for evaluation of suspected neuropathy. Imaging is mainly performed when there is concern over a proximal lesion. • Nerve conduction studies may reveal slight slowing and decreased amplitudes with mild distal denervation on electromyography. However, in mild cases, electrophysiologic studies often are normal.
Diagnosis	• Diabetic neuropathy is suspected when a patient presents with any of the clinical findings of the types of neuropathy. The most common is distal sensory-motor neuropathy with numbness and pain on the feet and later, the hands. Weakness can develop with this, but this initially is not noticed. • NCS and EMG confirm the diagnosis of neuropathy. • Measurement of markers of diabetes, including glycosylated hemoglobin and an abnormal glucose tolerance test, confirms the presence of diabetes if the diagnosis has not already been made.

DIABETIC NEUROPATHY—cont'd	
Differential diagnosis	• *Neuropathy.* Neuropathy due to factors other than diabetes can occur in patients with diabetes. Therefore, the mere presence of diabetes should not cause one to jump to the conclusion that this is the cause of the condition. • *Immune-mediated neuropathies.* Including CIDP, AIDP, and MMN, can develop in patients with diabetes, yet these are not predisposed in patients with diabetes.
Management	• There are no treatments that alter the course of the disease. • Pain from diabetic neuropathy usually is treated with tricyclic antidepressants and/or selected anticonvulsants. Amitriptyline and gabapentin are two of the most commonly used agents. • New treatments for neuropathic pain include selected antidepressants, other anticonvulsants, and light-emitting diode therapy.
Clinical course	• Diabetic mononeuropathies can wax and wane, but become chronic problems. They do not remain painful for the duration, but rather can become less problematic later in the course of the disease. • Diabetic polyneuropathy results in distal loss of sensation, but usually and eventually, the pain abates.

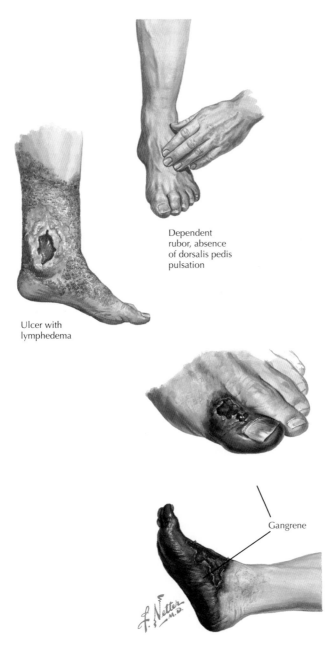

Dependent
rubor, absence
of dorsalis pedis
pulsation

Ulcer with
lymphedema

Gangrene

ACUTE INFLAMMATORY DEMYELINATING POLYNEUROPATHY (AIDP)/ GUILLAIN-BARRE SYNDROME	
Description	Also known as *acute inflammatory demyelinating polyneuropathy, Guillain-Barré syndrome* is seen with some regularity at most major medical centers.
Pathophysiology	The cause is unknown, but viral or bacterial gastroenteritis or occasionally surgery or injury seems to be a common preceding event.
Clinical findings	• The most common pattern is one of ascending, painless weakness and sensory loss, evolving to maximum severity over a period of 14 days or less. • Weakness can be extreme, with complete paralysis and ventilator dependence often noted. • Typical findings on examination include weakness, which is usually worst distally; loss of reflexes; and variable sensory loss.
Laboratory studies	• Neurophysiologic studies show evidence of demyelination, with slowing of nerve conduction velocities and often conduction block. • CSF studies show elevated albumin levels with normal glucose and no elevation in white cell count.
Diagnosis	• AIDP is suspected when a patient presents with subacute weakness and is found on examination to have areflexia. • EMG shows slowing of nerve conduction. Initially, the slowing may be subtle, and mainly of proximal portions of the nerves. • CSF is obtained in most patients, and the elevated protein without increased numbers of white blood cells supports the diagnosis.
Differential diagnosis	• *Chronic inflammatory demyelinating polyneuropathy.* Always considered, and is thought of by some as a chronic form of AIDP, although the immunology is different. CIDP has a slower progression. • *Botulism.* Considered in patients with progressive weakness. There are no sensory symptoms, and EMG findings differ. Also, there is no elevated CSF protein in botulism.
Management	• Two types of treatment have shown reasonable efficacy in shortening the length of disability and ventilator dependency—IVIG and plasma exchange. • High-dose IVIG is relatively more available and easier to administer than several cycles of plasma exchange, although there are little data comparing the two approaches. • Steroids are of no benefit. • Rehabilitation is needed for most patients. Although spontaneous improvement is expected, PT and OT can help with strengthening and self-care issues. Speech therapy is needed for some patients with prominent bulbar symptoms.
Clinical course	Most patients experience significant recovery of function, with as many as 85% having a relatively full return of function. A multidisciplinary approach, including physical and occupational therapy, is recommended.

─── Pathogenesis ───

Stage I. Lymphocytes migrate through endoneural vessels and surround nerve fiber, but myelin sheath and axon not yet damaged

Stage II. More lymphocytes extruded and macrophages appear. Segmental demyelination begins; however, axon not yet affected

Stage III. Multifocal myelin sheath and axonal damage. Central chromatolysis of nerve cell body occurs, and muscle begins to develop denervation atrophy

Stage IV. Extensive axonal destruction. Some nerve cell bodies irreversibly damaged, but function may be preserved because of adjacent less-affected nerve fibers

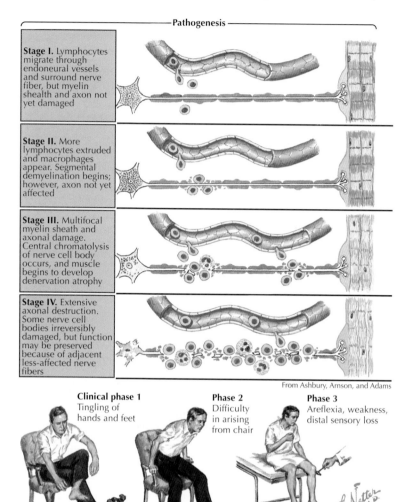

From Ashbury, Arnson, and Adams

Clinical phase 1
Tingling of hands and feet

Phase 2
Difficulty in arising from chair

Phase 3
Areflexia, weakness, distal sensory loss

CHRONIC INFLAMMATORY DEMYELINATING POLYNEUROPATHY (CIDP)	
Description	A relatively uncommon autoimmune neuropathy of unclear cause
Pathophysiology	Immune-mediated demyelination results in block of nerve conduction. This produces weakness and sensory change.
Clinical findings	Clinical deficits include weakness, reflex loss, and sensory loss that is often asymmetric, with the weakness evolving over the course of several weeks to even years.
Laboratory studies	• Routine labs typically are normal. • NCS and EMG shows findings of widespread demyelination and conduction block. • LP shows elevated CSF albumin levels, but the remainder of the CSF profile is normal.
Diagnosis	• CIDP is suspected when a patient presents with motor and/or sensory loss and is found to have demyelinating changes on EMG. Acute onset of this presentation suggests AIDP; chronic suggests CIDP. • Diagnosis is supported by the electrophysiologic findings of widespread demyelination and conduction block. CSF albumin levels often are elevated. • Nerve biopsy is sometimes performed.
Differential diagnosis	• *Acute inflammatory demyelinating polyneuropathy.* Can be acute or subacute. The presentation is similar to CIDP, but the findings are more acute. • *Critical illness polyneuropathy.* A subacute to chronic neuropathy that presents with weakness in the ICU setting. The development of profound weakness in these patients may suggest AIDP or CIDP.
Management	• Treatment with IVIG often is helpful. • Corticosteroids are the most useful for long-term treatment. It is important to make the distinction between CIDP and AIDP, because AIDP is not treated with corticosteroids.
Clinical course	• Most patients improve over time; however, many require persistent treatment. • Residual weakness is common.

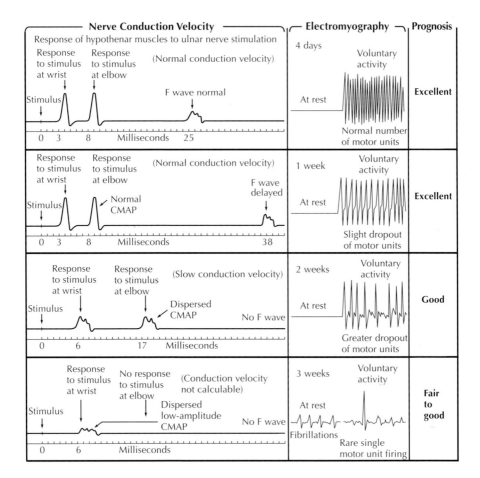

— Nerve Conduction Velocity —	— Electromyography —	Prognosis

Row 1:
Response of hypothenar muscles to ulnar nerve stimulation
Response to stimulus at wrist — Response to stimulus at elbow — (Normal conduction velocity)
Stimulus — F wave normal
0 3 8 Milliseconds 25
4 days — Voluntary activity — At rest — Normal number of motor units
Excellent

Row 2:
Response to stimulus at wrist — Response to stimulus at elbow — (Normal conduction velocity)
Stimulus — Normal CMAP — F wave delayed
0 3 8 Milliseconds 38
1 week — Voluntary activity — At rest — Slight dropout of motor units
Excellent

Row 3:
Response to stimulus at wrist — Response to stimulus at elbow — (Slow conduction velocity)
Stimulus — Dispersed CMAP — No F wave
0 6 17 Milliseconds
2 weeks — Voluntary activity — At rest — Greater dropout of motor units
Good

Row 4:
Response to stimulus at wrist — No response to stimulus at elbow — (Conduction velocity not calculable)
Stimulus — Dispersed low-amplitude CMAP — No F wave
0 6 Milliseconds
3 weeks — Voluntary activity — At rest — Fibrillations — Rare single motor unit firing
Fair to good

MULTIFOCAL MOTOR NEUROPATHY (MMN)	
Description	• A progressing disorder affecting motor nerves, resulting in weakness • The disorder is autoimmune, and as such, often responds to immune-modulating therapy.
Pathophysiology	• MMN is an autoimmune disorder, although the cause of the immune attack is not known. Ganglioside antibodies have been implicated in some cases. • Demyelinating changes predominate in the motor nerves, although there is some axonal drop-out. Conduction block is an important differentiating feature of MMN.
Clinical findings	• MMN presents with progressive weakness, often with cramping that affects peripheral nerve distributions in a patchy and asymmetric fashion, e.g., radial distribution producing wrist drop and peroneal distribution producing foot drop. • Sensory symptoms are absent. • Fasciculations can be seen along with the cramps. • Reflexes are normal or slightly reduced initially, but become absent with progressive disease.
Laboratory studies	• Routine labs are normal. • GM1 ganglioside antibodies are seen in about half of patients, and are supportive of the diagnosis but not required. • Imaging is normal and often not needed. • NCS and EMG show conduction block—where there is attenuation of conduction of the motor nerves through selected nerve segments. Sensory conduction through the same regions is normal. Fasciculations may be seen, but denervation is not prominent.
Diagnosis	• MMN is suspected when a patient presents with progressive asymmetric weakness without sensory abnormalities. ALS is usually the first thought in the clinician's mind, but exam does not show corticospinal tract signs (hyperactive tendon reflexes and up-going plantar responses), and NCS and EMG show conduction block rather than extensive denervation. • GM1 antibodies are supportive of the diagnosis, but not diagnostic and not required for diagnosis.
Differential diagnosis	• *Amyotrophic lateral sclerosis.* The main differential diagnosis presents with progressive asymmetric weakness, but there are signs of corticospinal tract dysfunction, and NCS and EMG show widespread denervation without significant conduction abnormalities. • *Mononeuropathy multiplex.* From many causes, can present with asymmetric weakness.
Management	• IVIG is first-line therapy for most patients. • Cyclophosphamide is used when patients cannot take IVIG or do not respond. • Corticosteroids are not effective and are not used.
Clinical course	Patients can have substantial improvement with IVIG treatment, so it is important to differentiate this from ALS, which essentially is untreatable.

CERVICAL RADICULOPATHY	
Description	Cervical nerve root damage can result in any combination or sensory loss, pain, or motor loss confined to a single nerve root distribution.

Pathophysiology	• Causes of cervical radiculopathy are multiple, and include:
	
	  • Disc disease
	
	  • Osteophyte formation
	
	  • Tumor
	
	  • Infection
	
	  • Diabetes
	
	• The common pathophysiology is nerve root impingement or infiltration with resultant damage to the myelin and axons.

Clinical findings	• Clinical findings depend on the level of the lesion. Most patients have neck pain that radiates down the arm in the dermatomal distribution. Weakness may be present, but is not invariable.
	
	• Rash over a portion of the involved dermatome suggests herpes zoster. This usually has a characteristic vesicular appearance.
	
	• Individual nerve root symptoms and signs are as follows:
	
	  • *C5 radiculopathy* produces sensory deficit in the radial forearm. Motor loss is in the deltoid and biceps. Biceps reflex is decreased.
	
	  • *C6 radiculopathy* produces sensory deficit in digits 1 and 2 of the hand. Motor deficit is in the biceps and brachioradialis. Biceps reflex often is decreased, and brachioradialis reflexes may be as well.
	
	  • *C7 radiculopathy* produces sensory deficit on digits 3 and 4 of the hand. Motor deficit is in the wrist extensors and triceps. Triceps reflex may be depressed.
	
	  • *C8 radiculopathy* produces sensory deficit on digit 5 of the hand. Motor deficit is in the intrinsic hand muscles—both median and ulnar innervated. Reflexes are normal.

Laboratory studies	• Routine labs are normal. • Imaging with MRI can show nerve root impingement or inflammation. • NCS is normal. EMG may show denervation in the distribution of the nerve root, but is not always present. • LP can be performed for neoplastic meningitis, but is of extremely low yield in patients without known cancer.
Diagnosis	• Cervical radiculopathy is suspected when a patient presents with pain and/or sensory loss in the arm with neck pain. • Imaging can show a structural cause in many patients. In others, diabetes and herpes zoster have to be considered. • Zoster is supported by the development of the rash, which may be minimal and may occur days after the onset of symptoms. • Diabetic radiculoneuropathy is suggested by the diagnosis of diabetes and the absence of a structural cause seen on studies.

CERVICAL RADICULOPATHY—cont'd	
Differential diagnosis	• *Brachial plexopathy.* Can produce motor and sensory findings in one or both arms. However, the symptoms span dermatomal distribution. • *Peripheral mononeuropathy.* Especially the radial nerve, peripheral mononeuropathy can mimic cervical radiculopathy, e.g., C7 lesion. However, examination of proximal and distal musculature helps to differentiate a peripheral from a nerve root lesion. Also, most peripheral nerve lesions span root distributions.
Management	*Nerve root compression* from disc or bony element usually can usually be treated conservatively. Treatment options include: • *Physical therapy* is extremely helpful for reducing pain and restoring function. This should be offered to almost all patients. • *Muscle relaxants* are used if there is paraspinal muscle spasm that contributes to the pain. • *Anti-inflammatory agents* are given to most patients and can reduce pain. • *Epidural corticosteroid injections* are considered if conservative measures are not helpful. • *Surgical decompression* is considered especially if there is weakness or refractory pain. *Herpes zoster* is treated with analgesics and antiviral medications. Anticonvulsants often are often used as an adjunct for control of the neuropathic pain. *Tumor infiltration* is treated with local or neuraxis radiation. Intrathecal and systemic chemotherapy also often are given. Corticosteroids also are helpful for the pain of tumor infiltration. *Diabetic radiculoneuropathy* produces neuropathic pain, which can be treated not only with analgesics but also by anticonvulsants such as gabapentin. These agents are less helpful for the mechanical pain than the neuropathic pain.
Clinical course	Most patients improve with treatment, although not all. If the cause is compressive, there is a high remission rate with medications and therapy, although there is the possibility of recurrence of the pain at a later time.

Dermatomes and Myotomes of Upper Limb

Note: Schematic demarcation of dermatomes (according to Keegan and Garrett) shown as distinct segments. There is actually considerable overlap between adjacent dermatomes. An alternative dermatome map is that provided by Foerster.

A. C2 to T1 Sensory Representation

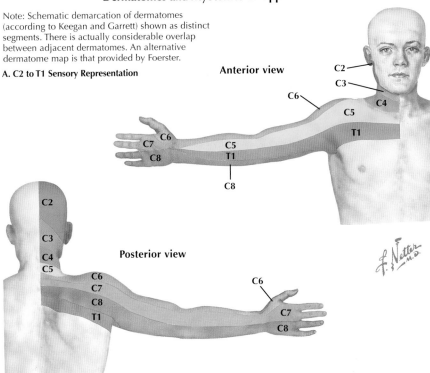

B. Motor Impairment Related to Level of Cervical Root Lesion

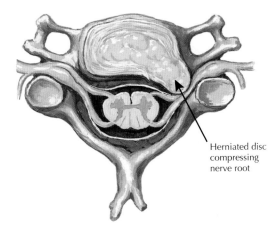

Herniated disc compressing nerve root

THORACIC RADICULOPATHY	
Description	Thoracic nerve root damage can result in pain, predominantly in the chest.
Pathophysiology	• All of the pathologies that can affect the cervical spine can affect the thoracic spine. In general, disc disease and osteophyte formation are less common than they are in the cervical and lumbar spine. • Herpes zoster and diabetic radiculoneuropathy are more important causes.
Clinical findings	• Thoracic radiculopathy commonly produces unilateral chest wall pain, which begins near the spine and radiates toward the front, following the dermatome. • Rash in the distribution suggests herpes zoster, especially when vesicular. • Motor deficit is not expected with thoracic radiculopathy. • Reflex abnormalities are not expected, unless there are myelopathic findings due to the cause of thoracic radiculopathy, e.g., disc or tumor with nerve and spinal cord compression.
Laboratory studies	• Routine labs are normal. • Imaging with MRI shows a structural cause in most patients. When imaging is normal, diabetes and herpes zoster have to be considered. • NCS and EMG are of little value in diagnosis of thoracic radiculopathy and are not routinely performed.
Diagnosis	• Thoracic radiculopathy is suspected when a patient presents with sensory loss and/or pain in the chest. Careful exam confirms the distribution of the symptoms within one nerve or dermatome distribution. • MRI can show a structural lesion. If this is normal, diabetes and herpes zoster have to be considered. • LP can be performed to look for neoplastic meningitis, but is of extremely low yield in patients without known cancer.
Differential diagnosis	• *Lung disorders.* Can produce pain that may be mistaken for thoracic radiculopathy, especially pleural-based lesions, e.g., mesothelioma and other tumors, infections, or inflammation. • *Cardiac pain.* Rarely confused with thoracic radiculopathy.
Management	• Treatment of thoracic radiculopathy does not greatly differ from treatment of cervical radiculopathy. • Thoracic radiculopathy is not associated with perceptible motor deficit, and, therefore, pain is the main symptom to be addressed.
Clinical course	Most patients improve with time, regardless of cause. Long-term use of agents for neuropathic pain occasionally is needed.

Spinal Nerve Origin: Cross Section

Section through thoracic vertebra

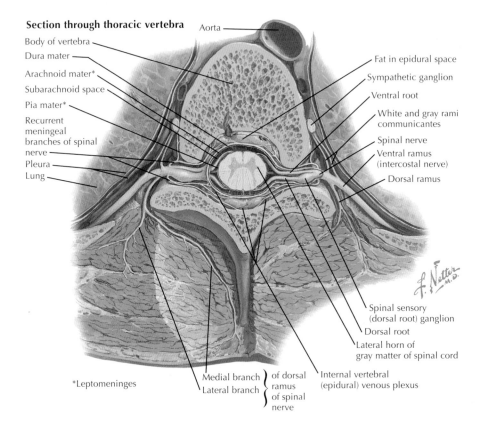

Aorta

Body of vertebra

Dura mater

Arachnoid mater*

Subarachnoid space

Pia mater*

Recurrent meningeal branches of spinal nerve

Pleura

Lung

Fat in epidural space

Sympathetic ganglion

Ventral root

White and gray rami communicantes

Spinal nerve

Ventral ramus (intercostal nerve)

Dorsal ramus

Spinal sensory (dorsal root) ganglion

Dorsal root

Lateral horn of gray matter of spinal cord

*Leptomeninges

Medial branch ⎱ of dorsal
Lateral branch ⎰ ramus ⎱ of spinal nerve

Internal vertebral (epidural) venous plexus

LUMBOSACRAL RADICULOPATHY	
Description	Damage to the lumbar or sacral nerves can produce sensory or motor deficit affecting the lower back, pelvis, and legs.
Pathophysiology	• The same causes of cervical radiculopathy can affect the lumbosacral nerve roots. • Disc disease and osteophyte formation are the most common. Tumor and infection are less likely.
Clinical findings	Lumbosacral radiculopathy causes pain in the back that can radiate down the hip and legs in a dermatomal distribution. Weakness can be present, and of great localizing value. Findings with individual nerve roots are as follows: • *L2 radiculopathy*—sensory deficit on the lateral and anterior upper thigh. Motor deficit in the psoas and quadriceps. No reflex abnormality. • *L3 radiculopathy*—sensory deficit on the lower medial thigh. Motor deficit in the psoas and quadriceps. Knee reflex is reduced. • *L4 radiculopathy*—sensory deficit on the medial lower leg. Motor deficit in the tibialis anterior and quadriceps. Knee reflex is decreased. • *L5 radiculopathy*—sensory deficit on the lateral lower leg. Motor loss of the peroneus longus, tibialis anterior. No reflex abnormality. • *S1 radiculopathy*—sensory deficit on the lateral foot involving digits 4 and 5. Motor deficit involving the gastrocnemius. Ankle reflex is decreased. The unlisted roots—L1 and S2-S4—can be involved, but much less commonly than the ones listed.
Laboratory studies	• Routine labs are normal. • MRI shows a structural cause in most patients. If this is negative, diabetes, herpes zoster, and tumor are considered. • CT of the lumbar spine is less sensitive than MRI, but has to be performed when MRI cannot be done (e.g., pacemaker). Intrathecal contrast dye improves the diagnostic sensitivity of the CT. • NCS is normal. EMG may show denervation in the appropriate nerve root distribution if there has been significant involvement of the motor nerves. • Lumbar puncture (LP) can be done to look for neoplastic meningitis, especially with polyradiculopathy, but is of low yield in the absence of known cancer.

LUMBOSACRAL RADICULOPATHY—cont'd	
Diagnosis	• Lumbosacral radiculopathy is suspected when a patient presents with sensory and/or motor symptoms in the leg. The presence of back pain is supportive, especially of structural causes.
	• MRI shows a structural lesion in most cases. If this is normal, diabetes, herpes zoster, and tumor are considered.
	• A vesicular rash in a dermatomal distribution suggests herpes zoster.
	• Laboratory signs of diabetes support the diagnosis of diabetic radiculoneuropathy, although this does not mean that some other cause is not present.
	• NCS and EMG can support the diagnosis of radiculopathy if there is localized denervation.
Differential diagnosis	• *Lumbosacral plexopathy.* Can produce pain in the leg, which can also involve the hip and back. Weakness is common. This disorder affects muscles of more than one dermatome, however. Examination and EMG can make this distinction.
	• *Peripheral mononeuropathy.* Can mimic radiculopathy, e.g., peroneal neuropathy and L5 radiculopathy can both produce foot drop without reflex changes. Differentiation is by examination and EMG.
Management	Management of lumbosacral radiculopathy does not differ from that of cervical radiculopathy.
Clinical course	Most patients improve. At least 75% of patients with lumbosacral radiculopathy improve with conservative care, although some will eventually still come to surgery.

Pain Patterns in Lumbar Disease

Radicular pain due to nerve root compression

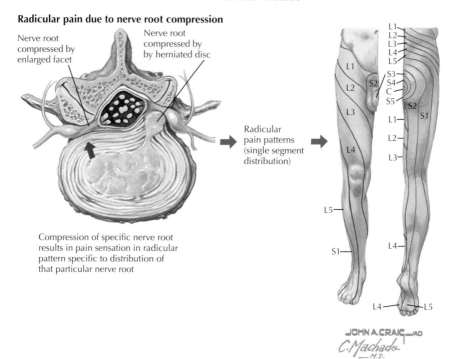

Nerve root compressed by enlarged facet

Nerve root compressed by by herniated disc

Radicular pain patterns (single segment distribution)

Compression of specific nerve root results in pain sensation in radicular pattern specific to distribution of that particular nerve root

JOHN A. CRAIG—AD
C. Machado
—M.D.

BRACHIAL PLEXOPATHY	
Description	Damage to the brachial plexus can produce pain, sensory loss, and/or weakness in one arm. Some plexopathies can be bilateral.
Pathophysiology	• The brachial plexus is formed from the individual cervical and upper thoracic nerve roots. The nerves diverge and reconnect to form the nerves of the arm, especially median, ulnar, radial, and musculocutaneous. There also are other minor nerves supplying shoulder muscles, and these are shown in the diagram. • Causes of brachial plexopathy include: trauma, plexitis, tumor, radiation, and bleeding.
Clinical findings	Clinical findings depend on the cause of the lesion and the precise location. Generally, there is pain and/or sensory loss in the arm. Weakness can develop in muscles innervated by the involved portion of the plexus. • *Upper plexus lesions* produce sensory and/or motor deficits affecting the distributions of the C5 and C6 nerve roots. Deltoid and biceps are especially affected, with sensory change that extends below the elbow to the hand. • *Lower plexus lesions* produce sensory and/or motor deficits affecting especially the C8 and T1 nerve roots. Median and ulnar-innervated muscles are affected, with hand weakness, and sensory symptoms involve much of the palmar hand, ulnar aspect of the dorsal hand. Specific findings with individual causes include: • *Trauma* produces variable damage to the plexus. Stab wounds can affect almost any portion, but the upper plexus is more exposed. Weakness is prominent early, soon followed by neuropathic pain. Upward traction of the shoulder can stretch the lower plexus. Downward traction of the shoulder can stretch the upper plexus. • *Brachial plexitis* presents with pain in the shoulder and arm that eventually improves. During this phase, weakness develops, which has slower improvement. Upper plexus is mostly affected. • *Tumor* can be compressive from the lung or infiltrating from cervical lymph nodes. Tumor presents with severe pain, often weakness, and Horner's syndrome. Lower plexus is mainly affected. • *Radiation therapy* to the neck and chest produces dysesthesias that are uncomfortable, but not really painful. Weakness can develop. The upper plexus is predominantly involved due to thinness of the tissues in the region of the upper plexus. • *Bleeding* into the neck and plexus from trauma and from bleeding disorder presents with weakness and motor loss in the arm, often with a palpable hematoma in the supraclavicular area. Pain may be present, but is less prominent than with tumor or plexitis.

BRACHIAL PLEXOPATHY—cont'd	
Laboratory studies	• Routine labs are normal. There are no reliable markers for brachial plexitis, although antinuclear antibodies (ANA) and ESR often are checked. • MRI is able to show structural cause in a minority of patients, chiefly tumor or signs of trauma. Brachial plexitis and radiation plexopathy are not associated with reproducible findings on studies. • NCS usually is normal, although the sensory and motor action potential can become reduced in amplitude after 1–2 weeks. EMG can show signs of denervation after 3–4 weeks.
Diagnosis	• *Trauma* as a cause for brachial plexopathy is evident from the inciting event. EMG can help to localize the lesion. Imaging may be normal with stretch/traction injuries but may show denervation hematoma and tissue disruption with penetrating trauma. • *Brachial plexitis* is suspected when a patient develops pain in an arm and no structural cause is identified. Subsequent development of weakness as the pain improves supports the diagnosis. • *Tumor infiltration* is suspected with severe shoulder and arm pain with or without weakness. Imaging shows tumor compression or infiltration in the region. • *Radiation plexopathy* is suspected when a patient develops dysesthesias in the arm months after known radiation therapy. Imaging does not show a structural cause. • *Bleeding* into the plexus can be seen on imaging and suspected from exam.
Differential diagnosis	• *Cervical radiculopathy* produces pain in the arm, but the lesion affects only a single nerve root, unless there is polyradiculopathy. • *Mononeuropathy* of the upper extremity can produce pain and weakness, but the deficit is distal to the plexus, which may be evident on exam or EMG.
Management	• Tumor can be treated with surgery, chemotherapy, and/or radiation therapy. Surgery can make the plexus damage worse, so this is less commonly used than radiation therapy and chemotherapy. • Brachial plexitis often is treated with corticosteroids, although this has not definitively been proven to be helpful. • Management for the other causes is supportive.
Clinical course	Improvement depends on the cause of the plexopathy. Idiopathic plexitis commonly improves, with most having resolution of the pain and eventual improvement in strength.

Brachial Plexus: Schema

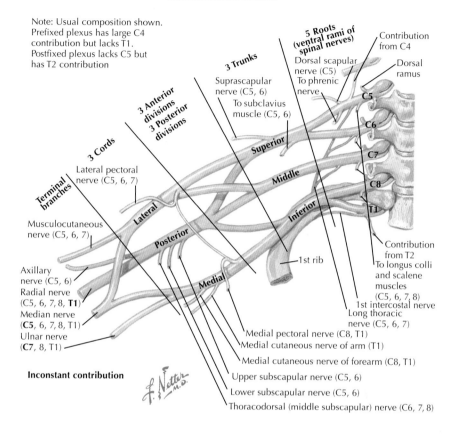

Note: Usual composition shown.
Prefixed plexus has large C4
contribution but lacks T1.
Postfixed plexus lacks C5 but
has T2 contribution

5 Roots
(ventral rami of
spinal nerves)

Contribution
from C4

3 Trunks

Dorsal scapular
nerve (C5)

Dorsal
ramus

Suprascapular
nerve (C5, 6)

To phrenic
nerve

3 Anterior
divisions

3 Posterior
divisions

To subclavius
muscle (C5, 6)

C5

C6

3 Cords

Superior

C7

Lateral pectoral
nerve (C5, 6, 7)

Middle

C8

Terminal
branches

Lateral

Inferior

T1

Musculocutaneous
nerve (C5, 6, 7)

Posterior

Contribution
from T2

To longus colli
and scalene
muscles
(C5, 6, 7, 8)

1st intercostal nerve

Long thoracic
nerve (C5, 6, 7)

Axillary
nerve (C5, 6)

1st rib

Radial nerve
(C5, 6, 7, 8, **T1**)

Median nerve
(**C5**, 6, 7, 8, T1)

Medial

Ulnar nerve
(**C7**, 8, T1)

Medial pectoral nerve (C8, T1)

Medial cutaneous nerve of arm (T1)

Medial cutaneous nerve of forearm (C8, T1)

Inconstant contribution

Upper subscapular nerve (C5, 6)

Lower subscapular nerve (C5, 6)

Thoracodorsal (middle subscapular) nerve (C6, 7, 8)

9 Lumbosacral Plexopathy

LUMBOSACRAL PLEXOPATHY	
Description	Damage to the lumbosacral plexus in the abdomen can produce leg sensory and motor symptoms. The differential diagnosis is similar to that of brachial plexitis.
Pathophysiology	• Lumbosacral plexitis has similar causes to brachial plexitis; however, radiation plexopathy is uncommon, and idiopathic plexitis is less likely. • Diabetic amyotrophy is sometimes discussed under plexopathy, but is really a polyradiculopathy
Clinical findings	Lumbosacral plexopathy is most commonly due to tumor. Bleeding, trauma, and idiopathic also are considered. Clinical features of individual entities are as follows: 　• *Tumor* compression or infiltration of the lumbosacral plexus presents with severe local and radiating pain into the leg. Patients typically have a known history of renal or gastrointestinal cancer. 　• *Trauma* can produce direct damage to the plexus, although in this case, there is likely to be significant direct abdominal organ damage. Pain in the abdomen and legs can be seen. 　• *Lumbar plexitis* is uncommon, and presents with hip and leg pain, followed by weakness. 　• *Bleeding* into the plexus from femoral stick for angiography or trauma produces a block of axonal transmission, resulting in decreased sensation and often weakness that spans dermatomal distributions.
Laboratory studies	• Routine labs are normal. • MRI can show a structural lesion or layered blood, if present, in the paraspinal region. • EMG can show denervation in a distribution appropriate to the deficit; however, 3–4 weeks may elapse before the EMG becomes abnormal, and a normal EMG does not rule out the diagnosis.
Diagnosis	• Lumbosacral plexopathy is suspected when a patient presents with pain and/or weakness of one leg, often associated with pain in the flank region or abdomen. • Imaging can confirm a structural lesion. If structural imaging is normal, then tumor infiltration is less likely, but not ruled out. • EMG is initially normal, but subsequently becomes abnormal 3–4 weeks later, and the distribution of the findings can confirm the localization to the lumbosacral plexus.
Differential diagnosis	• *Lumbosacral radiculopathy.* Can present with weakness and/or sensory deficit in one leg. The pain can radiate, suggesting radiculopathy, but the symptoms and signs are confined to one nerve root distribution. • *Diabetic amyotrophy.* Presents with pain and subsequent weakness involving, mainly, the quadriceps. The clinical presentation can be indistinguishable from lumbosacral plexitis.

LUMBOSACRAL PLEXOPATHY—cont'd	
Management	• Management of lumbosacral plexopathy is largely supportive unless treatable tumor is identified.
	• Lumbosacral plexitis often is treated with corticosteroids, although the benefits have not been proven.
	• Hematoma eventually absorbs, resulting in return of the function of the plexus. Evacuation seldom is necessary.
Clinical course	Most patients improve, but the prognosis depends on the cause. Idiopathic plexitis results in significant improvement in most patients.

Lumbar Plexus

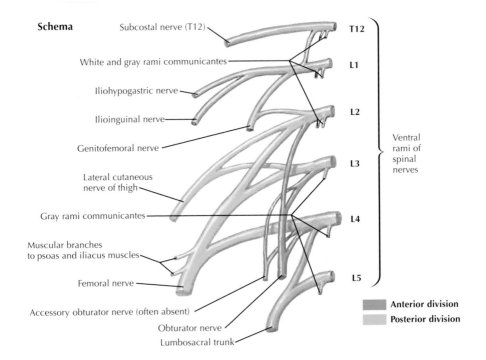

Schema

Subcostal nerve (T12)

White and gray rami communicantes

Iliohypogastric nerve

Ilioinguinal nerve

Genitofemoral nerve

Lateral cutaneous nerve of thigh

Gray rami communicantes

Muscular branches to psoas and iliacus muscles

Femoral nerve

Accessory obturator nerve (often absent)

Obturator nerve

Lumbosacral trunk

T12
L1
L2
L3
L4
L5

Ventral rami of spinal nerves

Anterior division
Posterior division

Sacral and Coccygeal Plexuses

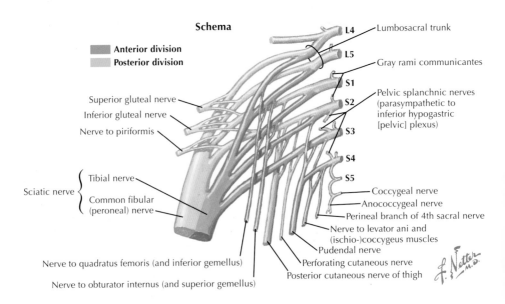

Schema

Anterior division
Posterior division

Superior gluteal nerve
Inferior gluteal nerve
Nerve to piriformis

Sciatic nerve { Tibial nerve
Common fibular (peroneal) nerve

Nerve to quadratus femoris (and inferior gemellus)
Nerve to obturator internus (and superior gemellus)

L4 — Lumbosacral trunk
L5
Gray rami communicantes
S1
S2 — Pelvic splanchnic nerves (parasympathetic to inferior hypogastric [pelvic] plexus)
S3
S4
S5
Coccygeal nerve
Anococcygeal nerve
Perineal branch of 4th sacral nerve
Nerve to levator ani and (ischio-)coccygeus muscles
Pudendal nerve
Perforating cutaneous nerve
Posterior cutaneous nerve of thigh

CRITICAL ILLNESS POLYNEUROPATHY (CIP)	
Description	A common cause of weakness and failure to wean ICU patients from their ventilator
Pathophysiology	The etiology of CIP likely is multifactorial. ICU care, critical illness, corticosteroid administration, and paralytic administration are all risk factors, although they are not all necessary for CIP development.
Clinical findings	• Patients develop weakness with decreased tone after at least 1 week, and usually 2 weeks, of ICU care. There may be sensory symptoms reported when the patients are questioned; however, pain is not a common feature. • The weakness often manifests as a failure to wean from the ventilator.
Laboratory studies	• Routine labs are normal, or only show abnormalities associated with the underlying disease. Creatine Kinase (CK) often is measured to look for myopathy, and is normal or only mildly increased. • Imaging is normal, and often not necessary when electrophysiologic studies have demonstrated the neuropathy. • NCS and EMG show polyneuropathy with mainly axonal features; widespread denervation is seen. • CSF is normal or shows mildly elevated protein.
Diagnosis	• CIP is suspected when a patient recovering in the ICU has slow weaning and is noted to have flaccid weakness, even in the absence of sedatives and paralytics. • Diagnosis is supported by lack of markedly elevated CK, axonal neuropathy identified on NCS and EMG, and absence of other identified abnormality from study.
Differential diagnosis	• *Critical illness myopathy.* A closely related condition with some of the same features. This is difficult to distinguish from CIP without biopsy. EMG can give some guidance, but may not be definitive, especially early in the disease process. Sensory examination in this clinical setting is imperfect, and many patients have other medical reasons to have polyneuropathy confounding the use of this as a distinguishing feature. • *Acute inflammatory demyelinating polyneuropathy (Guillain-Barré syndrome).* Presents with weakness, which can develop in an ICU setting. This occasionally is missed when a patient with known congestive heart failure (CHF) or chronic obstructive pulmonary disease (COPD) presents with weakness that is presumed to be due to their medical illness, and the neuropathy is not noticed. NCS and EMG show demyelinating changes, and CSF protein is elevated.
Management	• Treatment is supportive. If AIDP has been eliminated as a possibility, immune-modulating therapy is not of proven value. • Physical therapy and occupational therapy are of tremendous help. • Medical management includes minimizing corticosteroids and paralytics. This general approach may not only be helpful for the patient but also for lowering the risk in other patients.
Clinical course	• Patients make a dramatic recovery from CIP. Patients who are quadriplegic regain strength, and ultimately ambulation, with time and care. • About 50% have total recovery.

Weakness in the ICU

- Patient with illness and weakness
- Pain is uncommon
- Sensory loss may occur; when present suggests neuropathy
- Myopathic and neuropathic damage may coexist

↓

History

- Progressive weakness in the ICU
- Ask about sensory symptoms
- Ask about a history of DM, cancer, or other causes of neuropathy
- Ask about medications and other exposures that can cause neuropathy or myopathy (certain antibiotics, statins, alcohol)

Exam

- Motor exam – weakness may be proximal (myopathy), distal (neuropathy), or both.
- Sensory exam – any sensory loss and distribution – distal, proximal, or spinal level.
- Reflex exam – absent DTRs suggests AIDP, CIDP, CIP; increased suggests spinal or cerebral cause

↓

Tests may include:

- Lab: CPK, aldolase, myoglobin, TFTs, B_{12}, antibody tests
- NCS & EMG: can differentiate neuropathy, myopathy, neuromuscular transmission defect
- Muscle biopsy: confirmation of certain myopathies and supportive of some neuropathies
- Nerve biopsy: confirmation of certain neuropathies

Neuropathies	Myopathies	Neuromuscular transmission disorders
Critical illness polyneuropathy • Weakness, decreased tone • Loss of DTRs • Dx by NCS, EMG, lab. Bx?	**Critical illness myopathy** • Weakness and decreased tone • Dx by EMG and lab • Confirmed by biopsy	**Myasthenia** • Weakness, fatigue • No sensory deficit • Dx by NCS and lab
AIDP • Weakness, decreased tone • Often with pain • Loss of DTRs • Dx by NCS, lab, LP	**Rhabdomyolysis** • Weakness often with muscle pain • Dx by lab (including ↑CPK)	**Botulism** • Weakness and fatigue • No sensory deficit • Dx by NCS and lab
CIDP • Weakness, decreased tone • Loss of DTRs • Dx by NCS, lab • May need nerve bx +/o LP	**Inflammatory myopathy** • Weakness ± muscle pain • Dx by EMG and lab • Confirmed by muscle biopsy	**Lambert-Eaton Myasthenic syndrome** • Weakness, fatigue dry mouth. No sensory loss • Dx by NCS and lab

OVERVIEW OF MOTOR NEURON DISEASES (MND)	
Description	• Motor neuron diseases produce weakness through degeneration of the upper and/or the lower motor neuron. • They are pure motor disorders, without sensory symptoms or signs.
Upper motor neuron diseases	• The upper motor neurons are those whose axons make up the corticospinal and corticobulbar tracts. Their cell bodies lie predominately in primary and secondary motor cortices. They directly activate lower motor neurons, which primarily lie in the anterior horn of the spinal cord gray matter and in brainstem motor nuclei. • These disorders typically are painless and slowly progressive. Symptoms of weakness, spasticity, and increased deep tendon reflexes predominate.
Lower motor neuron diseases	• The lower motor neurons have their cell bodies in the anterior horns of the spinal cord and in the brainstem. They form the long motor axons, which supply the muscles of the entire body. • Lower motor neuron disorders cause weakness without spasticity, unless combined with upper motor neuron dysfunction. Decreased tone and decreased reflexes are seen.
Combined upper and lower motor neuron disease	• Degeneration of both the upper and lower motor neurons is usually idiopathic. ALS is the principle. • The upper motor neuron degeneration causes weakness especially distally with atrophy of the intrinsic muscles of the hands. • The lower motor neuron degeneration causes spasticity of the legs with impaired coordination. There are no sensory deficits. • The differential diagnosis consists of simultaneous unrelated upper motor neuron damage (e.g. spondylosis) plus lower motor neuron damage (e.g. neuropathy).

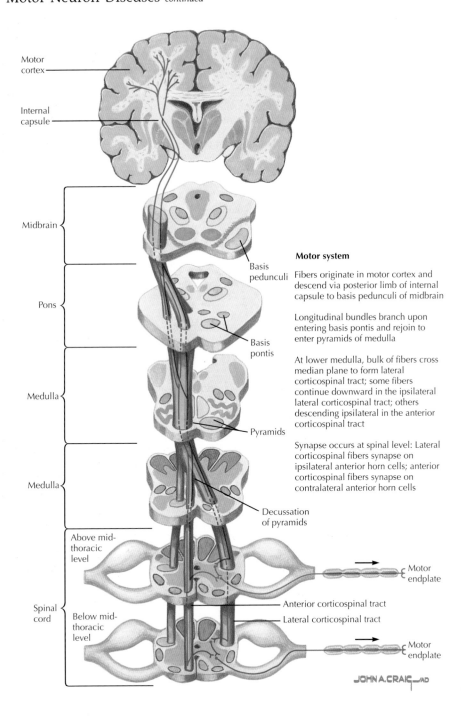

Motor cortex

Internal capsule

Midbrain

Pons

Medulla

Medulla

Spinal cord

Above mid-thoracic level

Below mid-thoracic level

Basis pedunculi

Basis pontis

Pyramids

Decussation of pyramids

Anterior corticospinal tract

Lateral corticospinal tract

Motor endplate

Motor endplate

Motor system

Fibers originate in motor cortex and descend via posterior limb of internal capsule to basis pedunculi of midbrain

Longitudinal bundles branch upon entering basis pontis and rejoin to enter pyramids of medulla

At lower medulla, bulk of fibers cross median plane to form lateral corticospinal tract; some fibers continue downward in the ipsilateral lateral corticospinal tract; others descending ipsilateral in the anterior corticospinal tract

Synapse occurs at spinal level: Lateral corticospinal fibers synapse on ipsilateral anterior horn cells; anterior corticospinal fibers synapse on contralateral anterior horn cells

JOHN A. CRAIG—AD

PRIMARY LATERAL SCLEROSIS (PLS)	
Description	Rare progressive spastic paraparesis, not due to focal structural lesion
Pathophysiology	Cause is unknown, but is a degenerative condition with no known triggers
Clinical findings	• This rare disorder usually presents as slowly progressive spastic paraparesis, which eventually progresses to include the upper extremities. • It sometimes is considered a variant of ALS. In many cases that are followed for long periods of time, some lower motor neuron involvement eventually develops. • Age of onset usually is in the fifth or sixth decade and equal incidence between the sexes.
Laboratory studies	• Routine labs are normal, multiple labs are performed to look for reversible causes. • Imaging of the spine is normal. MRI usually is performed. Myelography can occasionally show structural abnormalities not seen on MRI.
Diagnosis	• PLS is considered with a patient has progressive paraparesis and imaging studies do not show a structural cause. • PLS is a diagnosis of exclusion, only after ruling out multiple sclerosis, hydrocephalus, cervical spondylotic myelopathy, B_{12} deficiency, adrenomyeloneuropathy, HTLV-1 infection, Lyme disease, and other identifiable causes of gradually progressive myelopathy.
Differential diagnosis	• *Amyotrophic lateral sclerosis.* Considered in the differential diagnosis. Some patients, when followed over long period of time, will eventually develop lower motor neuron findings. Before this, PLS patients do not have denervation on EMG. • *Spinal cord lesion.* Always in the differential diagnosis. Spondylotic myelopathy features prominently in the differential diagnosis. Other causes include tumors, vascular malformations, and disc disease. The absence of back pain and imaging abnormalities favors PLS. • *Transverse myelitis.* A demyelinating disorder related to multiple sclerosis. Myelopathy can occur with TM or MS, and typically progresses over a few days without a later progression.
Management	There is no known treatment for the disorder itself, but spasticity may be partially ameliorated with the use of baclofen or tizanidine.
Clinical course	Patients progress slowly. In most, the symptoms remain confined to those of the spinal cord. However, in some individuals, there is later development of lower motor neuron degeneration.

Second thoracic

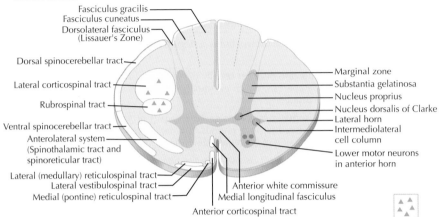

Fasciculus gracilis

Fasciculus cuneatus

Dorsolateral fasciculus (Lissauer's Zone)

Dorsal spinocerebellar tract

Lateral corticospinal tract

Rubrospinal tract

Ventral spinocerebellar tract

Anterolateral system (Spinothalamic tract and spinoreticular tract)

Lateral (medullary) reticulospinal tract

Lateral vestibulospinal tract

Medial (pontine) reticulospinal tract

Marginal zone

Substantia gelatinosa

Nucleus proprius

Nucleus dorsalis of Clarke

Lateral horn

Intermediolateral cell column

Lower motor neurons in anterior horn

Anterior white commissure

Medial longitudinal fasciculus

Anterior corticospinal tract

J. Perkins
MS, MFA

Descending monoamine axons (noradrenergic, serotonergic)

Descending fibers from hypothalamus and brain stem to spinal cord

Eighth thoracic

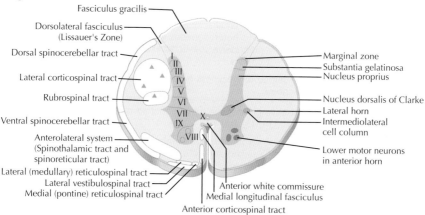

Fasciculus gracilis

Dorsolateral fasciculus (Lissauer's Zone)

Dorsal spinocerebellar tract

Lateral corticospinal tract

Rubrospinal tract

Ventral spinocerebellar tract

Anterolateral system (Spinothalamic tract and spinoreticular tract)

Lateral (medullary) reticulospinal tract

Lateral vestibulospinal tract

Medial (pontine) reticulospinal tract

Marginal zone

Substantia gelatinosa

Nucleus proprius

Nucleus dorsalis of Clarke

Lateral horn

Intermediolateral cell column

Lower motor neurons in anterior horn

Anterior white commissure

Medial longitudinal fasciculus

Anterior corticospinal tract

First lumbar

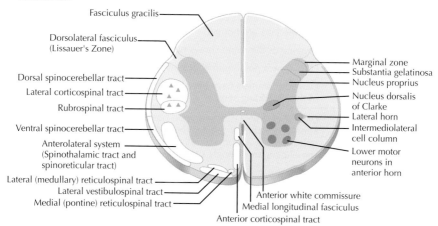

Fasciculus gracilis

Dorsolateral fasciculus (Lissauer's Zone)

Dorsal spinocerebellar tract

Lateral corticospinal tract

Rubrospinal tract

Ventral spinocerebellar tract

Anterolateral system (Spinothalamic tract and spinoreticular tract)

Lateral (medullary) reticulospinal tract

Lateral vestibulospinal tract

Medial (pontine) reticulospinal tract

Marginal zone

Substantia gelatinosa

Nucleus proprius

Nucleus dorsalis of Clarke

Lateral horn

Intermediolateral cell column

Lower motor neurons in anterior horn

Anterior white commissure

Medial longitudinal fasciculus

Anterior corticospinal tract

Third lumbar

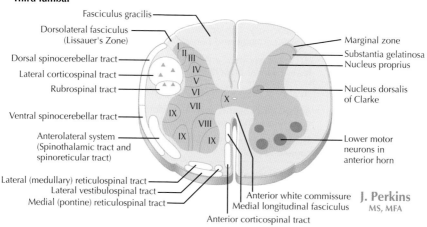

Fasciculus gracilis

Dorsolateral fasciculus (Lissauer's Zone)

Dorsal spinocerebellar tract

Lateral corticospinal tract

Rubrospinal tract

Ventral spinocerebellar tract

Anterolateral system (Spinothalamic tract and spinoreticular tract)

Lateral (medullary) reticulospinal tract

Lateral vestibulospinal tract

Medial (pontine) reticulospinal tract

Marginal zone

Substantia gelatinosa

Nucleus proprius

Nucleus dorsalis of Clarke

Lower motor neurons in anterior horn

Anterior white commissure

Medial longitudinal fasciculus

Anterior corticospinal tract

J. Perkins
MS, MFA

HEREDITARY SPASTIC PARPARESIS (HSP)	
Description	• Also known as familial spastic paraparesis and Strumpell-Lorraine syndrome, this heterogeneous group of disorders produces gradually progressive spastic weakness, usually confined to the lower extremities. • The degree of weakness is variable. Numerous families have been described.
Pathophysiology	• Causative genes have been identified on chromosomes X, 2, 3, 8, 11, 12, 14, 15, and 19. • The most common mode of inheritance is autosomal dominant, although X-linked and autosomal recessive inheritance has been described.
Clinical findings	• Patients present with progressive weakness, usually confined to the legs. • Exam shows spasticity, with increased tone in the legs and upgoing plantar responses. Gait is stiff and awkward. Balance clearly is impaired.
Laboratory studies	• Routine labs are normal. • Imaging of the spine shows no abnormalities. • EMG shows no abnormalities on routine testing. • Evoked potentials have been reported to show impaired conduction of the ascending sensory axons through the cord.
Diagnosis	• Diagnosis largely is based upon positive family history in the appropriate clinical setting. The clinical finding of extremely brisk leg reflexes, brisk abdominal reflexes, and downgoing toes to plantar stimulation are strongly suggestive of this disorder. • MRI of the spine is performed to look for structural cause and is negative. • Labs for other causes of myelopathy, including B_{12} deficiency and HTLV-1, are commonly performed and would be negative in HSP.
Differential diagnosis	• *Cord compression.* From any cause, can have identical clinical presentation; although this would not be expected to be familial. • *B_{12} deficiency.* Can produce myelopathy. Not all patients will have other neurologic and hematologic stigmata of B_{12} deficiency. • *HTLV-1–associated myelopathy.* A progressive myelopathy that can have a similar presentation.
Management	• Treatment is symptomatic and family counseling is advisable. • Antispasticity agents such as baclofen, tizanidine, and the benzodiazepines, are helpful for management of the spasticity. • Therapy and continued activity are important for maintenance of continued mobility.
Clinical course	The neurologic deficit is progressive. There are no treatments that alter the course of the weakness.

HTLV-I ASSOCIATED MYELOPATHY (HAM) TROPICAL SPASTIC PARESIS (TSP)	
Description	A paralyzing illness endemic in the Caribbean and Asian tropics
Pathophysiology	• HTLV-1 is the causative agent for adult T-cell leukemia and for TSP. Infection results in inflammatory infiltration and degeneration affecting the spinal cord and brain white matter.
Clinical findings	• HAM presents as a gradually progressive, often dysesthetic spastic paraparesis, with age of onset typically after 30. The arms can be affected, as well, although less so than the legs. • In contrast to most other pure upper motor neuron conditions, bladder dysfunction commonly is seen.
Laboratory studies	• Routine labs usually are normal. • HTLV-1 testing is confirmatory of infection.
Diagnosis	• HAM is suspected in a patient with myelopathy without a structural cause having been identified. In these patients, MS, B_{12} deficiency, and HAM should be considered and tested for. • Diagnosis rests upon HTLV-1–specific antibody or PCR testing of blood and CSF. • Imaging is normal. • CSF often is obtained and shows no specific abnormalities.
Differential diagnosis	• *Multiple sclerosis.* Can present with myelopathy with a subacute onset. • *B_{12} deficiency.* Can produce myelopathy, and the patient may have none of the other hematologic or neurologic stigmata of B_{12} deficiency.
Management	• Although there are a plethora of agents now available for treatment of HTLV-III, there is no known treatment for HTLV-I. • Immune-modulating therapy occasionally is helpful—plasma exchange and corticosteroids have been tried with only temporary benefit. • Management of spasticity is supportive. Baclofen, tizanidine, and diazepam commonly are used.
Clinical course	Progressive symptoms are expected, and there is no treatment that alters the course of the disease.

SPINAL MUSCULAR ATROPHY (SMA)	
Description	Progressive lower motor neuron degeneration, predominantly in childhood
Pathophysiology	• SMA is a genetically transmitted disease with predominantly autosomal recessive transmission, although rare X-linked and autosomal-dominant cases have been described. • The primary causative gene is the *SMN-1* gene on chromosome 5, a gene unique to humans. Absence of SMN-1 protein function leads to premature death of spinal motor neurons.
Clinical findings	Spinal muscular atrophy is one of the leading causes of childhood neurologic disability—with an incidence of 1/6000–1/9000 births. Age of onset is correlated with amount of protein function and is divided into four broad categories: • *Early-onset type 1*, usually evident in infancy, also is known as *Werdnig-Hoffmann disease*. Severe generalized flaccid weakness is noted, leading to death by the age of two—usually as a complication of respiratory failure. • When symptoms arise in childhood after the age of 18 months, type III, or *Kugelberg-Welander disease*, is diagnosed. Symptoms are identical, but severity is milder and patients usually survive well into adulthood. • *Type II* is intermediate in onset and severity between types I and III, but there is no corresponding eponym. In Type II SMA, onset is between 6 and 18 months. Patients never walk, but survival into adulthood is common. • SMA type IV, or *adult-onset spinal muscular atrophy*, is exceedingly rare and not associated with the *SMN-I* gene. Gradually progressive limb-girdle weakness with onset after age 20 is seen, along with prominent fasciculations and lack of respiratory muscle involvement. None of the patients have upper motor neuron findings.
Laboratory studies	• Routine labs are normal. • Imaging is normal. MRI often is done to look for a spinal cause of lower motor neuron degeneration. • EMG shows denervation, commonly with acute and chronic features. • Muscle biopsy shows denervation, and commonly is done to look for myopathies, which occasionally can be difficult to distinguish from SMA, especially in the very young.
Diagnosis	Electrodiagnostic testing, muscle biopsy, and genetic assays are very helpful in diagnosing these disorders.

SPINAL MUSCULAR ATROPHY (SMA)—cont'd	
Differential diagnosis	• *Amyotrophic lateral sclerosis.* A degeneration of the upper and lower motor neurons. ALS is not seen in youth. Also, corticospinal tract signs are not seen in SMA. • *Metabolic myopathies.* Can present in childhood with weakness. They are mainly differentiated by muscle biopsy, although some have manifestations on blood testing.
Management	• Treatment is supportive. Patients will have the need for therapy, training in adaptive skills, and medical devices later in the course. • There have been no treatments found effective for limiting the neuronal degeneration.
Clinical course	Weakness is progressive, although very slowly for some.

Werdnig-Hoffmann Disease

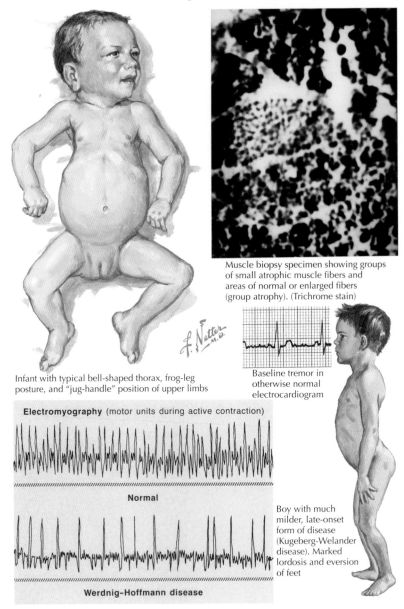

Infant with typical bell-shaped thorax, frog-leg posture, and "jug-handle" position of upper limbs

Muscle biopsy specimen showing groups of small atrophic muscle fibers and areas of normal or enlarged fibers (group atrophy). (Trichrome stain)

Baseline tremor in otherwise normal electrocardiogram

Electromyography (motor units during active contraction)

Normal

Werdnig-Hoffmann disease

Boy with much milder, late-onset form of disease (Kugeberg-Welander disease). Marked lordosis and eversion of feet

AMYOTROPHIC LATERAL SCLEROSIS (ALS)	
Description	Also known as "Lou Gehrig's disease," this is the prototypic motor neuron disease.
Pathophysiology	Degeneration of the upper and lower motor neurons is of unknown cause.
Clinical findings	• The usual clinical pattern is one of progressive painless generalized weakness, often asymmetric at least at onset. Fasciculations and muscle cramping are often seen both clinically and electrophysiologically. • Because motor neurons both in the brain and spinal cord are affected, there is a combination of upper-motor neuron and lower-motor neuron signs on neurologic examination. • Bowel and bladder functions are spared, but brainstem motor function and respiration are always eventually affected. • The disease typically strikes adults in the fifth decade and beyond, although age of onset varies. There is no difference in incidence between sexes. • As the disease progresses, significant weight loss occurs as a result of loss of muscle mass. Disease duration is a dismal 2–5 years, and if there is significant brainstem involvement at the time of diagnosis, duration is much shorter.
Laboratory studies	• Routine labs are normal. • Imaging shows no significant cord compression or lesion. • EMG shows widespread denervation changes, as does muscle biopsy. • Muscle biopsy shows denervation, but is not needed for diagnosis in most patients.
Diagnosis	• ALS is a clinical diagnosis. The combination of progressive weakness with fasciculations, atrophy, and upper motor neuron findings supports the diagnosis. • Imaging of the cord usually is needed to rule out cervical myelopathy. • EMG is needed to document the lower motor neuron degeneration in at least three extremities.
Differential diagnosis	• *Cervical spondylosis.* Can produce progressive weakness of the arms, with lower motor unit dysfunction in the hands and upper motor unit dysfunction in the legs from cord compression. Imaging is needed for diagnosis. Some patients with ALS undergo cervical decompressions when there is doubt about the diagnosis, but at least some of this is unavoidable. • *Myasthenia gravis.* Considered in patients with progressive weakness without sensory symptoms. Ptosis and diplopia are not expected in ALS, whereas they are common in MG. • *Multifocal motor neuropathy.* An autoimmune disorder characterized by weakness without sensory changes.

AMYOTROPHIC LATERAL SCLEROSIS (ALS)—cont'd	
Management	• Riluzole is the only medication approved for treatment of ALS in the United States. Not all patients take riluzole, due to uncertainty that the balance of benefit, cost, and adverse effects favors administration.
	• The remainder of treatment is supportive and palliative.
Clinical course	• Progression is expected, with patients losing independence.
	• Patients should decide about whether they want tube feedings and intubation with mechanical ventilation prior to these issues approaching crisis. Some patients may decide that they want to have complete support, whereas others will decide to withhold some or all of these supports. Most physicians feel these decisions are within the rights of the patient, and it is wrong to impose decisions on them.

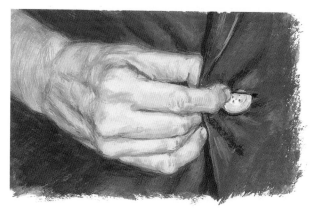

Fine movements of hand impaired; prominent metacarpal bones indicate atrophy of interossei muscles

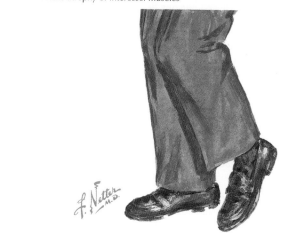

Weak, dragging gait; foot drop or early fatigue on walking

Clinical signs

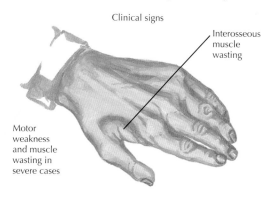

Interosseous muscle wasting

Motor weakness and muscle wasting in severe cases

PARALYTIC POLIO AND POST-POLIO SYNDROME	
Description	Paralytic polio has virtually vanished. Patients present with acute asymmetric paralysis.
Pathophysiology	*Paralytic polio.* Essentially eradicated from the world as an infectious disease, it is caused by a picornavirus transmitted by the fecal-oral route. Remaining polio outbreaks usually are due to politically motivated boycotts of worldwide vaccination programs. Extremely rare cases of polio occur as a result of the oral polio vaccine at a rate of about 1 case per 2.5 million exposures.
	Post-polio syndrome. The exact cause of this syndrome is unknown. There is no reported evidence of viremia in these cases. Acceptance that the syndrome exists is not universal.
Clinical findings	*Paralytic polio:*
	• Greater than 95% of persons infected with polio will experience asymptomatic viremia and spontaneous clearing. Fewer than 1% of exposed persons develop neurologic symptoms, although 2%–3% will develop a viral meningitis, and another 10% will have a brief flulike illness.
	• When neurologic symptoms develop, they do so following a brief flulike prodrome; followed by severe generalized myalgias with focal, often asymmetric, fasciculations; which is then followed by weakness that often is severe. The legs often are most affected, although any muscle or region can be involved, including diaphragm and bulbar muscles.
	• Recovery typically is incomplete, with atrophy and asymmetric weakness that often is permanent. The remaining motor neurons will undergo axonal sprouting so that partial reinnervation occurs, leading to some degree of recovery. This results in very large motor units noted in electromyographic testing.
	Post-polio syndrome:
	• Occasionally a syndrome develops in former paralytic polio victims several years following the initial attack.
	• Patients typically complain of diffuse myalgias and recurrence of weakness in muscles that were affected in the initial attack.
	• The lag between the initial attack and development of so-called post-polio syndrome often is measured in decades.
Laboratory studies	*Paralytic polio.* Routine labs are normal. Imaging is normal or shows inflammatory changes in the spinal cord with high-resolution images. CSF shows pleocytosis, which is initially polymorphonuclear, then evolves to lymphocytic.
	Post-polio syndrome. The diagnosis is more secure when new denervation can be discovered by electromyography in the absence of any other cause. This finding has suggested the hypothesis that the remaining pool of motor neurons has begun to age, fatigue, or otherwise wear out prematurely as a result of dramatically increased workload. In the absence of definitive EMG abnormalities, there is hesitation to suggest this diagnosis.

PARALYTIC POLIO AND POST-POLIO SYNDROME—cont'd	
Diagnosis	*Paralytic polio* is suspected when a patient presents with muscle pain followed by asymmetric weakness in association with a febrile illness, which begins days to weeks prior to the neurologic symptoms. This prodromal phase is typical of a viral illness with fever, sore throat, headache, nausea, and muscle aches. A virus can be detected in stool samples and also can be obtained from throat culture done early in the course. Isolation of virus from the CSF is rare.
	Post-polio syndrome is suspected when a patient with a history of polio has progressive weakness. EMG shows denervation. No other cause of neuronal degeneration is identified.
Differential diagnosis	• *Peripheral neuropathy.* In a patient with previous polio, it can produce what appears to be the post-polio syndrome. AIDP, CIDP, other immune-mediated neuropathies, and idiopathic peripheral neuropathies superimposed on the chronic axonal damage all have to be considered.
	• *Motor neuron diseases.* Including ALS, are considered in the differential diagnosis of post-polio syndrome. Corticospinal tract signs suggest the more ominous diagnosis.
Management	*Paralytic polio.* There is no treatment for the underlying infection. Therapy and support are the mainstays of management.
	Post-polio syndrome. Support and therapy are needed for these patients, with an aim to maintain mobility and functionality. Some have expressed concern that exercise may worsen the function in these patients, but there is no evidence of this.
Clinical course	• Most patients with paralytic polio eventually improve, although the recovery is protracted and incomplete.
	• Post-polio syndrome is a chronic condition and requires continued activity.

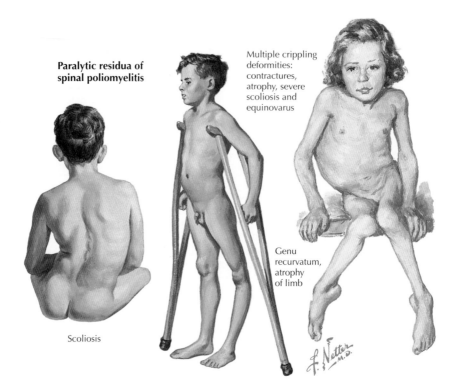

Paralytic residua of spinal poliomyelitis

Multiple crippling deformities: contractures, atrophy, severe scoliosis and equinovarus

Genu recurvatum, atrophy of limb

Scoliosis

OVERVIEW OF NEUROMUSCULAR JUNCTION DISORDERS	
Description	These disorders cause weakness by interfering with the transmission from the motor axon to the muscle fiber.
Pathophysiology	Three disorders comprise the most important neuromuscular transmission problems: • Myasthenia • Myasthenic (Lambert-Eaton) syndrome • Botulism
Common clinical features	• Patients present with weakness and often autonomic symptoms, indicating a deficit in cholinergic transmission. • Fatigability is common, with a significant drop-off in strength with repetitive activity.
Common laboratory features	• There are lab tests for these disorders, discussed on the following pages. • NCS shows abnormal responses to repetitive stimulation, with changes that differ depending on the disorder.
Disorder	**Essential Features**
Myasthenia	• Antibodies to the acetylcholine receptor produce impaired neuromuscular transmission. • Ocular myasthenia is weakness confined to the extraocular muscles and eyelids. • Myasthenia gravis is generalized weakness in addition to ocular weakness.
Myasthenic (Lambert-Eaton) syndrome	• Lambert-Eaton myasthenic syndrome (LEMS) often is related to cancer, particularly of the lung. Patients present with weakness and fatigability, and typically have autonomic symptoms.
Botulism	• Exposure to the toxin *Clostridium botulinum* produces failure of neuromuscular transmission. • Patients have weakness that progresses rapidly and has a slow recovery.

Neuromuscular Transmission

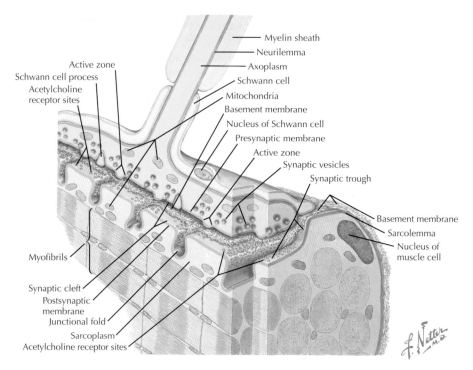

MYASTHENIA	
Description	Autoantibodies against the acetylcholine receptor produce weakness that can affect the entire body or only eye movement.
Pathophysiology	• Autoantibodies bind to the acetylcholine receptor and cause increased receptor degradation. The combination of the binding and the turnover effects results loss of receptor so that an action potential in the motor neuron does not always result in an action potential in the muscle fiber. The normal 1-to-1 transmission from motor axon to muscle fiber breaks down.
	• The cause of the autoantibodies is not known. The thymus is implicated in the inception and generation of the autoantibodies.
	• Thymoma is present in some patients with myasthenia.
Clinical findings	• Myasthenia presents in two ways—ocular and generalized (myasthenia gravis).
	• *Ocular myasthenia* is characterized by ptosis and weakness of eye movement that cannot be explained by a single ocular motor nerve or muscle lesion. Both eyes are affected, although not equally so. Patients with pure ocular involvement at onset usually remain pure ocular; however, some will progress to generalized myasthenia.
	• *Myasthenia gravis* (MG) is characterized by weakness not only of the ocular muscles, but also of bulbar and extremity muscles. Dysarthria, dysphagia, and weakness with arising from a chair are some of the common symptoms.
	• There are no sensory findings.
	• Weakness tends to be better in the morning and worse later in the day.
Laboratory studies	• Routine labs are normal. Myasthenia antibody testing shows abnormalities in most patients.
	• EMG often shows no abnormalities on routine testing, but repetitive stimulation usually shows a decremental response from the muscle with stimulation rates of 3/sec. Single fiber EMG shows increased jitter.
	• CT of the chest may show thymoma.
Diagnosis	• Myasthenia is suspected when a patient presents with diplopia and ptosis. Bilateral symptoms are more commonly myasthenia than unilateral.
	• Generalized weakness, especially with dysarthria and dysphagia, along with the bulbar weakness, supports the diagnosis of myasthenia gravis.
	• Myasthenia antibodies can confirm the diagnosis.
	• Chest CT is done on patients with myasthenia to look for thymoma.

MYASTHENIA—cont'd	
Differential diagnosis	• *Myasthenic (Eaton-Lambert) syndrome.* A paraneoplastic syndrome characterized by diffuse weakness and autonomic deficits. Paraneoplastic antibodies can help to make this differentiation. EMG special testing also can suggest myasthenic syndrome rather than myasthenia, although not all EMG machines have the capability of this testing.
	• *Inflammatory myopathy.* Patients with polymyositis can present with weakness and fatigue without sensory deficit. EMG shows myopathic features. CPK is elevated.
Management	• Weakness is managed by aceytlcholinesterase inhibitors. Long-term therapy is with immune suppression. Crisis is managed with plasma exchange or IVIG.
	• Immune suppression is a cornerstone of treatment with myasthenia, and mainly is used for people with generalized myasthenia—myasthenia gravis. Corticosteroids, such as prednisone, are begun as daily dosing, and ultimately adjusted to an alternating-day dosing schedule. The dose is tapered, so that most patients are able to get to a low alternating-day dosing schedule. Stronger agents, such as azathioprine and other chemotherapy agents, also are used, but are less common.
	• Acetylcholinesterase inhibitors are used for most patients with ocular myasthenia and myasthenia gravis. These are purely symptomatic and not disease-altering. They inhibit the breakdown of acetylcholine at the neuromuscular junction, thereby improving transmission.
	• Thymectomy is performed for patients with thymoma, and in patients who have not had adequate response to immune modulation treatment.
	• Intravenous immuoglobulin (IVIG) is used for some patients in crisis, and can help to improve strength. The risk is relatively low with close monitoring of the patients.
	• Plasma exchange (PE) is used for patients with crisis, and can be of tremendous benefit. PE often is often used if IVIG is not tolerated, contraindicated, or ineffective.
Clinical course	• Improvement is expected, although most patients are maintained on a low-dose corticosteroid after their initial tapering.
	• Crisis may develop requiring hospitalization, administration or IVIG or PE, and/or transient increases in corticosteroids.

Myasthenia Gravis: Clinical Manifestations

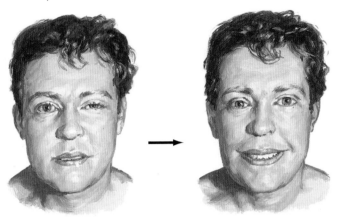

Ptosis and weakness of smile
are common early signs

Improvement after
edrophonium chloride

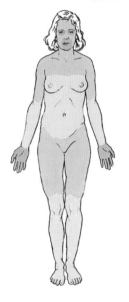

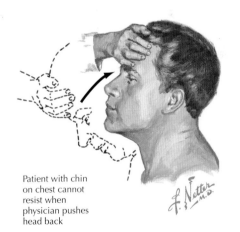

Patient with chin
on chest cannot
resist when
physician pushes
head back

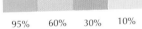

95%   60%   30%   10%

Regional distribution
of muscle weakness

LAMBERT-EATON MYASTHENIC SYNDROME (LEMS)	
Description	• Autoimmune disease affecting the neuromuscular junction • Associated with cancer, especially small cell lung cancer
Pathophysiology	• LEMS is a prototypic paraneoplastic condition. The most commonly associated cancer is small cell lung cancer. • Most patients have antibodies to voltage-gated calcium channels (VGCC). • The deficit is in transmitter release.
Clinical findings	• LEMS presents with a weakness and fatigue, mainly affecting proximal muscles. • Autonomic symptoms, including dry mouth, constipation, impotence, and bladder dysfunction, are common. • Tendon reflexes are decreased.
Laboratory studies	• Routine labs are normal. • Paraneoplastic panel shows antibodies to the voltage-gated calcium channel. • Imaging of the brain and spine is normal. Imaging of the chest is done to look for neoplasm, and often is positive. • NCS and EMG show an incremental response to repetitive stimulation at high rates. • Positron emission tomography (PET) can be performed to look for cancer.
Diagnosis	• LEMS is considered when a patient presents with proximal weakness. Myopathy usually is considered first, but EMG does not show myopathic features and CK typically is not elevated. Paraneoplastic panel is ordered, whether or not there is a known cancer. • Diagnosis is confirmed by NCS, EMG, and the VGCC antibodies. • Vigilance for cancer must continue after diagnosis—many months may elapse between development of any paraneoplastic condition and diagnosis of the cancer.
Differential diagnosis	• *Myasthenia gravis.* The main differential diagnosis. Patients present with weakness and abnormal response to repetitive stimulation, but the pattern of abnormality is different. Also, there are different results of antibody testing with MG, as opposed to LEMS. • *ALS.* Considered in patients with progressive weakness, although the weakness is more prominent distally. Also, corticospinal tract signs are seen in ALS, but not LEMS.
Management	• Diaminopyridine and pyridostigmine are used to improve strength of patients with LEMS, especially for disease that is not associated with malignancy. Guanidine is used but has significant toxicity. • Immune-modulating therapy often is used, including corticosteroids, IVIG, or plasma exchange.
Clinical course	• LEMS is a chronic condition, requiring continuing treatment. • Vigilance for the late development of cancer is needed.

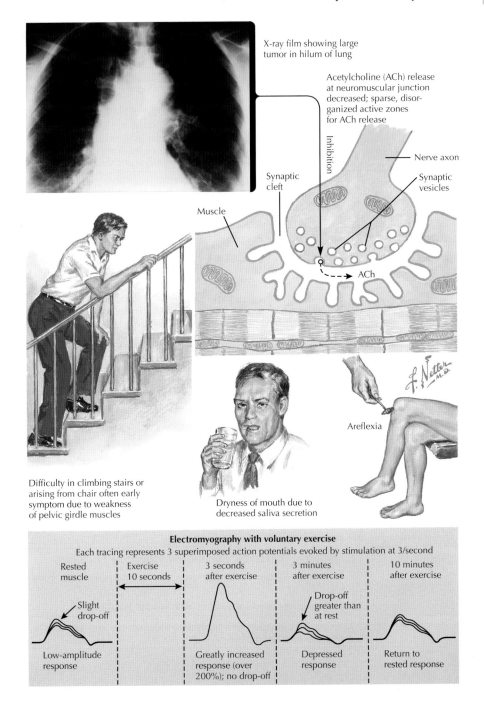

X-ray film showing large tumor in hilum of lung

Acetylcholine (ACh) release at neuromuscular junction decreased; sparse, disorganized active zones for ACh release

Inhibition

Nerve axon

Synaptic cleft

Synaptic vesicles

Muscle

ACh

Areflexia

Difficulty in climbing stairs or arising from chair often early symptom due to weakness of pelvic girdle muscles

Dryness of mouth due to decreased saliva secretion

Electromyography with voluntary exercise

Each tracing represents 3 superimposed action potentials evoked by stimulation at 3/second

Rested muscle	Exercise 10 seconds	3 seconds after exercise	3 minutes after exercise	10 minutes after exercise
Slight drop-off			Drop-off greater than at rest	
Low-amplitude response		Greatly increased response (over 200%); no drop-off	Depressed response	Return to rested response

BOTULISM	
Description	Paralyzing illness due to toxin of *C. botulinum* strains
Pathophysiology	• Botulinum toxin is produced by clostridium strains in anaerobic conditions. • The toxin binds to the presynaptic terminal and prevents release of acetylcholine from the terminal. • Exposure to botulinum toxin is from food or wound infection. Injections of botulinum toxin can produce localized weakness, but systemic botulism does not occur at therapeutic doses.
Clinical findings	• Botulism presents with autonomic symptoms, including nausea, abdominal cramps, diarrhea or constipation, followed by generalized weakness. Weakness of ocular motor and bulbar muscles also is present. Pupillary constriction is impaired as well.
Laboratory studies	• Routine labs are normal. • Imaging of the brain and spine is normal. Imaging often is performed of the brain when there are bulbar signs; of the spine when extremity weakness predominates. • NCS and EMG show reduced amplitude of the compound motor action potential. Special testing may show an incremental response to high rates of repetitive stimulation and an augmentation of response with exercise. The response often is patchy, with some muscles being normal.
Diagnosis	• Botulism is suspected when a patient presents with rapidly progressive weakness in the setting of autonomic symptoms shortly predating the weakness. • Diagnosis is supported by the typical electrophysiologic studies. • Toxin can be assayed in body fluids and foods. Isolation of the bacterium without the toxin does not make the diagnosis.
Differential diagnosis	• *Myasthenia gravis.* Presents with ocular motor weakness and generalized muscle weakness. Autonomic symptoms are not prominent. Also, the NCS and EMG findings differ with slow and fast repetitive stimulation. • *Lambert-Eaton myasthenic syndrome.* Presents with weakness and autonomic symptoms, although this is not a fulminant presentation as with botulism.
Management	• Supportive treatment is essential and typically can be difficult. • Antitoxin is administered whenever possible, and is available from the CDC. • Antibiotics are used for patients with wound botulism.
Clinical course	Most patients improve with treatment, although the improvement is protracted and incomplete.

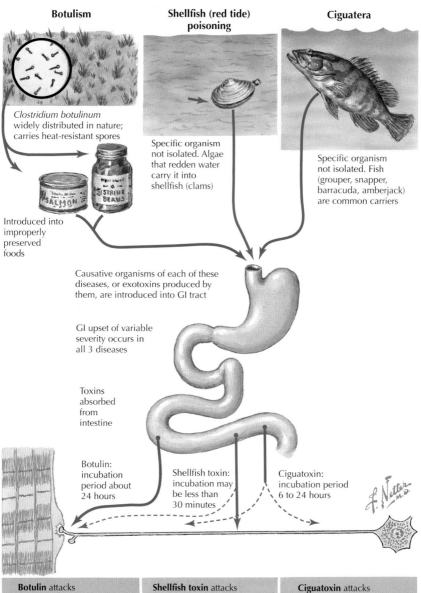

Botulism

Clostridium botulinum widely distributed in nature; carries heat-resistant spores

Introduced into improperly preserved foods

Shellfish (red tide) poisoning

Specific organism not isolated. Algae that redden water carry it into shellfish (clams)

Ciguatera

Specific organism not isolated. Fish (grouper, snapper, barracuda, amberjack) are common carriers

Causative organisms of each of these diseases, or exotoxins produced by them, are introduced into GI tract

GI upset of variable severity occurs in all 3 diseases

Toxins absorbed from intestine

Botulin: incubation period about 24 hours

Shellfish toxin: incubation may be less than 30 minutes

Ciguatoxin: incubation period 6 to 24 hours

Botulin attacks neuromuscular junction. Weakness, paralysis, respiratory distress occur. Prognosis variable, may be fatal	**Shellfish toxin** attacks peripheral motor neuron. Weakness, paralysis, respiratory distress, paresthesias occur. Prognosis variable, better than in botulism	**Ciguatoxin** attacks peripheral nerve, exact site unknown. Weakness, paralysis, radicular pain occur. Prognosis generally good

OVERVIEW OF MYOPATHIES	
Description	Myopathies are muscle degenerations, which can be congenital or acquired
Pathophysiology	The final common pathway to myopathies is muscle degeneration, which is caused by metabolic abnormalities in the muscle, toxins, or inflammation.
Clinical findings	• Myopathies present with weakness that is most prominent proximally. • There are no sensory findings.
Laboratory studies	• Muscle enzymes are elevated in most myopathies. Creatine kinase (CK) and aldolase are usually markedly elevated. Mild elevation can occur with neuropathy or motor neuron disease or in patients with "burned-out" late state myopathies. • Imaging is normal. • NCS and EMG show myopathic features. • Biopsy often can be specific about the diagnosis, whether type of dystrophy or inflammatory myopathy is determined.
Diagnosis	• Myopathy is suspected when a patient presents with generalized weakness that is most prominent proximally. The absence of sensory involvement and the absence of corticospinal tract signs argue in favor of myopathy. • Elevated CK and aldolase is supportive of myopathy. • NCS is normal. EMG shows myopathic features. • Muscle biopsy often is needed to give the definitive diagnosis.
Important Myopathies	**Essential Features**
Inflammatory myopathies	• Present with weakness, usually without pain • Have an association with neoplasms and other autoimmune diseases • Rash with inflammatory myopathy is dermatomyositis. • Muscle biopsy is diagnostic of the inflammatory component.
Muscular dystrophies	• Degenerative conditions characterized by weakness and often hypertrophy of the muscles • Occur in younger patients more than inflammatory myopathies • Muscle biopsy is diagnostic.
Toxic myopathies	• Present with weakness and elevated CK • The list of possible offending agents is large. Alcohol is one of the most important ones.
Periodic paralyses	• A group of disorders that present with attacks of weakness. Other features differ between subtype. • Patients usually have normal examination between attacks, although development of static weakness can occur.

Myopathy suspected
- Weakness, fatigue
- No sensory symptoms

NCS & EMG
- *Myopathy* – myopathic features on EMG. NCS is normal or reduced amplitudes
- *Neuropathy* – neuropathic features on EMG. NCS usually shows slowing +/o reduced amplitudes, depending on the type (axonal, demyelinating)
- *Neuromuscular transmission disorder* – EMG often normal. NCS special testing shows impaired transmission

Myopathy confirmed
- Determine the type
- Consider: dystrophy, inflammatory, metabolic, toxic disorder

Myopathy not confirmed
- Still could be myopathy
- Normal (e.g., FMS/CFS)
- Neuropathy
- Neuromuscular transmission defect

Labs may include
- TFTs, ANA, ESR, Cortisol, CPK, aldolase
- Muscle biopsy is confirmatory

Labs may include
- B$_{12}$, Folate, TFTs, ANA, ESR, Cortisol, CPK, aldolase, SIEP
- Antibody studies for myasthenia, myasthenic syndrome

Myopathy	No evidence of myopathy	
Muscular dystrophy • Weakness often with muscle hypertrophy • ↑CPK, aldolase • Dx: muscle biopsy	**ALS** • Weakness without sensory symptoms, but with corticospinal tract signs • Dx: Clinical and EMG	**Normal** • Weakness reported with normal exam • Labs are normal
Inflammatory myopathy • Weakness, occurs +/– muscle pain • ↑CPK, aldolase • Dx: muscle biopsy	**Myasthenia** • Weakness and fatigue without sensory symptoms • Dx: Lab and NCS special studies	**Neuropathy** • Weakness often with sensory symptoms • Labs and EMG show the diagnosis
Metabolic myopathy • Weakness and fatigue • Labs may show metabolic defect • Dx: muscle biopsy	**Lambert Eaton Myasthenic syndrome** • Weakness with autonomic symptoms • Dx: Lab and NCS special studies	**Multifocal motor neuropathy** • Weakness without sensory symptoms • Dx: Clinical and EMG

INFLAMMATORY MYOPATHIES—POLYMYOSITIS AND DERMATOMYOSITIS	
Description	Inflammatory myopathies produce weakness, mainly of proximal muscles. They can be idiopathic or due to other systemic disease.
Pathophysiology	Autoimmune disease, characterized by inflammatory degeneration of skeletal muscles. The cause of the immune attack is usually unknown, but cancer and connective tissue disease are present in some individuals.
Clinical findings	• There are three basic types—idiopathic polymyositis, idiopathic dermatomyositis, and inflammatory myopathy associated with connective tissue or cancer. • Weakness is the most prominent symptom, mainly of proximal muscles. Dysarthria and dysphagia are common, as is weakness of neck muscles; head instability is a common presenting sign. • Pain is not common, despite the inflammatory pathophysiology. Muscle pain without weakness is not polymyositis. • Reflexes are normal or slightly depressed. • Sensory function is normal. • Rash is seen in patients with dermatomyositis, and can be variable. Rash across the cheeks, bridge of the nose, and dorsum of the hands can be seen. • If the inflammatory myopathy is due to connective tissue disease, the common associations are lupus, rheumatoid arthritis, mixed connective tissue disease, and scleroderma. • Inflammatory myopathy due to cancer may be due to lung, breast, ovarian, or colon neoplasms.
Laboratory studies	• Routine bloods are normal, but CK and aldolase are increased. • Imaging is usually not needed, but if the inflammatory myopathy is thought to be due to malignancy, then body PET may be revealing. • Paraneoplastic panel may be positive, and search for cancer should always be considered. • EMG shows myopathic features in the vast majority of patients. • Muscle biopsy shows inflammatory changes in most patients.
Diagnosis	• Polymyositis is suspected when a patient presents with proximal weakness without pain or sensory abnormality. • Diagnosis can be confirmed by elevated CK and aldolase, myopathic changes on EMG, and characteristic features of muscle biopsy. However, not all of these features will be present, but the diagnosis is secure with three of the four basic features. • Dermatomyositis is diagnosed by making the diagnosis of polymyositis plus the characteristic rash.

INFLAMMATORY MYOPATHIES—POLYMYOSITIS AND DERMATOMYOSITIS—cont'd	
Differential diagnosis	• *Muscular dystrophy.* Presents with proximal muscle weakness, but the onset is slow. Onset in middle-aged or late adult life is not expected. • *Myasthenia gravis.* Presents with weakness but also with ocular motor weakness, which is not expected with polymyositis. • *ALS.* Can present with dysarthria and dysphagia in addition to generalized weakness. The weakness is more prominent distally than proximally. EMG findings are neuropathic rather than myopathic.
Management	• Immune suppression results in complete remission for some patients. Others need continued suppressive therapy. First-line treatment is with corticosteroid such as prednisone. Initial daily dosing is followed by alternate day dosing with a gradual taper. • Chemotherapy with azathioprine or methotrexate is used for patients who do not respond to corticosteroids.
Clinical course	Most patients improve with corticosteroids and/or chemotherapy. Some patients have complete response and are able to eventually get off meds, whereas others continue to require medications.

Dermatomyositis and Polymyositis

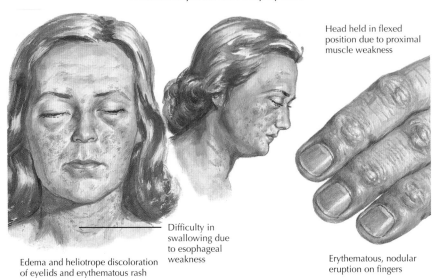

Head held in flexed position due to proximal muscle weakness

Difficulty in swallowing due to esophageal weakness

Edema and heliotrope discoloration of eyelids and erythematous rash

Erythematous, nodular eruption on fingers

Muscle biopsy: atrophy of muscle fibers and lymphocyte infiltration

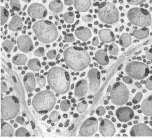

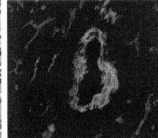

Fluorescence slide of muscle revealing gammaglobulin deposition in blood vessel

MUSCULAR DYSTROPHIES	
Description	• Muscular degeneration results in progressive weakness. • The muscular dystrophies are hereditary and the responsible genes and gene products have been identified for some.
Pathophysiology	• Muscular dystrophies are due to genetic errors. The most common is dystrophin deficiency, responsible for Duchenne and Becker dystrophy. • The responsible products for many other types have not been identified, but a common thread is genetic defect leading to metabolic derangement leading to muscular degeneration.

Clinical findings	There are many types of muscular dystrophies. Among the most important are:
	  • Duchenne muscular dystrophy
	  • Becker muscular dystrophy
	  • Myotonic dystrophy
	  • Limb-girdle dystrophy
	  • Facioscapulohumeral dystrophy
	  • Scapuloperoneal dystrophy
	The common features are weakness most prominent in proximal muscles and absence of sensory abnormalities. Depending on the subtype, other findings may include facial and bulbar weakness, muscle hypertrophy, myotonia, and/or cramps.

Laboratory studies	• Routine labs are normal for most patients. CK and aldolase are elevated for most muscular dystrophies. • Imaging is normal, and not needed for most patients. • EMG shows myopathic features. • Muscle biopsy shows myopathic features, and special studies for dystrophin and other gene products can help with the diagnosis.
Diagnosis	• Muscular dystrophy is suspected in a patient with progressive weakness, especially with onset in childhood. • Elevated CK and aldolase and myopathic changes on EMG support the diagnosis. • Muscle biopsy confirms the diagnosis.
Differential diagnosis	• *Spinal muscular atrophy.* Considered in a child with weakness. The weakness is more distal than with MD. Also, EMG and muscle biopsy show neuropathic findings rather than myopathic features. • *Inflammatory myopathies.* Can present with weakness without sensory signs. These can occur in youth, but are more common in older patients.
Management	• Corticosteroids have recently been shown to be effective in preserving muscle function in children with Duchenne muscular dystrophy. • No other treatments have been shown to alter the course of the disease. • Physical therapy is helpful and is combined with braces, when needed.

MUSCULAR DYSTROPHIES—cont'd	
Clinical course	• Progression is expected. Muscles become weaker. • The calves may show progressive hypertrophy, especially with dystrophin deficiency; however, this muscle is ineffectual, and weakness is present.

Individual Dystrophies	Essential Features
Duchenne	• An X-linked disorder related to dystrophin deficiency • Patients present with weakness, pseudohypertrophy of the calves, Gower's sign (climbing up self to stand erect). • Onset is in young childhood, and patients live into late adolescence. • Corticosteroids have recently been shown to maintain mobility, and are offered to most patients.
Becker-type	• Also a dystrophinopathy with abnormal dystrophin. This is also X-linked. • Onset is later than with Duchenne dystrophy and patients live to adult life. • The role of corticosteroids in treatment has not been established.
Myotonic	• An autosomal dominant disorder that presents with weakness that is more prominent distally. Hatchet facies, cataracts, and glucose intolerance are other important features.
Limb-girdle	• A family of disorders with mainly autosomal dominant inheritance. The biochemical defects have largely been identified. • Patients present with weakness that can be predominantly arm, leg, scapular, and/or pelvic weakness, depending on the disorder. The limb weakness can be more prominent proximally and distally, depending on the disorder.
Facio-scapulo-humeral (FSH)	• An autosomal dominant disorder that presents with facial weakness followed by arm and shoulder girdle weakness. Despite the name, proximal weakness of the legs is common.
Scapuloperoneal	• This is a group of disorders that present with weakness that is prominent in the scapular muscles and in the region of the tibialis anterior—anterior compartment of the lower leg. Inheritance is autosomal dominant or X-linked recessive.

Duchenne Muscular Dystrophy

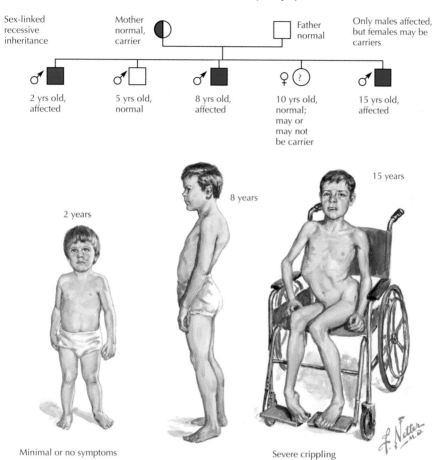

Sex-linked recessive inheritance

Mother normal, carrier

Father normal

Only males affected, but females may be carriers

♂ 2 yrs old, affected

♂ 5 yrs old, normal

♂ 8 yrs old, affected

♀ (?) 10 yrs old, normal; may or may not be carrier

♂ 15 yrs old, affected

2 years

8 years

15 years

Minimal or no symptoms

Severe crippling deformities and contractures

TOXIC MYOPATHIES	
Description	Muscle inflammation and degeneration can develop in response to toxins, which may be drugs.
Pathophysiology	• The most common toxic myopathy is due to alcohol intoxication. • Statins have been implicated in causing toxic myopathies. • Types of abnormalities can range from myalgia without overt pathology to focal ischemic myopathy to chronic myopathy to acute rhabdomyolysis.
Clinical findings	• *Myalgia* is muscle pain and can develop in almost any cause of myopathy. However, myalgia can occur without pathologic change in the muscle. Myalgia is common in patients with statin therapy, and the incidence in placebo-treated controls is almost the same. Exam is normal. • *Rhabdomyolysis* presents with muscle pain and swelling. Muscles are weak, partly due to pain and partly due to decreased contractile ability if the myopathy is severe. • *Focal myopathy* presents with focal muscle pain and swelling.
Laboratory studies	• Routine labs are usually normal, although alcoholics often have chemical signs including hyponatremia, hypomagnesemia, increased LFTs, and others. • Myoglobinuria is seen in patients with rhabdomyolysis. • EMG is abnormal in patients with rhabdomyolysis, and often shows signs of acute muscle destruction. • CK is elevated in patients with myopathy. • Muscle biopsy shows myopathic changes. In some patients, focal ischemic changes can be seen. • Imaging is usually not needed.
Diagnosis	• *Myalgia* is a clinical diagnosis and often has no pathologic correlate. CK is performed, but is usually normal or only mildly increased—even minor trauma can increase CK. • *Chronic myopathy* is suspected with weakness with or without pain in the absence of sensory findings. • *Rhabdomyolysis* is suspected when a patient develops swollen and tender muscles. Elevated CK, renal insufficiency, and myoglobinuria support the diagnosis.
Differential diagnosis	• *Critical illness myopathy.* Considered in a sick patient with weakness and increased CK, but this occurs usually after at least 7 days of hospital care. • *Benign elevation in CK.* Seen in some patients and is not associated with muscle destruction or risk of renal failure. • *Polyneuropathy from any cause.* Can be associated with mild elevation in CK, but EMG shows neuropathic changes rather than myopathic changes. Also, there are usually signs of sensory involvement in symptoms, signs, or NCS.

TOXIC MYOPATHIES—cont'd	
Management	• Treatment is supportive with discontinuation of the offending agent. • Statins should be discontinued, if possible. However, the incidence of myopathy due to statins is generally overstated.
Clinical course	Most patients improve, with the degree of residual deficit depending on magnitude of the problem. Rhabdomyolysis may result in incomplete recovery.

Effects of Alcohol on End Organs

Cellular damage

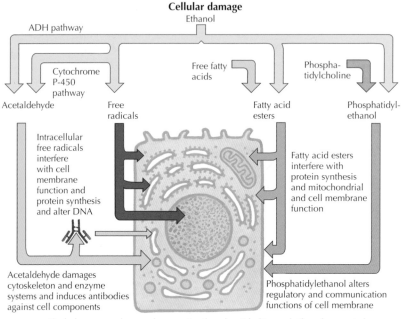

Ethanol

ADH pathway

Cytochrome P-450 pathway

Acetaldehyde

Free fatty acids

Phospha-tidylcholine

Free radicals

Fatty acid esters

Phosphatidyl-ethanol

Intracellular free radicals interfere with cell membrane function and protein synthesis and alter DNA

Fatty acid esters interfere with protein synthesis and mitochondrial and cell membrane function

Acetaldehyde damages cytoskeleton and enzyme systems and induces antibodies against cell components

Phosphatidylethanol alters regulatory and communication functions of cell membrane

Alcohol causes end-organ damage via ethanol metabolites and ethanol-generated compounds, which alter structure and function of cell components

Organ damage

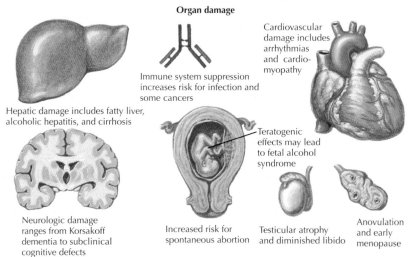

Immune system suppression increases risk for infection and some cancers

Cardiovascular damage includes arrhythmias and cardio-myopathy

Hepatic damage includes fatty liver, alcoholic hepatitis, and cirrhosis

Teratogenic effects may lead to fetal alcohol syndrome

Neurologic damage ranges from Korsakoff dementia to subclinical cognitive defects

Increased risk for spontaneous abortion

Testicular atrophy and diminished libido

Anovulation and early menopause

JOHN A. CRAIG—AD

PERIODIC PARALYSIS	
Description	A group of disorders with a common feature of episodic weakness due to electrical inexcitability of the muscle fiber membrane
Pathophysiology	Basic types of periodic paralysis are hyperkalemic, hypokalemic, and normokalemic. All are inherited as autosomal dominant: • *Hyperkalemic periodic paralysis* features a marked increase in potassium increases markedly during the attack. • *Hypokalemic periodic paralysis* shows a fall in potassium during an episode. • *Normokalemic periodic paralysis* is associated with no change in potassium but is thought to be related to hyperkalemic periodic paralysis. Potassium loading can cause an attack in some individuals.
Clinical findings	• Periodic paralysis presents with episodic weakness without pain. The pattern differs between elements. • Hyperkalemic periodic paralysis presents with diffuse weakness that is most prominent after exercise. • Hypokalemic periodic paralysis presents with weakness that is most prominent after heavy carbohydrate meal or strenuous exercise. Patients may awaken from sleep with paralysis after a precipitating event. • Normokalemic periodic paralysis presents similarly to hypokalemic periodic paralysis.
Laboratory studies	• Routine labs are usually normal between attacks. During attacks, there may be an increase or decrease in serum potassium, depending on the subtype of the disorder. • Imaging is normal. • NCS usually is normal. EMG is normal between attacks, unless fixed myopathic changes develop.
Diagnosis	• Periodic paralysis is suspected when a patient presents with complaints of episodic weakness. • Exam is normal. • EMG is normal between attacks, although late in the condition, myopathic findings clinically and on EMG can develop.
Differential diagnosis	Other causes of myopathy have to be considered, although there are few disorders with episodic weakness.
Management	• Hyperkalemic periodic paralysis is treated by hydrochlorothiazide, with or without acetazolamide. • Hypokalemic periodic paralysis is treated by daily administration of potassium.
Clinical course	• Most patients improve with treatment, although recurrent attacks are common. • Persistent myopathic changes are seen subsequently.

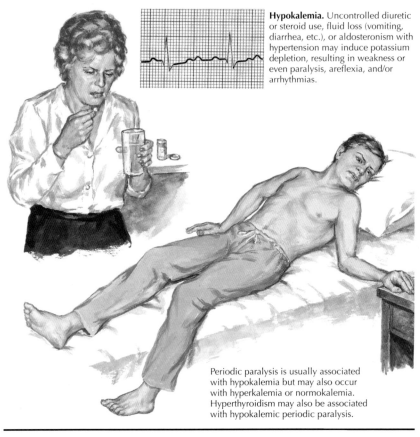

Hypokalemia. Uncontrolled diuretic or steroid use, fluid loss (vomiting, diarrhea, etc.), or aldosteronism with hypertension may induce potassium depletion, resulting in weakness or even paralysis, areflexia, and/or arrhythmias.

Periodic paralysis is usually associated with hypokalemia but may also occur with hyperkalemia or normokalemia. Hyperthyroidism may also be associated with hypokalemic periodic paralysis.

Hyperkalemia. Addison's disease (primary adrenocortical insufficiency), characterized by bronzing of skin, weakness, weight loss, and hypotension, is associated with elevated serum potassium. Manifestations may be mild in early stages, with weakness predominating.

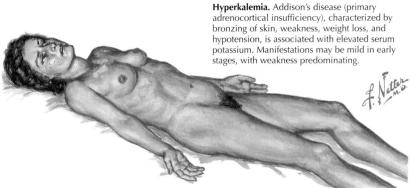

CRITICAL ILLNESS MYOPATHY	
Description	Patients in critical care units have an increased incidence of myopathy.
Pathophysiology	• The same risk factors for critical-illness polyneuropathy are risk factors for critical-illness myopathy—bed rest with disuse, corticosteroid therapy, and paralytic agents.
Clinical findings	• Diffuse weakness and depressed reflexes is the most common clinical presentation. Patients often have failure to wean quickly from the ventilator. • Sensory symptoms are absent.
Laboratory studies	• Routine labs are normal. CK and aldolase are typically elevated. • EMG show normal sensory conduction but compound motor action potentials are very small. Electrical stimulation of the motor nerves may not activate the muscles. • Muscle biopsy shows necrosis in severe cases, atrophy most prominent of type 2 fibers in milder cases. • Imaging is normal and usually not needed.
Diagnosis	• Diagnosis is clinical, with weakness, hyporeflexia, hypotonia, and elevated muscle enzymes. • EMG can be supportive of the diagnosis. • Muscle biopsy is definitive, although it is not needed in most patients, because in the appropriate clinical setting, supportive care is satisfactory for ruling out other diagnoses that would alter management.
Differential diagnosis	• *Critical illness polyneuropathy.* Presents with diffuse weakness, hypotonia, and hyporeflexia. CIP is difficult to distinguish from CIM. Sensory findings are identified in CIP, but because there are few sensory complaints, the diagnosis can be missed. • *AIDP.* Presents with weakness and areflexia, and can be of increased incidence around the time of a serious illness. • *Rhabdomyolysis.* Can present with weakness and a myopathic pattern on EMG. CPK is extremely high, and there is risk for renal failure. • *Myasthenia.* Can present as diffuse weakness that may initially be attributed to CHF, DM, or some other medical illness.
Management	Treatment is supportive. There is no intervention other than avoiding precipitating events.
Clinical course	Patients typically have improvement, but necrotizing damage to the muscles may not recover.

OVERVIEW OF INFECTIONS OF THE NERVOUS SYSTEM	
Description	Infections are one of the cardinal mechanisms of neurologic disease. Infections of the nervous system mainly include meningitis and encephalitis.
Pathophysiology	• Infections of the nervous system can be bacterial, viral, fungal, parasitic, or prion. • Viral syndromes are most common, with bacterial meningitis being fairly common in busy emergency departments.

Methods of involvement	Include:
	  • Abscess
	  • Meningitis
	  • Encephalitis
	  • Sepsis syndrome
	  • Post infectious effects

Infectious agents affecting the nervous system	Include:
	  • Bacteria
	  • Fungus
	  • Virus
	  • Parasite
	  • Prion

Type of Infection	Essential Features
Bacterial meningitis	• Fulminant meningitis with headache, nuchal rigidity, and fever. Appears toxic. • Occurs in a normal host • Prominent leukocytosis in the cerebrospinal fluid (CSF) • Requires antibiotics for improvement
Viral meningitis	• Subacute to acute meningitis with headache and some nuchal rigidity. May have fever. • Mild to moderate lymphocytic pleocytosis in the CSF
Fungal meningitis	• Subacute to chronic meningitis with any of headache, cranial nerve palsies, and cognitive changes. Meningeal signs often are absent. • More common in immunocompromised host • Mild to moderate lymphocytic pleocytosis in the CSF • Antifungal treatment is required for improvement.
Viral encephalitis	• Acute to subacute encephalitis with headache, confusion, and sometimes fever • Mild lymphocytic pleocytosis, with increased red cells with HSV encephalitis • HSV encephalitis responds to antiviral agents, but most viruses do not.

Type of Infection	Essential Features
Prion encephalitis	• Chronic dementing disease, often with myoclonus • CSF may be normal, and specific testing for prion products is needed. • There is no effective treatment.
Brain abscess	• Most brain abscesses are bacterial, although fungi and parasites can produce solid foci of infection. • Abscess is diagnosed by biopsy, and treatment may include medication with or without resection, depending on the etiology and location.
SECONDARY EFFECTS OF INFECTIONS	

- Infections of the nervous system can produce secondary effects in a number of ways. These include mass effect, edema, post infectious autoimmune syndromes, and neurologic consequences of sepsis syndrome.
- Mass effect and edema can develop from infection and can produce damage to otherwise uninvolved neurons through compression and secondary ischemia.
- Post infectious autoimmune syndromes include acute disseminated encephalomyelitis (ADEM), acute inflammatory demyelinating polyneuropathy (AIDP), and a few others. In these conditions, there are central or peripheral demyelinating changes, respectively.
- Immune deficiency associated with HIV increases the incidence of neurologic disorders as well.

Bacterial meningitis

Inflammation and suppurative process on surface of leptomeninges of brain and spinal cord

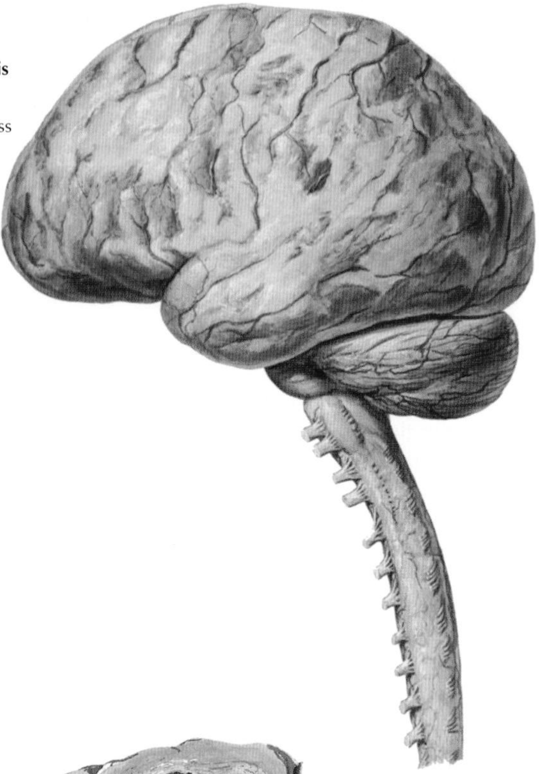

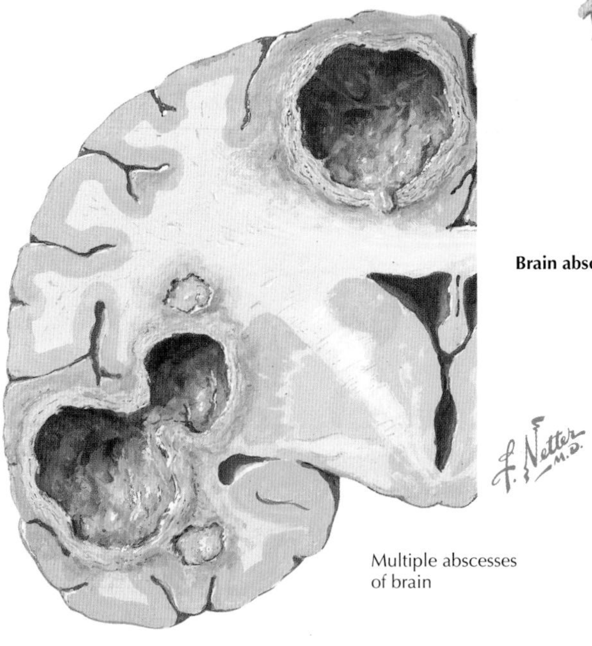

Brain abscess

Multiple abscesses of brain

EVALUATION OF SUSPECTED CENTRAL NERVOUS SYSTEM (CNS) INFECTION	
Symptoms of CNS infection	• Fever with headache • Confusion of subacute onset • Development of seizures with mental status changes
Clinical Scenario	**Synopsis and Approach**
Fever with headache without other neurologic signs	• Bacterial meningitis could cause this manifestation, although viral meningitis and noncentral nervous system (CNS) infections also can do this. • Neurologic evaluation usually is normal in this scenario. • In the absence of signs of CNS dysfunction, blood testing, and urgent lumbar puncture (LP) can be done.
Fever with confusion or focal signs or seizure, with or without headache	• Meningitis, brain abscess, and encephalitis all can produce this presentation. • LP should be delayed because of the risk for herniation if there is mass lesion. Therefore, emergent imaging with CT is indicated prior to LP. Antibiotics are given prior to the imaging, and, therefore, there is no delay in treatment. • LP is performed if the imaging is normal.
Focal deficit with imaging suggesting abscess	• Patients being evaluated for an indication other than suspected infection may have a scan that suggests abscess. Magnetic resonance imaging (MRI) and computed tomography (CT) are not specific enough to make the differentiation of abscess vs. tumor; however, there are guidelines. • The urgency of evaluation is greater if the patient is thought to have potential for abscess, and biopsy usually is indicated if the lesion is at all accessible.
Confusion in a patient with known immunodeficiency	• Direct effects of the immunodeficiency virus and opportunistic infections have to be considered. • Imaging with CT or MRI usually is done first, because brain abscess is common, especially in patients with AIDS, where toxoplasmosis predominates.

CNS infection suspected
- Fever with headache, or
- Altered mental status of subacute onset
- Seizures and altered mental status

Evaluation
- CT usually first
- MRI if possible
- Labs: CMP. CBC, CRP, ANA, ESR, blood cultures
- Echo: for suspected bacterial abscess
- LP: if no mass lesion for possible meningitis, encephalitis
- Brain biopsy: for abscess and occasionally for encephalitis

Abscess
- Focal or multifocal infection of the brain
- Cause is usually bacterial and related to sinus or dental disease. Consider cardiac emboli. Consider immune disorder
- Abscess may be in spine.
- Specific entity determined by surgery – aspiration, biopsy, or excision

Meningitis
- Infection of the CSF usually viral, may be bacterial or fungal
- *Viral:* CSF ↑ WBC, ↑ protein.
- *Bacterial:* CSF ↑↑ WBC, ↑ protein, ↓ glucose
- *Fungal:* CAF ↑ WBC, ↑ protein, may be ↓ glucose

Encephalitis
- Viral or prion infection of the brain
- CT and MRI may show regions of edema, enhancement
- LP may show mild elevation in protein, WBC, or RBC
- EEG often slow, with characteristic periodic pattern in HSV encephalitis

Abscess

Bacterial abscess
- MRI/CT shows enhancing lesion(s)
- Bacteria identified on biopsy

Fungal abscess
- MRI/CT shows enhancing lesion(s)
- Biopsy shows fungi

Parasitic abscess
- MRI/CT shows enhancing lesion(s); often multiple
- Biopsy makes the diagnosis

Meningitis

Bacterial meningitis
- MRI/CT normal or meningeal enhancement
- LP shows CSF leukocytosis; glucose often reduced

Viral meningitis
- MRI/CT are normal
- LP shows moderate lymphocytic pleocytosis
- Viral serologies may be positive

Fungal meningitis
- MRI may show meningeal enhancement, may be hydrocephalus
- LP shows fungal element and often positive serology

Encephalitis

Herpes encephalitis
- MRI often shows focal temporal lesions
- EEG may show periodic discharges
- LP may show positive serology

Non-HSV viral encephalitis
- MRI normal or multifocal abnormality
- LP may show mild–moderate pleocytosis, mononuclear
- EEG usually slow

Prion encephalitis
- MRI may give specific abnormalities
- EEG often shows periodic discharges
- LP can be supportive

BACTERIAL MENINGITIS	
Description	• A bacterial infection of the spinal fluid • This is a serious infection with a fulminant course.

Pathophysiology	Strains of bacterial meningitis include:
	  • *Haemophilus influenzae*
	  • *Streptoccus pneumoniae*
	  • *Neisseria meningitidis*
	  • *Listeria monocytogenes*
	Medical conditions that predispose to meningitis include sinusitis, immune-deficiency states, skull fractures, or other reasons for skull defects, such as neurosurgery, shunts, implanted stimulation and recording electrodes, sickle cell disease, and splenectomy.

Clinical findings	• Headache, fever, and neck pain are common presenting symptoms. • Mental status changes often develop, ranging from confusion to coma. • Seizures can develop. • Meningeal signs commonly are commonly seen, in addition to the neck pain and stiffness.
Laboratory studies	• Routine labs show elevated white blood cells (WBCs) in most patients. C-reactive protein (CRP) may be elevated. The remainder of the labs is normal. • Imaging with MRI or CT usually is normal, although MRI may show meningeal enhancement. Cerebral edema can be seen. Regions of cerebritis also can be seen. • CSF shows a polymorphonuclear pleocytosis that is in the thousands, unless there is an immune deficit. Protein is often elevated and glucose is reduced. Very low glucose is a poor prognostic sign. • Identification of the organism depends on microscopic examination and culture of the CSF. Counter-immune electrophoresis (CIE) is a rapid test performed on CSF that can identify the most common causes of bacterial meningitis; however, the identification must be confirmed by culture.
Diagnosis	• Bacterial meningitis is suspected when a patient presents emergently with fever, headache, and is found on exam to have neck stiffness. • Imaging often is done to look for abscess, because LP should be avoided with cerebral mass lesions. This is especially important if the patient presents with mental status changes or seizures. • LP is the definitive test, and shows yellow cloudy fluid, usually under increased pressure. Perfectly clear and colorless fluid argues against bacterial meningitis even before analysis of the fluid. CIE can suggest a specific organism, but is not definitive, and there occasionally are false positives. Microscopic examination can identify the organism in some patients. Culture is definitive.

BACTERIAL MENINGITIS—cont'd	
Differential diagnosis	• *Brain abscess.* Can present with fever and headache, and focal signs are not always present. Imaging is required for the diagnosis.
	• *Aseptic meningitis.* Can present with headache and may be associated with fever. The toxic appearance of most patients with bacterial meningitis is not mirrored in most patients with aseptic meningitis. CSF analysis makes the diagnosis.
	• *Encephalitis.* Can present with fever and headache, and some alteration of mental status or seizures is common. The meningeal signs seen with bacterial meningitis are not typical. CSF may show some inflammatory change, but not to the degree of bacterial meningitis.
Management	Antibiotic treatment is begun as soon as the diagnosis of bacterial meningitis is suspected. For best identification of the organism, the LP should be performed prior to start of antibiotics course; however, this is not always feasible. Patients who need an imaging study prior to LP should have antibiotics begin so that treatment is not delayed. The risk for administration of unneeded antibiotics is small in comparison to the risk of delay in treatment.
	Dexamethasone has been shown to have some benefit so is usually recommended starting immediately before the first dose of antibiotics.
Clinical course	Most patients with bacterial meningitis improve, although this is not invariable. Some patients will develop cerebral edema, herniation, and brain death despite prompt medical treatment. Others will be left with neurologic deficits and/or seizures.

Most common causative organisms

H. influenzae still causes ~25-50% of meningitis in developing countries (90% reduction in U.S. with Hib vaccine)

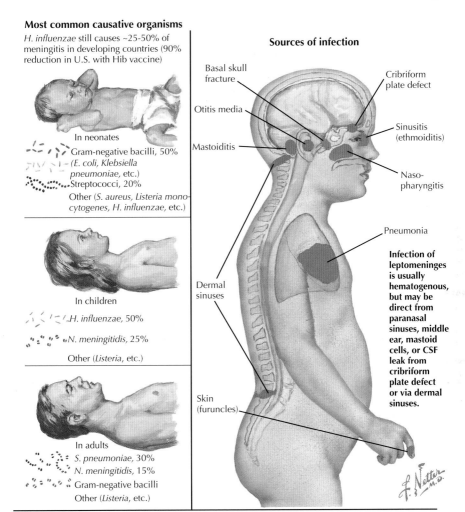

Sources of infection

In neonates
Gram-negative bacilli, 50%
(E. coli, Klebsiella pneumoniae, etc.)
Streptococci, 20%
Other (*S. aureus, Listeria monocytogenes, H. influenzae,* etc.)

In children
H. influenzae, 50%
N. meningitidis, 25%
Other (*Listeria,* etc.)

In adults
S. pneumoniae, 30%
N. meningitidis, 15%
Gram-negative bacilli
Other (*Listeria,* etc.)

Basal skull fracture

Otitis media

Mastoiditis

Dermal sinuses

Skin (furuncles)

Cribriform plate defect

Sinusitis (ethmoiditis)

Naso-pharyngitis

Pneumonia

Infection of leptomeninges is usually hematogenous, but may be direct from paranasal sinuses, middle ear, mastoid cells, or CSF leak from cribriform plate defect or via dermal sinuses.

Brain Abscess

BRAIN ABSCESS	
Description	• Loculated infection of the brain • Most are due to bacteria, although fungal and parasitic infections also can create abscesses

Pathophysiology	The most common bacteria to produce brain abscesses include:
	  • *S. aureus*
	  • Streptococci
	  • *Enterobacter*
	  • *Pseudomonas* and other anaerobes
	• Fungi and parasites form a small proportion of brain abscesses.
	• Many brain abscesses develop from contiguous spread from sinuses and other tissues. Neurosurgical procedures, skull defects, trauma, and other breaches of the skull increase the risk for brain abscess.

Clinical findings	• Fever is present in patients, especially with bacterial abscesses. The fever may be mild and overlooked. • Headache is common, and can be generalized or localized. • Mental status changes can include confusion, lethargy, and even coma if severe. • Seizures can develop. • Focal signs can include hemiparesis, hemianopia, frontal lobe deficits, aphasia, neglect. • Onset of the symptoms is within days to a few weeks, depending on the organism.
Laboratory studies	• Routine labs are normal, but peripheral WBC usually is elevated. CRP and erythrocyte sedimentation rate (ESR) also are commonly elevated. • Imaging is normal, except for MRI, which occasionally may show enhancement of the meninges. • LP usually is not done when brain abscess is suspected; however, if performed it has a polymorphonuclear pleocytosis with elevated protein, but normal glucose. Organisms typically do not grow out of the CSF. • Brain biopsy can reveal the organism on microscopic examination. Culture is needed for confirmation of the precise organism.
Diagnosis	• Brain abscess is suspected when a patient presents with fever and focal neurologic deficits or seizures. • Imaging shows an enhancing lesion that may have the radiographic appearance of an abscess; however, biopsy is needed to make the definitive diagnosis of abscess.
Differential diagnosis	• *Bacterial meningitis.* Presents with headache and fever, and in patients who develop meningoencephalitis, there may be cognitive changes and seizures. Imaging can make the differentiation. • *Brain tumor.* Can present with headache and focal findings on exam or seizures. Cognitive changes are common. There are no outward signs of infection in these patients, and while imaging cannot be definitive about etiology, biopsy can.

BRAIN ABSCESS—cont'd	
Management	• Appropriate antimicrobial therapy for the eradication of the organism is needed. Before tissue is obtained, broad spectrum antibiotics with good CSF penetrance are given, followed by more directed therapy when an organism has been isolated and characterized.
	• Surgical resection of a brain abscess depends on the individual clinical situation. An accessible lesion in a patient with mass lesion of unknown etiology most likely needs, at the least, surgical biopsy. Total resection of a brain abscess usually is not needed, and, furthermore, can leave the patient with extended deficit.
Clinical course	Most patients improve, although abscess in patients with immune deficiency can be the opening of a variety of immune attacks.

Parameningeal Infections

Brain abscess

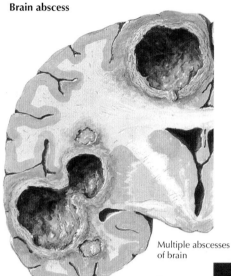

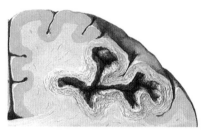

Scar of healed brain abscess with collapse of brain tissue into cavity

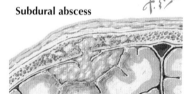

Multiple abscesses of brain

Subdural abscess

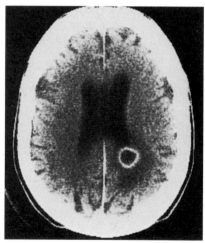

Osteomyelitis of skull, with penetration of dura to form subdural "collar button" abscess

CT scan shows brain abscess with thin enhancing rim and central necrosis

SPINAL EPIDURAL ABSCESS	
Description	A bacterial infection in the spinal canal, but outside of the dura
Pathophysiology	• Spinal epidural abscess usually develops from extension from surrounding tissues. Discitis is one potential cause. With time, the infection can migrate into the adjacent epidural space. Any form of spinal procedure or injury also can predispose to epidural infection, including spine surgery, lumbar puncture, and local spine trauma. Local skin infection also can predispose to infection. This is also of increased incidence in bacterial endocarditis. • Bacteria involved in epidural spinal abscess include *Staphylococcus* species.
Clinical findings	• Patients usually present with pain in the back, which may also manifest erythema, swelling, and warmth suggestive of local infection; however, these findings are not always present. Radiation of the pain in a root distribution is common. • Exam shows normal function if there is no compression of the cord or cauda equina. Rapidly expanding mass effect of the abscess can produce myelopathy or cauda equina syndrome, depending on the level of the lesion.
Laboratory studies	• Routine labs show signs of infection with elevated blood WBC, ESR, and CRP. • Blood cultures commonly are done, with suspected spinal epidural abscess to look for bacterial endocarditis. • Imaging urgently is performed when spinal epidural abscess is considered. MRI is most sensitive, but may miss a small developing infection. Contrast-enhanced MRI is most sensitive. CT is much less sensitive. Myelography can show the lesion, but the LP required for this procedure should be avoided if this diagnosis is suspected. • LP usually is not done, but if CSF is obtained, it shows mild-to-moderate pleocytosis with elevated protein. Glucose is normal. • Culture of the abscess gives definitive identification of the organism.
Diagnosis	• Spinal epidural abscess is suspected when a patient presents with back pain and has fever or other signs of infection. A history of spinal surgery, skin infection, or risk factors for SBE increases the level of suspicion. • Urgent MRI is the procedure of choice for demonstrating the abscess. Contrast-enhanced MRI is most sensitive, and must specifically be requested, because most routine spine studies do not use contrast dye. • Surgical exploration and drainage is not only therapeutic, but also provides substance for microscopic exam and culture.
Differential diagnosis	• *Meningitis.* Can present with spine pain and signs of infection, but the spine pain is less well localized and headache typically predominates over the spine pain. • *Discitis.* Infection of the disc space. Many of the same conditions that predispose to spinal epidural abscess can predispose to discitis. Differentiation rests on MRI. • *Extraspinal infection.* Can produce severe pain in the spine with signs of infection.

SPINAL EPIDURAL ABSCESS—cont'd	
Management	• Treatment begins with urgent administration of antibiotics when the diagnosis is suspected. • Surgical exploration and drainage of the abscess is the definitive treatment. Cultures and smears may alter the choice of antibiotics.
Clinical course	• Most patients with spinal epidural abscess are identified prior to the development of severe neurologic deficit, and, therefore, treatment of the abscess usually can halt the progression of symptoms. Immunocompromised hosts may present a challenge to antibiotic treatment. • If spinal cord or cauda equina compression has resulted in neurologic deficit at the time of diagnosis, then residual weakness and ataxia is common.

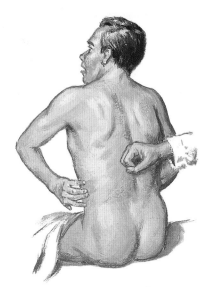

Pain on percussion of spine.
Local warmth may be noted.

Epidural abscess

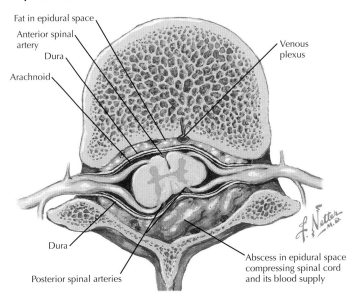

Fat in epidural space

Anterior spinal artery

Dura

Arachnoid

Venous plexus

Dura

Posterior spinal arteries

Abscess in epidural space compressing spinal cord and its blood supply

SEPTIC THROMBOPHLEBITIS	
Description	Infections of the sinuses can predispose to septic thrombosis of the intracranial veins. The clinical manifestations differ depending on which sinuses are affected.
Pathophysiology	• Infection of the ear and sinuses, including paranasal and mastoid, can result in venous thrombosis with resultant impairment in venous drainage. • Infectious occlusion of intracranial veins also can occur from other intracranial and cranial infections. • Occlusion can be of the cavernous sinus, lateral sinus, or sagittal sinuses. • Findings can be due to increased intracranial pressure or venous infarction.
Clinical findings	• Patients can present with combinations of fever, headache, altered mental status, or focal symptoms. • Exam may show papilledema; focal deficits, including weakness (although this usually is not complete); hemiparesis; or seizures. • Lateral sinus or sagittal sinus thrombosis can produce features of increased intracranial pressure with headache and papilledema. • Cavernous sinus thrombosis can produce orbital swelling and injection, often with cranial nerve palsies. Any ocular motor nerves can be affected, resulting in diplopia. Involvement of the first division of the trigeminal nerve (V_1) can produce pain and sensory deficit on the forehead, extending to the vertex. • Signs of ear or sinus infection may be evident.
Laboratory studies	• Routine labs may show elevated WBC, ESR, and/or CRP, but this is not invariable. • Imaging with CT or MRI may show the inflammatory changes in the ear, mastoid, and/or paranasal sinuses. MRI additionally may show venous infarctions in the brain, which can be multiple and smaller than most arterial cortical infarcts. • MRV or CTA can show lack of flow in the venous sinuses, and sometimes a clot even can be seen. There is significant variability in venous anatomy, so hypoplasia or aplasia should be differentiated from thrombosis. • LP sometimes is performed in patients with venous sinus thrombosis; however, there are some individuals who will have LP performed when bacterial meningitis is considered in the diagnosis. In these patients, there will be increased intracranial pressure and often a lymphocytic pleocytosis.
Diagnosis	Septic thrombophlebitis is considered when a patient presents with headache and signs of increased intracranial pressure. Presence of the signs of infection supports the diagnosis.
Differential diagnosis	• *Meningitis.* Can produce headache and signs of infection, and also is a potential consequence of sinus and ear infection. • *Brain abscess.* Can present with similar symptoms, but imaging shows enhancing lesion rather than venous infarction and venous occlusive disease.

SEPTIC THROMBOPHLEBITIS—cont'd	
Management	• Antibiotics are used for intracranial thrombophlebitis. Initial broad-spectrum therapy can be focused when an organism and sensitivities are known. • Anticoagulation often is often used, although there is some risk for facilitating intracranial hemorrhage. • Surgical treatment of the sinusitis or ear infection may be ultimately needed.
Clinical course	Most patients improve, although there is the possibility of increased intracranial pressure to the point that there is decreased brain-perfusion pressure.

Intracranial Complications

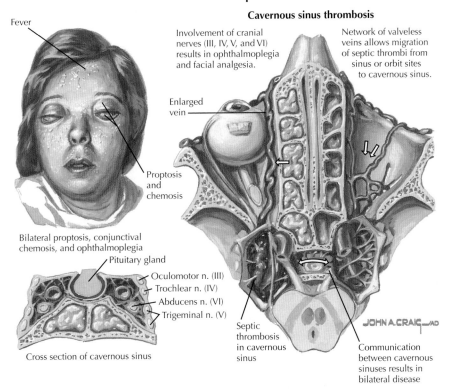

Cavernous sinus thrombosis

Fever

Involvement of cranial nerves (III, IV, V, and VI) results in ophthalmoplegia and facial analgesia.

Network of valveless veins allows migration of septic thrombi from sinus or orbit sites to cavernous sinus.

Enlarged vein

Proptosis and chemosis

Bilateral proptosis, conjunctival chemosis, and ophthalmoplegia

Pituitary gland

Oculomotor n. (III)
Trochlear n. (IV)
Abducens n. (VI)
Trigeminal n. (V)

Cross section of cavernous sinus

Septic thrombosis in cavernous sinus

Communication between cavernous sinuses results in bilateral disease

JOHN A. CRAIG—AD

FUNGAL MENINGITIS	
Description	Infection of the meninges is an uncommon cause of nonbacterial meningitis.
Pathophysiology	• *Cryptococcus* is the most common organism to cause fungal meningitis, although *Candida* and *Aspergillus*, as well as some others, can. • Fungal meningitis rarely is seen in immunocompetent hosts; patients with AIDS are particularly susceptible to cryptococcal meningitis.
Clinical findings	• Patients present with any combination of headache, confusion, visual difficulty, or ataxia. Fever may be present, but is an inconstant feature. • Meningeal signs commonly are not seen. • Exam may show confusion, ataxia, or papilledema.
Laboratory studies	• Routine labs usually are normal, although there may be signs of immunodeficiency. • Imaging with CT and MRI usually is normal. Contrast-enhanced MRI sometimes may show meningeal enhancement. Hydrocephalus may be seen on either imaging modality, and contributes to symptoms and signs. • LP shows increased CSF pressure, lymphocytic pleocytosis with 100–300 cells. Protein commonly is increased and glucose may be reduced. • Cryptococcal antigen is a rapid test for screening CSF for cryptococcal meningitis. Although therapy can be initiated on the basis of these results, final diagnosis depends on cultures. • Fungal cultures make the definitive diagnosis of all fungal meningitides.
Diagnosis	• Fungal meningitis is suspected in patients with headache and confusion, although the differential diagnosis is large. • Imaging is performed to look for mass lesions or subarachnoid hemorrhage; in fungal meningitis imaging may be normal or show enhancing meninges. Hydrocephalus is present in a small proportion of patients. • CSF analysis is confirmatory with the typical profile described above. Cryptococcal antigen is positive in most patients with cryptococcal meningitis. Fungal culture is the definitive diagnostic study.
Differential diagnosis	• *Bacterial meningitis*. Has a more fulminant course than fungal meningitis. The CSF profile differs substantially. • *Normal pressure hydrocephalus*. Presents with ataxia, dementia, and, often, urinary incontinence, with imaging showing communicating hydrocephalus. However, this especially is seen in elderly patients. CSF is normal with NPH. • *Encephalitis*. Presents with headache, confusion, and often ataxia. Imaging also may be normal. CSF can even look similar, and, therefore, specific antigen assays and cultures for fungi are done to help with the differentiation.

FUNGAL MENINGITIS—cont'd	
Management	Antifungal treatment depends on the agent and host factors. Amphotericin, flucytosine, and fluconazole are commonly used agents.
Clinical course	Prognosis is generally good if the host has adequate immune response to the infection. Patients with few CSF WBCs have a poorer outcome because they lack the robust immune response that is required along with the antifungal treatment.

Cryptococcosis

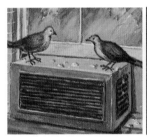 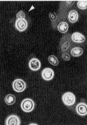 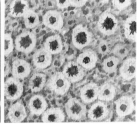

Infection is by respiratory route. Pigeon dung and air conditioners may be factors in dissemination.

India ink preparation showing budding and capsule

Accumulation of encapsulated cryptococci in subarachnoid space (PAS or methenamine-silver stain)

VIRAL MENINGITIS	
Description	Viruses can easily invade the meninges, producing an acute meningitis that can be difficult to distinguish from bacterial meningitis.
Pathophysiology	• A host of viruses can produce viral meningitis, including enteroviruses, HSV2, CMV, EBV, LCM, HIV, and adenoviruses. • HSV2 is more likely to cause meningitis than encephalitis, whereas the reverse is true for HSV1, which is more likely to cause encephalitis.
Clinical findings	• Patients present with headache and fever, often with neck pain. Confusion and seizures are not expected, and when present they indicate meningoencephalitis. • Neurologic exam often shows meningeal signs. Neck stiffness is common, although the severity of meningeal signs is not what is seen with bacterial meningitis.
Laboratory studies	• Routine labs are normal. • Imaging is normal. Usually, there is insufficient meningeal inflammation to be seen on MRI. • LP most commonly shows a lymphocytic pleocytosis in the CSF, usually less than 100 cells, although several hundred cells can be seen. Thousands of cells suggest bacterial infection. Protein may be elevated, but glucose is normal. • Specific titers for certain viruses can be performed. Culturing CSF for viruses has an extremely low yield.
Diagnosis	• Viral meningitis is suspected in a patient with headache and fever, especially in the absence of other signs of infection. • Imaging usually is performed to look for abscess. • LP is definitive for meningitis. The lower WBC, lymphocytic predominance, and absence of bacterial antigens argue in favor of viral meningitis.
Differential diagnosis	• *Brain abscess.* Can present with fever and headache, although focal signs commonly are seen. Imaging makes the differentiation. • *Bacterial meningitis.* Can present similarly to viral meningitis, although the onset is more fulminant with bacterial meningitis. CSF profile is different, with greater WBC and a polymorphonuclear predominance. • *Fungal meningitis.* Especially with *Cryptococcus*, it produces a syndrome of aseptic meningitis, which only reveals the organism with special testing. The CSF formula can look very similar.
Management	• There are no treatments for most viruses. • HSV can be treated with acyclovir.
Clinical course	Most patients improve, and in general, the prognosis is better for viral meningitis than for encephalitis.

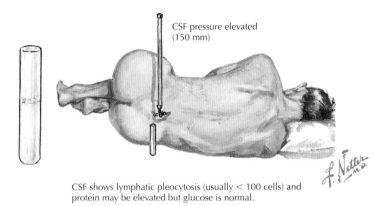

CSF pressure elevated
(150 mm)

CSF shows lymphatic pleocytosis (usually < 100 cells) and
protein may be elevated but glucose is normal.

ENCEPHALITIS	
Description	A diffuse infection of the brain. Most are viral, although rare cases of bacterial encephalitis can develop.
Pathophysiology	• Viruses are the most common cause of encephalitis, with a wide range of possible pathogens. Herpes encephalitis is a prototypic encephalitis, important to diagnose because it is treatable. • Bacterial encephalitis is uncommon, and is most likely related to SBE. In some patients with SBE, the bacteria produce extensive cerebral and meningeal inflammation without forming defined abscesses. • Cancers can be associated with a paraneoplastic encephalitis. This is autoimmune, and a remote effect of the cancer.
Clinical findings	• Encephalitis presents with rapid onset of confusion, often with headache. Fever is seen in some forms of encephalitis, but not all. • Focal neurologic signs may develop, especially with encephalitis that produces necrotizing changes, especially HSV. Hemiparesis and/or aphasia are common. • Seizures can develop with any encephalitis, especially HSV.
Laboratory studies	• Routine labs commonly are normal, although elevated blood WBC is sometimes seen. This is much less common with viral than bacterial infections. • Imaging can show diffuse or multifocal regions of edema and enhancement. HSV encephalitis shows changes most prominent in the temporal areas. • LP shows inflammatory changes in most patients, indicating that this is commonly a meningoencephalitis. The CSF profile differs depending on the type of encephalitis. • Electroencephalogram (EEG) shows slowing and disorganization of the record in most patients, consistent with encephalopathy. However, many patients with HSV encephalitis will have periodic discharges in the temporal regions.
Diagnosis	• Encephalitis is suspected when a patient presents with fever, headache, and confusion. The addition of focal neurologic findings and seizures supports the diagnosis and is most often seen with HSV. • Imaging is performed which may show focal or multifocal inflammatory changes. Predominant involvement of the temporal lobes with necrosis suggests HSV. • CSF analysis shows a profile similar to aseptic meningitis with lymphocytic pleocytosis and elevated protein. The elevation in WBC is moderate. • Rapid testing for HSV by polymerase chain reaction (PCR) is now available. West Nile virus (WNV) also is testable from the serum and CSF. • Blood tests for many forms of encephalitis are now available, including St. Louis, California, eastern equine, and western equine encephalitides.

ENCEPHALITIS—cont'd	
Differential diagnosis	• *Brain abscess.* Can present with confusion, seizures, and focal neurologic signs. Imaging shows a defined abscess. Imaging gives different results, with focal abscess formation rather than cerebritis. • *Meningitis.* Can present with confusion and seizures, although in this case, some cerebritis is implied.
Management	• Management of most patients with encephalitis is supportive. Routine medical management for seizures and cerebral edema, as well as fluid and nutritional support, are needed. • HSV encephalitis is treated with intravenous acyclovir. Treatment is begun as soon as the diagnosis is suspected, because treatment should not await the results of the HSV-PCR testing. Therefore, many patients are begun on treatment for HSV who will not ultimately be maintained on treatment when the labs return. Because MRI and EEG cannot definitively distinguish HSV from other meningitides, treatment of many encephalitis patients is needed.
Clinical course	• Most patients improve, though not all. Patients with necrotizing HSV encephalitis are often left with neurologic deficits including aphasia, focal weakness, and/or seizures. • Patients with WNV and many of the other encephalitides also can have neurologic deficit, with damage from edema or secondary infarction.

Clinical Features of HSV Encephalitis

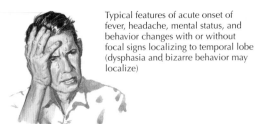

Typical features of acute onset of fever, headache, mental status, and behavior changes with or without focal signs localizing to temporal lobe (dysphasia and bizarre behavior may localize)

Seizure activity is common, often within 1 week of initial symptoms.

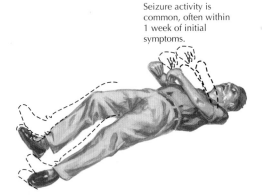

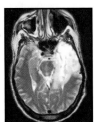

MRI demonstrating temporal lobe involvement is a diagnostic cornerstone.

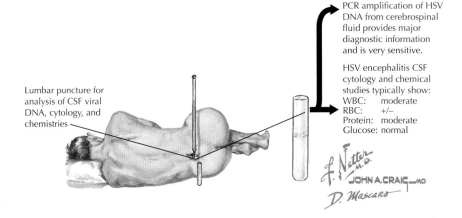

Lumbar puncture for analysis of CSF viral DNA, cytology, and chemistries

PCR amplification of HSV DNA from cerebrospinal fluid provides major diagnostic information and is very sensitive.

HSV encephalitis CSF cytology and chemical studies typically show:
WBC: moderate
RBC: +/–
Protein: moderate
Glucose: normal

PRION DISEASES	
Description	Chronic neurologic disorders producing mainly cognitive and motor symptoms
Pathophysiology	• Prions are proteins that alter native proteins to produce cellular degeneration. • Prion diseases can be transmitted or inherited, because both mechanisms can result in the abnormal prion proteins, which produce the disease. • The incubation period can be many years for prion diseases. Modes of transmission have included surgical procedures, such as brain instrumentation and corneal transplants, and ingestion of infected meat. Modern methods of handling and surveillance reduce the chance of prion transmission in foods, but safety cannot be ensured.
Clinical findings	• Creutzfeldt-Jakob disease (CJD) is the prototypic disorder. Patients present with rapidly progressive dementia, ataxia, myoclonus, and exaggerated startle. • This is termed myoclonic encephalopathy, which has a limited differential diagnosis in an adult.
Laboratory studies	• Routine labs are normal. • Imaging with MRI may show changes in the basal ganglia, particularly the globus pallidus and putamen, in patients with CJD. • CSF is normal. 14-3-3 protein and neuron-specific enolase have traditionally been assayed, but these are not helpful in solidifying the diagnosis. Assay of the *PrP* gene is more definitive. • EEG commonly shows slowing and disorganization of the background; however, periodic discharges can be seen in CJD that suggest and support the diagnosis; these findings are not present throughout the course of the disease.
Diagnosis	• Diagnosis of prion diseases is considered in patients with myoclonic encephalopathy. However, the myoclonus is not prominent in all cases, and in some forms of prion diseases, cognitive dysfunction is late. Therefore, suspicion is raised when a combination of cerebellar and corticospinal tract dysfunction develops.
Differential diagnosis	• *Multiple sclerosis.* Can present with multifocal signs with cerebellar and corticospinal tract dysfunction. MRI and CSF can distinguish this from CJD. • *Vasculitis.* Can present with multifocal CNS findings. MRI and lab studies can distinguish these possibilities.
Management	Treatment is supportive. Although medications have been tried, none have proven to alter the course of the disorder.
Clinical course	Prion diseases are progressive.

Specific Prion Disease	Features
Creutzfeldt-Jakob disease (CJD)	• Prototypic prion disease, presents with encephalopathy, often with myoclonus. • Diagnosed by biopsy, although immunoassay of the *PrP* gives strong indication of diagnosis.
Gerstman-Straussler-Scheinker (GSS)	• Autosomal dominant form of prion disease • Patients present with progressive ataxia and dementia, which progresses to death within a few years.
New variant CJD (nvCJD)	• Thought to be caused by the same agent that causes bovine spongiform encephalopathy (BSE) • Patients present with progressive dementia, which is often preceded by psychiatric disturbances and sensory complaints. • Patients with nvCJD are younger than patients with CJD. Most patients were in the United Kingdom, or at least were residing in the United Kingdom during the period of susceptibility to infection.
Fatal familial insomnia	• Patients present with insomnia plus other neurologic manifestations, including autonomic dysfunction, motor deficits, and dementia. The presentation is variable, and all patients do not develop all symptoms. • Patients progress to death within a few years. • Genotypic analysis makes the diagnosis.

Transmissible Spongiform Encephalopathy

Creutzfeldt-Jakob disease

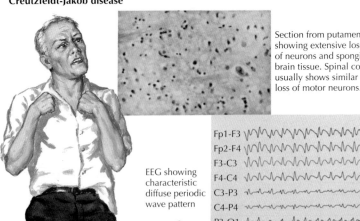

Section from putamen showing extensive loss of neurons and spongiform brain tissue. Spinal cord usually shows similar loss of motor neurons.

EEG showing characteristic diffuse periodic wave pattern

Fp1-F3
Fp2-F4
F3-C3
F4-C4
C3-P3
C4-P4
P3-O1
P4-O2

75 μV
1 sec

Demented patient exhibiting myoclonus

HUMAN IMMUNODEFICIENCY VIRUS	
Description	As the causative agent for AIDS, HIV has tremendous direct and indirect effects on the nervous system. Neurologic effects are related, yet supplement, the systemic non-neurologic effects of the virus.
Pathophysiology	• HIV is a retrovirus that mainly is passed through sharing of body fluids from sexual intercourse, blood transfusion, transplantation, and other significant fluid or tissue exposure. • HIV causes immune deficiency that predisposes to a number of opportunistic infections. • HIV also has direct effects on the nervous system, including AIDS-dementia.
Clinical findings	Clinical presentation depends on the specific entity, discussed below.

Disorder	Features
AIDS-dementia	• Progressive dementia develops due to the virus, itself, rather than an indirect by opportunistic organism. • Treatment is supportive. Medications commonly used for Alzheimer's disease are tried, but efficacy is unproved.
Toxoplasmosis	• *Toxoplasma gondii* is a protozoa that is almost exclusively seen in patients with immune deficiency. When a patient with AIDS presents with mass lesion, tumor is possible, but *Toxoplasma* is more likely. Immunocompetent individuals have asymptomatic infection. • MRI or CT shows multifocal enhancing lesions. • Toxoplasma serology is confirmatory in the appropriate clinical setting. • Treatment is successful for most patients with sulfadiazine and pyrimethamine, although sustained treatment is needed for many patients.
CNS Lymphoma	• The main disorder in the differential diagnosis of patients with multifocal lesions in a patient with AIDS. The lesions are focal or multifocal. • Lymphomatous meningitis can be seen with symptoms separate from parenchymal CNS lymphoma. • CSF shows a lymphocytic pleocytosis and sometimes positive cytology. • Treatment is with radiotherapy and chemotherapy, but response is typically incomplete.
Progressive multifocal leukoencephalopathy (PML)	• An opportunistic infection caused by the JC virus. Before the development of AIDS, PML mainly was seen in cancer patients, particularly those with lymphomas and leukemias and other disorders with immune suppression. • Demyelinating changes in the brain are focal or multifocal, and can be cerebral, cerebellar, and/or brainstem. • Aggressive retroviral treatment of AIDS patients can result in some improvement; otherwise, there is no effective treatment.

Disorder	Features
Cryptococcal meningitis	• Seldom seen in immunocompetent hosts • Treated successfully with antifungal agents in most patients, although those with markedly impaired immune response have a poorer outcome.
Polyneuropathy	• Has varying manifestations in AIDS patients. A painful sensory neuropathy is common. • Immune mediated neuropathy is commonly seen, resembling AIDP or CIDP. • Herpes zoster is common. • Cytomegalovirus polyradiculitis can be seen.
Myopathy	• Inflammatory myopathy equivalent to polymyositis can be seen. • Degenerative myopathies are seen.

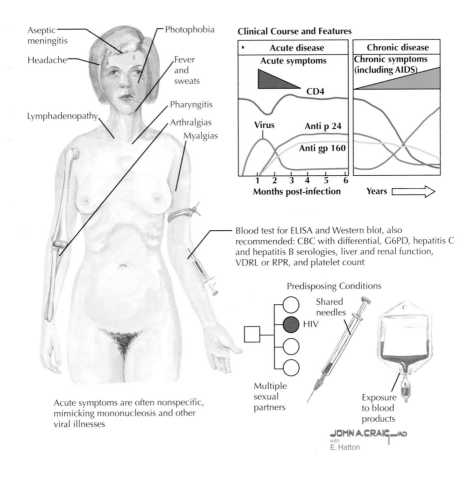

Aseptic meningitis

Photophobia

Headache

Fever and sweats

Lymphadenopathy

Pharyngitis

Arthralgias

Myalgias

Clinical Course and Features

Acute disease	Chronic disease
Acute symptoms	Chronic symptoms (including AIDS)

CD4

Virus   Anti p 24

Anti gp 160

1 2 3 4 5 6
Months post-infection   Years

Blood test for ELISA and Western blot, also recommended: CBC with differential, G6PD, hepatitis C and hepatitis B serologies, liver and renal function, VDRL or RPR, and platelet count

Predisposing Conditions

Shared needles

HIV

Multiple sexual partners

Exposure to blood products

Acute symptoms are often nonspecific, mimicking mononucleosis and other viral illnesses

JOHN A. CRAIG—AD
with
E. Hatton

OVERVIEW OF NEURO-ONCOLOGY	
Description	Neoplasia is one of the prime methods of neurologic disease.
	Neoplasms can be benign or malignant, have direct or indirect effects.
Pathophysiology	• Local effects of neoplasms include tumor infiltration and compression. Remote effects include paraneoplastic syndromes.
	• Benign and malignant tumors can all have compressive effects. Remote effects are only seen with malignant tumors.
Clinical features	• Local effects of neoplasia are suspected when a patient presents with clinical findings of a mass lesion of the brain or spine.
	• Remote effects of neoplasia are suspected when a patient presents with encephalopathy, ataxia, or weakness in the absence of local tumor identified as cause of these findings—paraneoplastic syndromes.
Neoplastic Syndrome	**Features**
Brain tumor	• Features of brain tumor include headache, papilledema, hemiparesis, aphasia with dominant hemisphere lesion, and/or seizures.
	• *Aggressive malignant tumors* are more likely to present with neurologic deficit.
	• *Benign and low-grade malignant tumors* are more likely to present with seizures.
	• *Primary brain tumors* are more likely to be solitary.
	• *Metastatic tumors* are more likely multifocal and usually have a known history of cancer, although brain "mets" can occasionally be the presenting sign of the cancer.
	• *Benign intraparenchymal tumors* usually are astrocytomas.
	• *Benign extra-axial tumors* usually are meningiomas.
	• *Malignant primary tumors* usually are gliomas.
	• *Malignant metastatic tumors* can be from anywhere, but are most commonly from lung, breast, gastrointestinal (GI) causes, melanoma, or lymphoma.
Cerebellar tumor	• Produces ataxia, which can affect gait and limbs. Brainstem involvement from direct extension or compression can produce diplopia with upper stem involvement, dysarthria, dysphagia with lower stem involvement, hemiparesis or quadriparesis with compression of the corticospinal tracts at any level.
	• Most common in children, especially cystic astrocytoma. Cerebellopontine angle lesion includes acoustic neuroma and meningioma.

Neoplastic Syndrome	Features
Spinal cord tumor	• Presents with pain at the level of the mass lesion. Weakness below the level is expected, with spasticity if the corticospinal tract is affected. Lumbar spine lesions affecting the conus medullaris and cauda equina produce flaccid paraparesis and sphincter disturbance. • *Extra-axial spinal cord tumors* can be benign or malignant. Benign include meningioma and neurofibroma. Malignant can be from extension from adjacent spine, include lung, breast, ovarian, renal, or other malignant tumor. Lymphoma can produce compression without destruction of adjacent tissue. • *Intramedullary tumors* include astrocytoma and ependymoma. Metastatic intramedullary tumors are not expected.
Neoplastic meningitis	• Can present with pain and neurologic deficit in the distribution of multiple cranial and spinal nerves. Diplopia, sensory disturbance with pain, weakness, and signs of increased intracranial pressure with headache, nausea, and vomiting is common. • Always malignant. Some common tumors to cause this are lung, breast, and GI.
Paraneoplastic syndrome	• Systemic symptoms not associated with structural lesion in a patient with known cancer suggests paraneoplastic syndrome. • *Limbic encephalitis* often is due to small cell lung cancer, and presents with cognitive changes. • *Peripheral neuropathy* can be due to small cell lung cancer, breast, or ovarian cancer. • *Myasthenia* can be related to thymoma or, less likely, lung cancer.

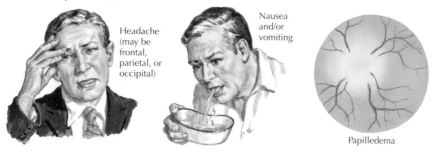

Some Common Manifestations of Brain Tumors

A. Intracranial pressure triad

Headache (may be frontal, parietal, or occipital)

Nausea and/or vomiting

Papilledema

B. Various focal manifestations

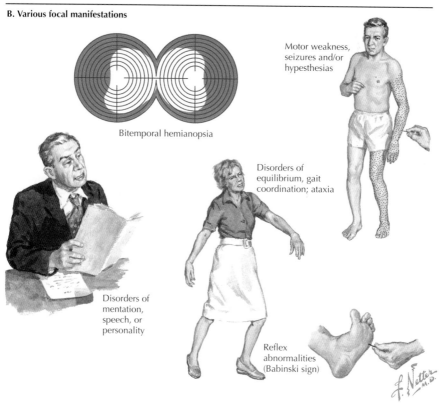

Bitemporal hemianopsia

Motor weakness, seizures and/or hypesthesias

Disorders of equilibrium, gait coordination; ataxia

Disorders of mentation, speech, or personality

Reflex abnormalities (Babinski sign)

11 Primary Brain Tumors

PRIMARY BRAIN TUMORS	
Description	Can be malignant or benign. Tumors produce symptoms mainly by mass effect and destruction of functioning brain tissue.
Pathophysiology	• Primary brain tumors can be of several causes. Exposure to radiation and genetic predisposition is responsible for some of tumors. • The most important primary brain tumors are: astrocytoma, oligodendroglioma, glioblastoma, lymphoma, meningioma, neurofibroma, and primitive neuroectodermal tumor (PNET).
Clinical findings	• Patients with brain tumors can present with any combination of headache, nausea/vomiting, mental status changes, focal weakness, papilledema, and/or seizures. • Patients with malignant tumors are more likely to have focal deficits. Patients with benign tumors are more likely to have seizures, although these generalizations are not always correct.
Laboratory studies	• Routine labs usually are normal. Syndrome of inappropriate antidiuretic hormone (SIADH) is occasionally seen, and may produce electrolyte abnormalities. • Imaging identifies a solitary mass lesion in most patients with primary brain tumors. Imaging features can usually differentiate between tumor and infection. Also, differentiation between malignant and benign can be suggested. • Definitive diagnosis depends on pathologic evaluation, which is performed on biopsy or resection.
Management	• Management depends on many features, including age and status of the patient, location and geometry of the lesion, and presumed type of lesion. • Resection is performed if possible. If not, then debulking is beneficial for most tumors. Biopsy is performed if surgical resection would be devastating. Central nervous system (CNS) lymphoma is often sensitive to radiation and medical therapy so if this is identified on frozen section, then resection is not performed. Resection can cure some lesions, especially benign tumors such as meningiomas. • Chemotherapy and/or radiation therapy is performed for some patients with malignant tumors. Unfortunately most malignant gliomas do not respond well to these treatments. PNETs and CNS lymphoma can respond quite well.
Specific Tumors	**Features**
Astrocytoma	• Tumors of astrocytic origin can be benign or malignant. Of the malignant tumors, anaplastic are less aggressive, whereas glioblastoma is the most aggressive. Glioblastoma multiforme (GBM) is the most malignant of the astrocytic series, and is discussed below. • Patients usually present with seizures, but may have focal deficits. Weakness and ataxia can develop. • Diagnosis is suspected by magnetic resonance imaging (MRI), which shows a lesion with variable levels of enhancement, depending on the grade of the lesion. Low-grade astrocytoma has little enhancement, whereas anaplastic astrocytoma enhances, although not as greatly as GBM.

Specific Tumors	Features
	• Treatment begins with proper diagnosis. Resection is performed if possible. But astrocytic tumors can infiltrate brain, resulting in expanded deficit if there is aggressive resection of the lesion. • Radiation therapy and chemotherapy are offered for patients with more malignant lesions.
Oligodendroglioma	• Much less common then astrocytoma. Can be low-grade or anaplastic. • Pathologic features make the diagnosis. • Patients present with focal deficit or seizures. If seizures are not present at the time of diagnosis, they commonly develop later. • Treatment is with resection. Chemotherapy is given especially for anaplastic oligodendrogliomas. Radiation therapy is given for most patients with anaplastic forms and patients with low-grade forms with incomplete resection.
Glioblastoma multiforme (GBM)	• The most malignant form of glioma. This is highly undifferentiated, aggressive, and infiltrative. GBM is a single lesion, although migratory character may give it a multicentric appearance. • Diagnosis is suspected when imaging identified an irregular infiltrative enhancing lesion. • Debulking helps treatment, although complete resection is not possible. • Radiation therapy is almost always given. Chemotherapy usually is performed as well. • Prognosis is poor. Response to treatment is incomplete and temporary. Progression is expected.
Meningioma	• Arises from the arachnoid layers, and begins extra-axially. Can extend into the substance of the brain. • Patients present with mental status change, focal deficit, seizures. Meningioma in the posterior fossa can produce hearing loss and ataxia. • Surgical resection is curative for many patients. If the tumor has extended into the brain, resection may not be complete. Rare patients with malignant meningiomas may require radiation therapy after debulking.

Specific Tumors	Features
Acoustic neuroma	• Benign tumors of CN-8. They are of increased incidence in patients with neurofibromatosis type 2. • Although acoustic neuroma is a common name, the term *vestibular schwannoma* is a more recently used term. • Patients present with hearing loss, tinnitus, and ataxia. It is easy to ascribe these findings to vestibulopathy, and, therefore, the diagnosis often is delayed. • Imaging with MRI is sensitive for most acoustic neuromas, although special views of the internal auditory canal may be needed to see the lesion. • Brainstem auditory evoked potential shows abnormalities that are suggestive, although not diagnostic, of acoustic neuroma. • Treatment is surgical if removal or debulking is needed. Some patients have lesions that can be followed. Stereotactic radiosurgery is another alternative.
Primitive neuroectodermal tumor (PNET)	• Includes the medulloblastoma, which is predominantly seen in children. • Patients present with typical features of mass lesion and often hydrocephalus. • MRI shows mass filling the 4th ventricle. • Surgery is performed to resect as much of the tumor as possible. • Radiation therapy and chemotherapy are given to reduce residual tumor. • Steroids are given to reduce edema before and after surgery. • Many children have a good response with long-term survival.
Craniopharyngioma	• Arises from Rathke pouch or the craniopharyngeal cleft near the sella. It is a slow-growing cystic lesion. • Patients present with headache, visual loss, and may have nausea/vomiting. Some patients are asymptomatic and the mass is found when a scan is performed for an unrelated reason. • MRI shows a cystic mass in the suprasellar region. Calcifications are seen. Significant mass effect and even hydrocephalus can be seen. • Surgical approach can be by a variety of methods, which would depend on size, location, and geometry of the tumor. • Radiation therapy can be performed. Chemotherapy is sometimes used, although the effectiveness is debatable. Neuro-oncologist consultation is needed.

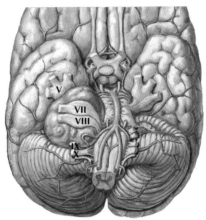

Large acoustic neurinoma filling cerebellopontine angle, distorting brainstem and cranial nerves V, VII, VIII, IX, X

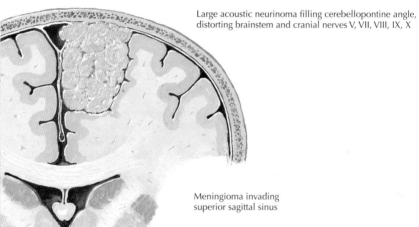

Meningioma invading superior sagittal sinus

Large, hemispheric glioblastoma multiforme with central areas of necrosis. Brain distorted to opposite side

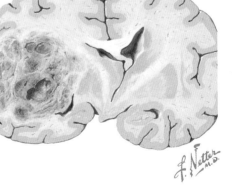

Metastatic Brain Tumors

METASTATIC BRAIN TUMORS	
Description	Brain metastases develop from malignant tumors. They have their effects by mass effect, vascular changes, and tissue destruction.
Pathophysiology	Spread of tumor to the brain can be hematogenously or via direct extension. Direct extension is more an issue with spine tumors than with brain tumors.
	Common tumors to produce brain metastases are:
	· Lung
	· Breast
	· Colon
	· Renal cell
	· Melanoma
	· Ovarian
Clinical findings	· Patients usually present with focal or multifocal lesions with their resultant symptoms. This can include headache, focal weakness, and coordination deficit.
	· Signs of increased intracranial pressure are common, especially with extensive cerebral edema, multiple lesions, or hydrocephalus.
Laboratory studies	· Routine labs are normal.
	· Imaging shows one or more enhancing lesions. MRI cannot definitively differentiate between tumor and abscess, but there are guidelines.
	· Biopsy with pathology gives definitive diagnosis.
Diagnosis	· Brain metastases are suspected when a patient presents with any combination of focal weakness, seizures, and headache. Onset is insidious.
	· Imaging suggests brain tumor. Clear differentiation between primary and metastatic lesion cannot be made, but multiple lesions suggest metastatic disease.
	· Pathology makes the diagnosis, from biopsy or resection.
Differential diagnosis	· *Primary brain tumor.* The main differential diagnosis. Multiple lesions suggest metastases.
	· *Abscesses.* Can be multiple and resemble metastases, especially in patients with SBE.
	· *CNS lymphoma.* Can be multifocal, and resemble metastases from distant tumor.

METASTATIC BRAIN TUMORS—cont'd	
Management	• Diagnosis by biopsy is the first step in management. Resection is performed if the lesion is solitary. Multiple lesions are not resected because of the possibility of extensive damage.
	• Steroids are used for edema.
	• Anticonvulsants are used for patients with seizures. Prophylactic anticonvulsants commonly are not used.
	• Chemotherapy and radiation therapy are used for some patients, depending on the type and location of the metastases and primary tumor.
Clinical course	Metastatic tumors to the brain seldom are the cause of death; patients more commonly die from their systemic disease.

Tumors Metastatic to Brain

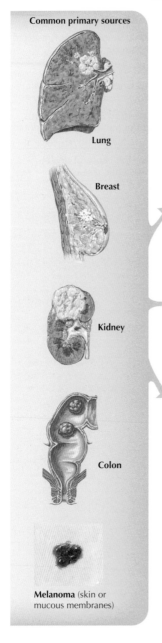

Common primary sources

Lung

Breast

Kidney

Colon

Melanoma (skin or mucous membranes)

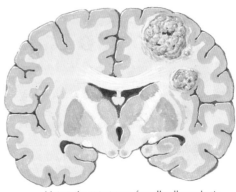

Metastatic metastases of small cell anaplastic (oat cell) carcinoma of lung to brain

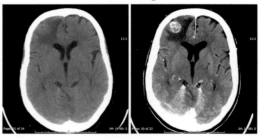

Axial CT demonstrates edema within the right frontal pole. An ill-defined heterogeneous region is seen peripherally, which enhances after iodinated contrast administration. Incidental small remote lacunar infarct is seen within the left putamen (arrowhead).

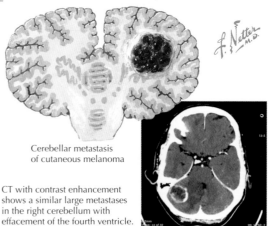

Cerebellar metastasis of cutaneous melanoma

CT with contrast enhancement shows a similar large metastases in the right cerebellum with effacement of the fourth ventricle.

SPINAL CORD TUMORS	
Description	• Can be primary or secondary • Primary tumors are usually benign, whereas tumors that spread from distant sites or contiguous regions are typically malignant.
Pathophysiology	• Primary tumors of the spinal sac include neurofibromas, meningiomas, ependymomas. Secondary neoplasms can spread by blood, cerebrospinal fluid (CSF), or contiguous extension from the tumor, which has metastasized to adjacent vertebrae.
Clinical findings	• Presenting findings usually are back pain and weakness. The weakness is most commonly seen in the legs, although cervical spine tumors can produce arm deficits; the pattern of weakness correlates with the level of the lesion. • Reflexes are increased in the legs with cervical and thoracic spine lesions; they can be reduced with lumbar spine disease and cauda equina compression. • Bowel and bladder control deficits are common.
Laboratory studies	• Routine labs are normal. • MRI shows a structural lesion in most circumstances. An enhanced study should be performed when neoplastic, infectious, or demyelinating causes of myelopathy are suspected. Intrinsic neoplasms of the spinal cord may have normal MRI unless contrast is used. • Computed tomography (CT) may show spinal column destruction but is much less sensitive for tumor in the canal.
Diagnosis	• Spinal cord tumor is suspected when patient with known cancer presents with back pain and leg weakness. Non-neoplastic causes can be suspected, and some patients will have disc disease or some other benign structural lesion. • Signs of myelopathy or cauda equina lesion support the diagnosis. • MRI confirms the diagnosis in most patients. If the MRI is normal at the level of the symptoms, then the MRI should be performed on more rostral spinal segments, because the lesion can be above the level of the deficit. • If MRI cannot be done because of artificial valve, pacemaker, or other implanted device, CT myelography can make the diagnosis. In this case, total myelography should be performed. • CSF analysis can be performed to look for neoplastic meningitis, but there is some risk for increasing the deficit when lumbar puncture (LP) is performed when there is a structural spinal lesion.

SPINAL CORD TUMORS—cont'd	
Differential diagnosis	• *Neoplastic meningitis.* Can present with radicular symptoms and spinal cord involvement occasionally can occur. • *Transverse myelitis.* As a component of MS or acute disseminated encelphalomyelitis (ADEM), can present with myelopathy with an intraparenchymal enhancing lesion. • *Degenerative changes of the spine.* Can produce cord compression, which can subsequently appear as cord changes on MRI—myelomalacia can be difficult to distinguish from inflammatory changes.
Management	• Surgical decompression is commonly done when spinal cord tumor is resulting in secondary compressive myelopathy. • Resection of extra-axial tumor can give the diagnosis. Biopsy or resection of intramedullary tumor is seldom done, and carries significant risk for neurologic deficit.
Clinical course	• Most patients improve with treatment, but the residual deficit is common. • Whether the lesion is curable is determined by the pathology and anatomy.

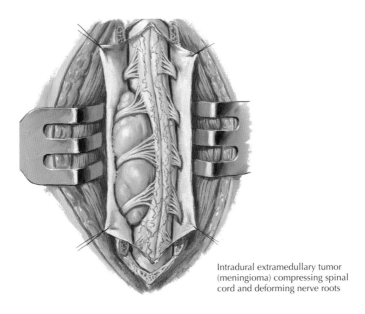

Intradural extramedullary tumor (meningioma) compressing spinal cord and deforming nerve roots

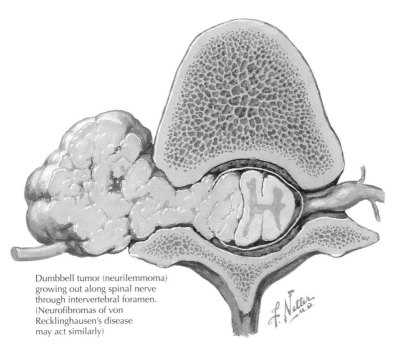

Dumbbell tumor (neurilemmoma) growing out along spinal nerve through intervertebral foramen. (Neurofibromas of von Recklinghausen's disease may act similarly)

Paraneoplastic Syndromes

PARANEOPLASTIC SYNDROMES	
Description	• Paraneoplastic syndromes are remote effects of cancer. There are several paraneoplastic syndromes and corresponding antibodies, and the numbers are increasing. • Can be described by the specific antibodies and the clinical syndromes
Pathophysiology	Antibodies are created in response to the tumor cells. They attack neurons of the CNS and parasympathetic nervous system (PNS), producing a host of clinical presentations.
Clinical findings	The most important clinical manifestations are: • Encephalomyelitis • Cerebellar ataxia • Opsoclonus-myoclonus syndrome • Polyneuropathy • Myasthenia gravis and LEMS • There are other disorders that can occur as well, but this is less likely. • Details of the specific entities are discussed below.
Laboratory studies	• Routine laboratory studies are normal. Specific assays for paraneoplastic antibodies often are revealing. • Imaging usually is normal. • CSF may show a mild pleocytosis and elevated protein. Paraneoplastic antibody testing on the CSF is available. • Imaging of body may reveal a cancer, with lung, breast, and ovarian being of specific interest. Positron emission tomography (PET) may help identify a neoplasm, in addition to MRI and CT.
Diagnosis	• Paraneoplastic syndrome is suspected when a patient with known cancer presents with neurologic symptoms that are not associated with a structural lesion. CSF shows pleocytosis without neoplastic meningitis. Paraneoplastic antibodies are positive. • Paraneoplastic syndrome is suspected in patients without known cancer when there is cerebellar ataxia or subacute onset of dementia or encephalopathy without identified cause. • Imaging is performed to look for structural lesions causing the symptoms. LP also is often done.
Differential diagnosis	• *Neoplastic meningitis.* Can produce weakness and multifocal neurologic deficits with no obvious abnormalities identified on imaging. • *Metastatic tumor.* Can produce ataxia and weakness, although it is usually identified on imaging with MRI.

PARANEOPLASTIC SYNDROMES—cont'd	
Management	• There is no proven treatment of paraneoplastic syndromes. Corticosteroids, intravenous immunoglobulin G (IVIG), or plasma exchange are used to suppress the autoimmune response. • Treatment of the tumor can produce improvement, although treatment does not always help the paraneoplastic syndrome.
Clinical course	Patients may improve with treatment with immune-modulation or treatment of the underlying tumor, but persistent symptoms are expected. Also, there often is progression of the causative tumor.
Specific Entity	**Features**
Encephalomyelitis	• Encephalopathy with cognitive changes, lethargy, and progressive functional decline can be seen with anti-Hu, APCA-2, ANNA-3. • Most common associated tumors are lung (especially small cell), breast, and testicular. • Seizures can develop, and may be the presenting sign.
Cerebellar ataxia	Progressive cerebellar ataxia with appendicular and axial manifestations can be seen with anti-Yo (APCA-1), APCA-2, Tr, and perhaps other antibodies.
Peripheral neuropathy	• Can be sensory and/or motor. • Small cell lung cancer can be associated. Anti-Hu and anti-Yo are most correlated.
Myasthenia gravis (MG)	• Associated with thymoma in some patients • Removal of thymoma can result in eventual improvement in the MG, although the improvement is delayed.
Lambert-Eaton myasthenic syndrome (LEMS)	• Produces weakness and autonomic insufficiency • Small-cell lung cancer is most commonly associated with LEMS. • Diagnosis is established by clinical symptoms, NCS and EMG findings, and antibodies to voltage-gated calcium channels.
Opsoclonus-myoclonus syndrome	• Characterized by rapid irregular eye movements (opsoclonus), myoclonus, often associated with ataxia or dysarthria. • Breast cancer often is associated, with anti-Ri antibody.

Antibody Target	Clinical Association
Hu (ANNA-1)	• Anti-Hu or antineuronal nuclear antibody-1 is associated with encephalopathy or neuropathy. Small cell lung cancer is the chief associated tumor.
Ri (ANNA-2)	• Associated with opsoclonus-myoclonus syndrome, and also is seen with breast cancer. Other cancer associations have been determined as well.
Ta (Ma1, Ma2)	• Anti-Ta antibodies can be associated with limbic encephalitis. Ma2 is associated with testicular cancer. Ma1 antibodies may contribute, but Ma2 appears to be the most important element.
Yo (APCA-1)	• Anti-Purkinje cell antibody is associated with paraneoplastic cerebellar degeneration or peripheral neuropathy. Myopathy and corticospinal tract degeneration also can be seen.
Voltage-gated calcium channel (VGCC)	• Antibodies to the VGCC are found in most patients with LEMS.
Tr	• Tr is an anti-Purkinje cell antibody seen in patients with subacute cerebellar ataxia associated with Hodgkin's lymphoma.
ANNA-3	• Antineuronal nuclear antibody-3 is yet another anti-Purkinje cell antibody associated with small cell lung cancer. • Patients may have cerebellar ataxia, brainstem or limbic encephalitis, or myelopathy.

Neuromuscular Manifestations of Bronchogenic Carcinoma

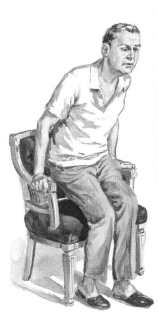

Lambert-Eaton syndrome: weakness of proximal muscle groups (often manifested by difficulty in rising from chair)

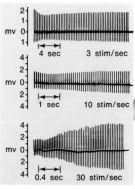

Electromyographic abnormality in Lambert-Eaton syndrome (readings from hypothenar muscles with stimulation of ulnar nerve at wrist). Note low amplitude and initial decline. (Normal = 5 mv or more with no initial decline)

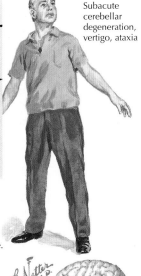

Subacute cerebellar degeneration, vertigo, ataxia

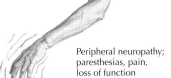

Peripheral neuropathy; paresthesias, pain, loss of function

Dementia may occur rarely (may predate onset of pulmonary symptoms)

APPROACH TO TOXIC/METABOLIC DISORDERS	
Description	• Toxins are suspected when a patient presents with mental status changes or weakness that is not related to identified structural, infectious, or immune mediated disease. • Withdrawal from many agents also can present with mental status changes.
Types of presentations	• Encephalopathy • Ataxia • Movement disorder • Myopathy • Neuropathy
Red flags for toxic/metabolic effects	• Toxic and metabolic abnormalities are suggested by development of neurologic deficits, which are diffuse, nonfocal, and without a structural cause. • Infectious and autoimmune etiologies must be considered.

Presentation	Features
Encephalopathy	• Mental status changes due to toxins usually have a subacute onset. Differentiation from dementia is the short duration and presence of disordered level of consciousness, from agitation to lethargy to coma. • Many toxins can produce encephalopathy, including analgesics, antidepressants, neuroleptics, anticonvulsants, and sedative/hypnotics.
Ataxia	• Can affect gait and/or limbs • Chronic alcohol intoxication can produce cerebellar degeneration with predominant gait ataxia. Any drug that can produce mental status alteration can produce ataxia. Anticonvulsants can produce ataxia and nystagmus even at doses that do not produce encephalopathy, especially phenytoin and carbamazapine.
Movement disorder	• Can be created by numerous drugs. Not all of these effects are at toxic doses. • An akinetic-rigid syndrome indistinguishable from Parkinson's disease can develop from neuroleptic administration. • Valproate and amiodarone can produce a tremor, but in rare cases also can give a parkinsonian appearance. • Chorea can develop from certain medications, including some anticonvulsants, levodopa, antipsychotics, oral contraceptives, amphetamines, cocaine, and tricyclic antidepressants. • Dystonia can develop from chronic use of neuroleptics. • Tardive dyskinesia develops from use of antipsychotics—the newer atypical neuroleptics have a lower incidence of TD.

Presentation	Features
Myopathy	• Can develop from alcohol intoxication, and frank rhabdomyolysis can occur
	• Statins have been described as producing myopathy, although the incidence of myalgia and myopathy attributed to statins is largely overstated.
	• Cocaine can produce myopathy and rhabdomyolysis.
	• Corticosteroids with chronic use can produce a myopathy characterized by atrophy of type 2 muscle fibers. Acute myopathy also can develop with rhabdomyolysis, although this is rare.
Neuropathy	• Several chemotherapeutic agents can produce peripheral neuropathy. Vincristine and cisplatin are two of the prominent agents, but there are others.
	• Phenytoin can produce a sensory neuropathy.
	• Gold can produce a motor neuropathy.

HEAVY METAL INTOXICATION	
Description	Heavy metals are an uncommon but important cause of neurotoxicity.
Pathophysiology	The most important elements to produce heavy metal intoxication are: • Lead • Mercury • Arsenic These elements interfere with the normal metabolism of the neurons.

Element	Findings
Lead	• Main sources of lead toxicity are paints in old houses, enamel on some imported toys and jewelry, and industrial exposure. • Clinical features include central and peripheral manifestations. Central symptoms are headache, irritability, lethargy, and associated cerebral edema. Peripheral symptoms include distal numbness and weakness due to neuropathy. Acute high-dose exposure is more likely to produce central findings, whereas chronic lower-level exposure is more likely to produce peripheral neuropathy. Non-neurologic findings in adults can include lead lines in the gingival tissue, which can be seen with any heavy metal intoxication. • Laboratory findings include elevated blood lead level. Some patients may have anemia, especially children. • Treatment is with cessation of exposure, chelation, and supportive therapy.
Mercury	• Mercury intoxication can be from organic or inorganic mercury. Minamata disease is an example of organic mercury intoxication. Inorganic mercury intoxication comes from contact or inhalation of the metallic mercury or the vapor. • The clinical features of mercury intoxication are varied, but can include cognitive difficulties, symptoms of peripheral neuropathy, ataxia, visual and hearing loss. Emotional instability is common. • Blood and urine mercury levels are increased. • Nerve conduction study (NCS) and electromyelogram (EMG) show axonal neuropathy. • Chelating agents are used for treatment.
Arsenic	• Arsenic poisoning usually is from exposure to certain insecticides and through intentional poisoning. Certain herbs may contain arsenic. Today, exposure from smelting is not expected. • Acute intoxication by ingestion produces pain with burning in the mouth, followed by gastrointestinal (GI) distress. • Chronic intoxication can produce peripheral neuropathy with sensory and motor symptoms. • Diagnosis is made by urine measurement and assay of hair and nails. • Treatment is avoidance of exposure and supportive. Chelating agents can be used, but their benefit is controversial.

Peripheral Neuropathy Caused by Heavy Metal Poisoning

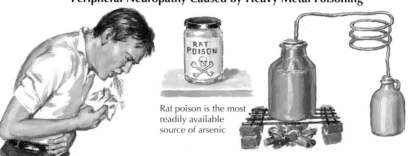

Rat poison is the most readily available source of arsenic

History of nausea and vomiting may suggest arsenic poisoning in patient with peripheral neuropathy

Antique copper utensils (e.g., still for bootleg liquor) and runoff waste from copper smelting plant may be sources of arsenic poisoning

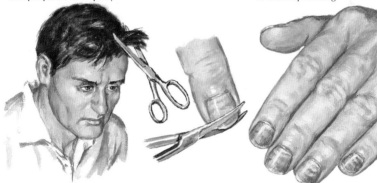

Although 24-hour urinalysis is best diagnostic test for arsenic, hair and nail analysis may also be helpful

Mees' lines on fingernails are characteristic of arsenic poisoning

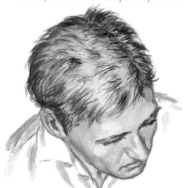

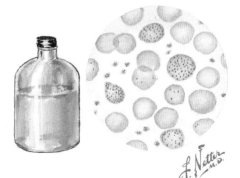

Spotty alopecia associated with peripheral neuropathy characterizes thallium poisoning

Lead poisoning, now relatively rare, causes basophilic stippling of red blood cells. 24-hour urinalysis is diagnostic test

CHOLINESTERASE INHIBITORS	
Description	• Used in weak form for patients with Alzheimer's disease and other dementias, as well for myasthenia • High-potency agents include some pesticides and nerve agents.
Pathophysiology	Binding and inhibition of the acetylcholinesterase produces increased availability of acetylcholine at the terminal, which is the basis for benefit in patients with dementia and myasthenia. Hyperstimulation results in damage to the nerve terminal with use of high-potency agents such as organophosphates.
Clinical findings	• Acute intoxication results in GI distress, confusion, seizures, cerebral edema (if severe), and can result in death. The acronym SLUDGE refers to salivation, lacrimation, urination, defecation, GI distress, and emesis. • Delayed neurotoxicity can be manifest as peripheral neuropathic symptoms, including weakness with cramps and sensory symptoms. The prominence of motor deficit is more suggestive of delayed neurotoxicity than sensory symptoms.
Laboratory studies	• Routine labs are normal. Red cell cholinesterase activity is reduced in patients with acute exposure. • Imaging is normal. • Electrocardiogram (ECG) can show arrhythmia. • There are NCS and EMG abnormalities; however, these special tests are not routinely performed.
Diagnosis	• Cholinesterase inhibition is suspected when a patient presents with salivation and GI distress. This suggests acute toxicity. • Delayed neurotoxicity is considered when a patient presents with neuronal degeneration without another identifiable cause. • Red cell cholinesterase assay only is helpful for identification of acute toxicity; delayed neurotoxicity depends on a history of significant exposure.
Differential diagnosis	• *Encephalitis.* Can present with seizures, mental status changes, and GI distress, although the profound salivation is not expected. • *Other causes of polyneuropathy* can present with distal sensory and motor findings, which can resemble the delayed neurotoxicity.
Management	• Treatment for acute intoxication is supportive. Seizures are treated with diazepam or other benzodiazepine. • 2-PAM is an antidote that often is given in addition to atropine, especially for patients with severe intoxication.
Clinical course	Most patients improve from the acute intoxication, although delayed neurotoxicity has no effective treatment.

The Pupils in Poisoning

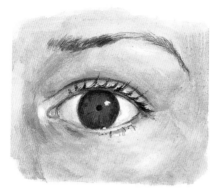

Miosis (pinhole pupils)

Seen in poisoning by morphine and morphine derivatives, some types of mushrooms, cholinesterase inhibitors, parasympathomimetics, nicotine, chloral hydrate, sympatholytics, and some other compounds

Action at the Neuromuscular Junction

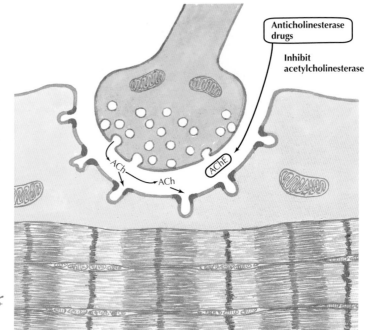

Anticholinesterase drugs

Inhibit acetylcholinesterase

WITHDRAWAL SYNDROMES	
Description	• Almost as much of a medical problem as intoxication • May develop because the patient runs out of money, decides to stop a habit, or is institutionalized (e.g., jail, hospital) and has no availability • If the patient has not been honest about their substance use, withdrawal will not be anticipated by others.
Pathophysiology	• The agents from which patients withdraw are so diverse that general pathophysiology cannot precisely be discussed. • In general, alcohol and drugs produce adaptive changes in the brain that can evoke dependency on several planes: molecular, neuronal, and/or psychologic. • Lack of "feeding" a dependency can create a craving for the substance, as well as autonomic symptoms common to withdrawal.
Clinical findings	• Common findings with withdrawal are anxiety, agitation, and craving. Adrenergic symptoms are common, including tachycardia, diaphoresis, abdominal pain, and nausea. • Alcohol withdrawal can produce confusion, seizures, fever, and hyperventilation. Delirium tremens (DTs) is progression of the withdrawal state to prominent cognitive change. Seizures may occur prior to the DTs. • Opiate withdrawal can produce many of the same symptoms, and commonly causes nausea, vomiting, diarrhea, and abdominal pain.
Laboratory studies	• Routine labs usually are normal. • Drug screen commonly is normal because patients have been off the agent(s) for several days. • Magnetic resonance imaging (MRI) and computer tomography (CT) are normal, except for atrophy, which is a common finding with chronic alcoholism. • Electroencephalogram (EEG) may be normal, but if there are mental status changes, slowing is common. • Cerebrospinal fluid (CSF) commonly is obtained to look for encephalitis or meningitis, but is normal.
Diagnosis	• Withdrawal syndrome is suspected when a patient presents with anxiety, agitation, diaphoresis, and tachycardia. • The presentation can suggest CNS infection, and, therefore, imaging and CSF analysis often are performed, especially if the diagnosis is not certain. • Normal studies and a history from the patient or associates of substance use make the diagnosis.

WITHDRAWAL SYNDROMES—cont'd	
Differential diagnosis	• *CNS infection.* With encephalitis or meningitis, can present in a similar fashion. • *Hyperthyroidism.* Can present with some of the same symptoms. • *Pheochromocytoma.* Can present with episodic hyperadrenergic symptoms, although the episodes are briefer than withdrawal syndromes, and blood pressures (BPs) are extremely high.
Management	• Supportive care is essential, with management of the autonomic instability and sedation when needed. Benzodiazepines are predominantly used. • Clonidine or propranolol often is used for cardiovascular protection.
Clinical course	• There is a real risk of death from withdrawal, mainly from cardiovascular causes. • With treatment, most patients do improve, although the risk for subsequent substance-use problems continues to be problematic.

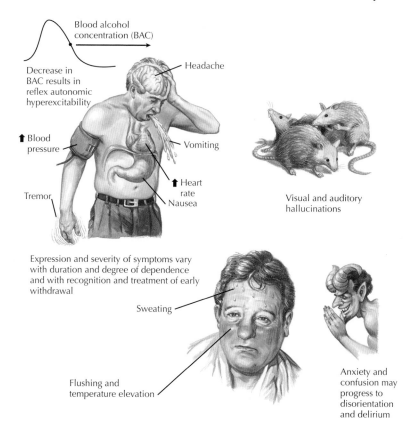

Blood alcohol concentration (BAC)

Decrease in BAC results in reflex autonomic hyperexcitability

Headache

↑ Blood pressure

Vomiting

Tremor

↑ Heart rate
Nausea

Visual and auditory hallucinations

Expression and severity of symptoms vary with duration and degree of dependence and with recognition and treatment of early withdrawal

Sweating

Flushing and temperature elevation

Anxiety and confusion may progress to disorientation and delirium

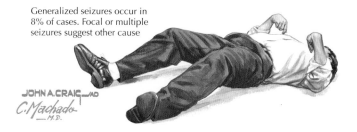

Generalized seizures occur in 8% of cases. Focal or multiple seizures suggest other cause

JOHN A. CRAIG—MD
C. Machado
—M.D.

Opiod Withdrawal
Signs and symptoms

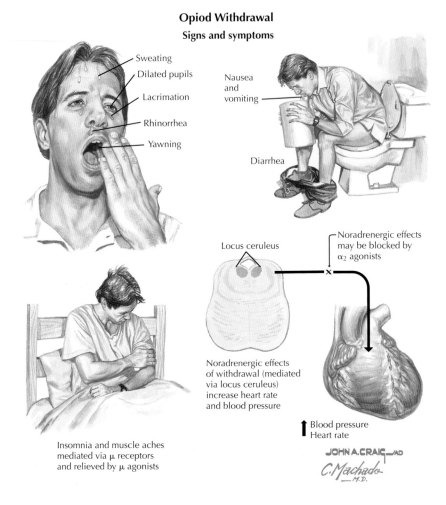

Sweating

Dilated pupils

Lacrimation

Rhinorrhea

Yawning

Nausea and vomiting

Diarrhea

Locus ceruleus

Noradrenergic effects may be blocked by α_2 agonists

Noradrenergic effects of withdrawal (mediated via locus ceruleus) increase heart rate and blood pressure

↑ Blood pressure Heart rate

Insomnia and muscle aches mediated via μ receptors and relieved by μ agonists

JOHN A. CRAIG—AD

C. Machado—M.D.

Benzodiazepine Withdrawal

High-dose withdrawal

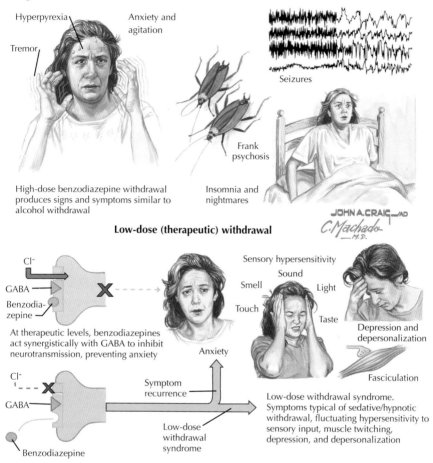

Hyperpyrexia

Anxiety and agitation

Tremor

Seizures

Frank psychosis

High-dose benzodiazepine withdrawal produces signs and symptoms similar to alcohol withdrawal

Insomnia and nightmares

JOHN A. CRAIG—MD

C.Machado—M.D.

Low-dose (therapeutic) withdrawal

Cl⁻

GABA

Benzodiazepine

At therapeutic levels, benzodiazepines act synergistically with GABA to inhibit neurotransmission, preventing anxiety

Anxiety

Sensory hypersensitivity

Sound

Smell

Light

Touch

Taste

Depression and depersonalization

Cl⁻

GABA

Benzodiazepine

Symptom recurrence

Low-dose withdrawal syndrome

Fasciculation

Low-dose withdrawal syndrome. Symptoms typical of sedative/hypnotic withdrawal, fluctuating hypersensitivity to sensory input, muscle twitching, depression, and depersonalization

Withdrawing long-term benzodiazepine causes loss of synergism with GABA inhibition, resulting in recurrence of original symptoms and low-dose withdrawal syndrome

ELECTROLYTE ABNORMALITIES	
Description	Numerous electrolyte abnormalities can produce neurologic manifestations. This discussion concentrates on neurologic manifestations of the electrolyte abnormalities.
Sodium Disorders	
Hypernatremia	• Hypernatremia is usually due to dehydration, with concentration of the blood sodium. • Clinical features are confusion, lethargy, and sometimes agitation. Seizures and/or myoclonus may occur. • Associated medical findings are tachycardia, oliguria, hypotension that is orthostatic, and generalized weakness. • Treatment is with hydration. Acute hypernatremia can be rapidly reversed. Chronic hypernatremia requires slow reversal because of the risk for cerebral edema. Nonsodium containing fluids usually are used; however, if the patient has marked hypovolemia in addition to hypernatremia, isotonic fluids often are administered initially.
Hyponatremia	• May be seen in alcoholics or in patients with certain medical conditions such as renal failure, hepatic failure, pneumonia, or congestive heart failure (CHF) • Clinical features are nausea, vomiting, confusion, and lethargy. • Seizures and coma may develop with profound hyponatremia. • Treatment depends on the clinical situation, including concurrent medical illness, tonicity, and volume status.
Potassium Disorders	
Hyperkalemia	• Usually related to renal insufficiency, potassium supplements, rhabdomyolysis, or other potassium-releasing injury • Clinical features are paresthesias and diffuse weakness. Cardiac arrhythmia may produce palpitations, although the incipient arrhythmias may not be symptomatic. • Treatment can include calcium supplements and glucose with insulin. Sodium bicarbonate especially is used with hyperkalemia cardiac arrest. Many diuretics can enhance excretion of potassium, and is all that is needed for many. • Binders usually are not needed.
Hypokalemia	• Usually is due to potassium-wasting diuretics and GI losses • Clinical features include generalized weakness that is due to impairment in muscle contraction. Associated symptoms include nausea, vomiting, abdominal cramping, and palpitations. ECG may show characteristic T-wave changes and arrhythmias. • Treatment is with potassium supplementation. If hypomagnesemia is concurrent, both need to be treated.

Calcium Disorders	
Hypercalcemia	• The most common cause is malignancy with bony erosion. Sarcoidosis and hyperparathyroidism also have to be considered.
	• Clinical findings are confusion, nausea, vomiting, abdominal pain, and weakness. With marked hypercalcemia, coma may ensue.
	• Diagnosis can usually be made by measurement of calcium, albumin, and parathyroid hormone (PTH) levels. A history of malignancy supports that diagnosis.
	• Treatment begins with hydration in most patients. Loop diuretics can help to reduce the calcium level. Dialysis may be needed for patients with renal failure, in whom aggressive hydration is not possible. Treatment of the parathyroid abnormality or malignancy also is done when possible.
	• Prognosis for patients with malignancy with hypercalcemia is not good, but because of the tumor—not the calcium abnormality.
Hypocalcemia	• A host of metabolic derangements can produce hypocalcemia. These can include cirrhosis, renal failure, sepsis syndrome, any cause of hypomagnesemia, rhabdomyolysis, malignancy, PTH deficiency, and certain medications.
	• Clinical features are muscle cramps and twitching, dysesthesias, and paresthesias. With severe hypocalcemia, confusion, lethargy or irritability, and coma can develop; seizures are also possible.
	• Treatment is with calcium replacement. Administration can be oral for patients with mild symptoms and modest hypocalcemia, and intravenous for more severely affected patients.
Magnesium Disorders	
Hypermagnesemia	• Some of the important causes are acute renal failure, rhabdomyolysis, malignancy, diabetic ketoacidosis (DKA), and excessive administration of magnesium (e.g., for eclampsia)
	• Clinical features are nausea, vomiting, and generalized weakness. Arrhythmia is common and can range from conduction delay to death.
	• Treatment is with hydration and supportive care. Diuretics can reduce magnesium levels, albeit slowly.
Hypomagnesemia	• Most commonly seen in alcoholics. Malnutrition from any cause also can produce hypomagnesemia. Certain drugs, including diuretics and chemotherapy agents, can be a cause.
	• Clinical features include generalized weakness, muscle cramps, and twitching. Severe cases may have confusion, lethargy or irritability, ataxia, and/or seizures.
	• Treatment is with magnesium replacement. Seizures can be treated with benzodiazepines.

Hypoglycemia and Hyperglycemia

HYPOGLYCEMIA AND HYPERGLYCEMIA	
Overview	• Both are associated with significant neurologic implications. • Patients with stroke have a poorer outcome with significant hyperglycemia or hypoglycemia.
Hypoglycemia	**Features**
Reactive hypoglycemia	• The reduction in glucose after a meal. It is most often seen in females, usually younger than age 45 and often overweight. • Patients can present with weakness and hyperadrenergic symptoms. Hunger, anxiety, tremulousness, and tachycardia are typical symptoms. • Patients with reactive hypoglycemia are at risk for diabetes, including both normal and overweight patients. • Treatment is with dietary manipulation, including frequent smaller meals, complex rather than simple carbohydrates, and exercise.
Insulin-induced hypoglycemia	• Insulin administration can result in hypoglycemia intentionally or unintentionally. Patients may not always notice the hypoglycemia, especially with long-standing diabetes, where the adrenergic response to hypoglycemia is blunted. • Treatment is with glucose replacement and supportive care. • Prognosis is usually good; however, profound and prolonged hypoglycemia can produce permanent damage.
Hyperglycemia	**Features**
Diabetic ketoacidosis (DKA)	• Hyperglycemia in the setting of insulin deficiency. DKA can be the presenting symptom of diabetes mellitus. • Clinical features are thirst, polydipsia, and polyuria. Associated symptoms are weakness, fatigue, nausea, vomiting, and anorexia. Exam shows tachycardia and signs of dehydration. • Patients may be confused or even comatose. Ketotic breath is characteristic. • Diagnosis is suspected when a patient presents with ill appearance, some of the typical features, and with glucose level >300 mg/dL. Acidosis also is present. • Treatment is with fluid replacement, balance of electrolytes, and insulin administration. Patients with DKA often are fragile.
Hyperosmolar hyperglycemia nonketotic coma (HHNC)	• Hyperglycemia with hyperosmolarity in the absence of ketosis. Unlike DKA, this is predominantly a disorder of patients with established diabetes, and is less likely to occur as a presenting manifestation. • Neurologic manifestations include confusion and lethargy progressing to coma. Focal signs, including hemiparesis and/or aphasia, can suggest stroke. Seizures can develop. • Glucose often is markedly increased, higher than with DKA, and <500$^+$ mg/dL. • Treatment is with hydration, critical care support, correction of electrolyte abnormalities, and insulin. If infection was a cause, appropriate antibiotic treatment is needed.

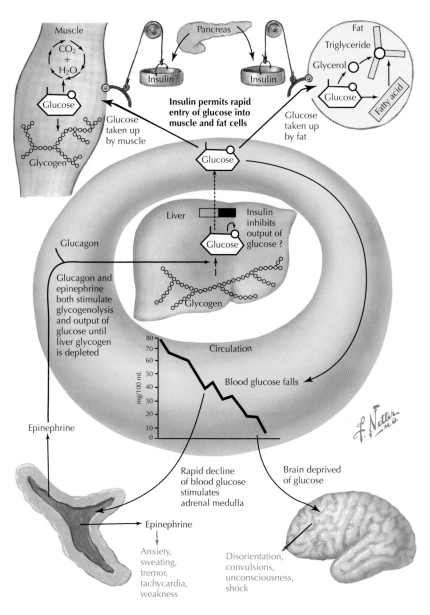

Muscle

CO_2 + H_2O

Glucose

Glycogen

Pancreas

Insulin

Insulin

Insulin permits rapid entry of glucose into muscle and fat cells

Glucose taken up by muscle

Fat

Triglyceride

Glycerol

Glucose

Fatty acid

Glucose taken up by fat

Glucose

Liver

Insulin inhibits output of glucose ?

Glucose

Glucagon

Glucagon and epinephrine both stimulate glycogenolysis and output of glucose until liver glycogen is depleted

Glycogen

Circulation

mg/100 mL

Blood glucose falls

Epinephrine

Rapid decline of blood glucose stimulates adrenal medulla

Brain deprived of glucose

Epinephrine

Anxiety, sweating, tremor, tachycardia, weakness

Disorientation, convulsions, unconsciousness, shock

B$_{12}$ DEFICIENCY	
Description	An important cause of weakness and ataxia because of central and peripheral effects
Pathophysiology	B$_{12}$ deficiency usually is due to impaired absorption rather than dietary deficiency. Long-term B$_{12}$ deficiency results in dysfunction of the posterior and lateral columns of the spinal cord. In addition, there often is polyneuropathy and central brain demyelinating changes.

Clinical findings	• Patients present with any combination of peripheral, central neural, or hematologic problems. Not all are present in all patients.
	
	• Important symptoms are:
	
	  • Ataxia
	
	  • Weakness
	
	  • Fatigue
	
	  • Sensory loss
	
	  • Neurologic symptoms commonly develop prior to development of hematologic abnormalities.
	
	• Exam may show cerebellar ataxia, corticospinal tract signs with increased tendon reflexes and upgoing plantar responses, decreased reflexes from polyneuropathy, confusion from cerebral involvement, and visual loss from optic neuropathy.

Laboratory studies	• Routine labs are normal, except some patients may have already developed a macrocytic anemia. B$_{12}$ level is low, but measurement of methylmalonic acid and homocysteine provides even greater diagnostic sensitivity. • Imaging with magnetic resonance imaging (MRI) may show abnormalities on T$_2$-weighted imaging consistent with the lesion. These lesions improve with treatment.
Diagnosis	• B$_{12}$ deficiency is suspected when a patient presents with a combination of clinical signs that cannot be explained by a single lesion. For example, cerebellar ataxia, myelopathy, and signs of neuropathy would suggest B$_{12}$ deficiency. • Diagnosis is confirmed by measurement of B$_{12}$, methylmalonic acid, and homocysteine levels.
Differential diagnosis	The main elements in the differential diagnosis are other conditions that produce multifocal abnormalities. • *Multiple sclerosis.* Can present with the combination of cerebellar and corticospinal dysfunction. Cognitive dysfunction can develop, although this is usually with advanced disease. Polyneuropathy is not expected. • *Vasculitis.* Can produce multifocal central and peripheral findings, and is considered in patients with B$_{12}$ deficiency. Differentiation is on labs and MRI appearance. Biopsy often is needed to make the definitive diagnosis of vasculitis.

B$_{12}$ DEFICIENCY—cont'd	
Management	B$_{12}$ replacement is key. Initial B$_{12}$ administration can be as often as daily, with reduction in frequency of injections as the B$_{12}$ has been replenished. Life-long replacement is needed. Injections are needed initially.
Clinical course	Most patients improve, although some deficit may persist. Although B$_{12}$, methylmalonic acid, and homocysteine levels normalize within 1–2 weeks, weeks to months are required for improvement in the neurologic condition.

Subacute Combined Degeneration

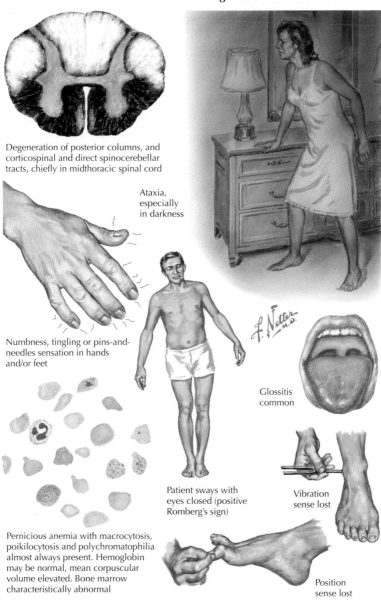

Degeneration of posterior columns, and corticospinal and direct spinocerebellar tracts, chiefly in midthoracic spinal cord

Ataxia, especially in darkness

Numbness, tingling or pins-and-needles sensation in hands and/or feet

Glossitis common

Pernicious anemia with macrocytosis, poikilocytosis and polychromatophilia almost always present. Hemoglobin may be normal, mean corpuscular volume elevated. Bone marrow characteristically abnormal

Patient sways with eyes closed (positive Romberg's sign)

Vibration sense lost

Position sense lost

THIAMINE DEFICIENCY	
Description	Can produce the combination of ocular motor abnormalities, polyneuropathy, ataxia, and mental status changes
Pathophysiology	• Thiamine deficiency usually is nutritional. Classic presentation is in patients with alcoholism, although thiamine deficiency syndromes are also seen in some patients with cancer. • There are multifocal degenerative changes with damage especially prominent in the mammary bodies and periaqueductal gray matter.
Clinical findings	• Thiamine deficiency has two distinct presentations—Wernicke's encephalopathy and Korsakoff's syndrome. Without treatment, Wernicke's encephalopathy progresses to Korsakoff's syndrome, and, therefore, they should be considered manifestations of the same disease process. • *Wernicke's encephalopathy* produces a combination of diplopia, nystagmus, confusion, and cerebellar ataxis. Patients may not have all the features. The ocular motor features often include loss of lateral gaze and horizontal nystagmus. The ataxia involves gait and trunk more than limbs. • *Korsakoff's syndrome* presents with confusion, confabulation, and psychotic features. • Most patients with chronic thiamine deficiency have some degree of polyneuropathy, giving distal sensory deficit with or without motor deficit.
Laboratory studies	• Routine labs are normal, although some patients will have findings consistent with chronic alcoholism, including hyponatremia and elevated liver function tests (LFTs). Transketolase and thiamine levels can be reduced. Pyruvate levels may be increased. • Imaging with MRI often shows abnormalities on T_2-weighted images in the thalamus and periaqueductal gray. • Lumbar puncture (LP) usually is normal, but is often obtained for study to look for infection, hemorrhage, demyelinating disease, and other conditions that may resemble Wernicke-Korsakoff syndrome.
Diagnosis	• Wernicke's encephalopathy is suspected when a patient presents with encephalopathy and has ocular motor defects. Abnormal labs, abnormal MRI, and determination of a history of predisposition by alcoholism or other chronic disease support the diagnosis. • Korsakoff's syndrome is suspected when a patient presents with confusion and confabulation, and is suspected of having a history of alcohol abuse or other chronic disease.
Differential diagnosis	• *Encephalitis and certain forms of meningitis.* Can present with confusion and ocular motor abnormalities. LP with cerebrospinal fluid (CSF) analysis can distinguish these diagnoses. • *Multiple sclerosis.* Can produce multifocal abnormalities on examination. However, cognitive abnormalities are not common early in the course.

THIAMINE DEFICIENCY—cont'd	
Management	• Administration of thiamine is the definitive treatment. Immediate injection of thiamine on suspicion of diagnosis is followed by daily oral thiamine.
	• Before the thiamine administration results in definitive improvement, psychosis and agitation may have to be treated. Neuroleptics and benzodiazepines commonly are used; the latter, in part, can treat the alcohol withdrawal, which commonly accompanies thiamine deficiency.
Clinical course	Most patients improve, especially if the patient is treated early. Fully-developed Korsakoff's psychosis often ends in incomplete recovery.

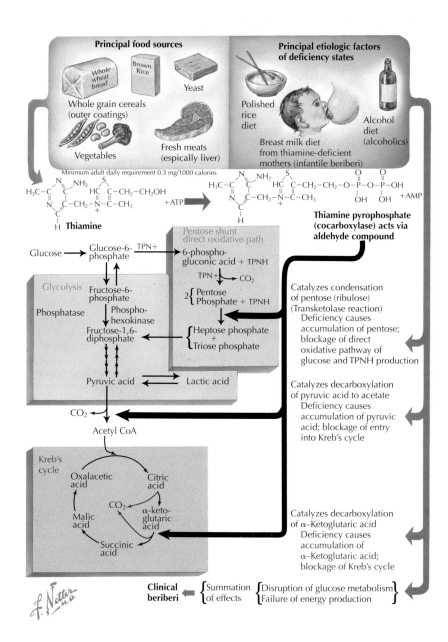

Principal food sources

Whole grain cereals (outer coatings)

Whole wheat bread

Brown Rice

Yeast

Vegetables

Fresh meats (espically liver)

Principal etiologic factors of deficiency states

Polished rice diet

Breast milk diet from thiamine-deficient mothers (infantile beriberi)

Alcohol diet (alcoholics)

Minimum adult daily requirement 0.3 mg/1000 calories

H_3C-C ... Thiamine

$+ATP$

Thiamine pyrophosphate (cocarboxylase) acts via aldehyde compound

$+AMP$

Glucose → Glucose-6-phosphate — TPN+ →

Pentose shunt direct oxidative path

6-phospho-gluconic acid + TPNH

TPN+ → CO_2

2{ Pentose Phosphate + TPNH

Glycolysis

Fructose-6-phosphate

Phosphatase

Phospho-hexokinase

Fructose-1,6-diphosphate

{ Heptose phosphate + Triose phosphate

Pyruvic acid ⇄ Lactic acid

CO_2

Acetyl CoA

Kreb's cycle

Oxalacetic acid — Citric acid

CO_2 — α-keto-glutaric acid

Malic acid

Succinic acid

Catalyzes condensation of pentose (ribulose) (Transketolase reaction) Deficiency causes accumulation of pentose; blockage of direct oxidative pathway of glucose and TPNH production

Catalyzes decarboxylation of pyruvic acid to acetate Deficiency causes accumulation of pyruvic acid; blockage of entry into Kreb's cycle

Catalyzes decarboxylation of α–Ketoglutaric acid Deficiency causes accumulation of α–Ketoglutaric acid; blockage of Kreb's cycle

Clinical beriberi ⇐ { Summation of effects { Disruption of glucose metabolism Failure of energy production }

DIABETES MELLITUS (DM)	
Description	• Divided into types 1 and 2 • *Type 1 diabetes* has a childhood onset and is due to impaired insulin control over glucose. Patients are insulin dependent. • *Type 2 diabetes* has an adult onset and is due to insulin resistance with some level of insulin production deficit.
Pathophysiology	• *Type 1 diabetes* is predominantly a genetic condition, with the possibility of environmental triggers. • *Type 2 diabetes* is more likely in obese patients, in pregnancy, and with a family history of adult-onset diabetes.
Clinical findings	• Patients may present with symptoms of hyperglycemia, including polydipsia and polyuria. • Patients may present with diabetic ketoacidosis (DKA) or hyperglycemic hyperosmolar nonketotic coma. • Patients may be asymptomatic for years prior to the diagnosis.
Laboratory studies	• Routine labs may show hyperglycemia, but this is not invariable, because the levels are erratic. Blood glucose commonly is high. • Hemoglobin A_{1C} (HbA$_{1C}$) is elevated in patients with diabetes, indicating persistence of deficits of glucose control. • Long-standing diabetes can produce laboratory findings of neuropathy, renal damage, and cardiac damage. Neuropathy commonly is present at diagnosis. • Imaging usually is not needed, because this is not a structural problem. If there are focal neurologic signs, magnetic resonance imaging (MRI) or computer tomography (CT) is needed to assess for stroke, etc.
Diagnosis	Diabetes is suspected when a patient has polyuria with polydipsia. With this history, random glucose often is found to be high. Glucose levels and HbA$_{1C}$ make the diagnosis.
Differential diagnosis	*Diabetes insipidis.* Can produce polyuria, but this is not associated with a disorder of glucose control.
Management	• Diabetes is managed with a host of treatments. Overall glucose is managed by proper diet, exercise, and medications to regulate glucose levels. • Management of DKA and hyperosmolar hyperglycemic nonketotic coma (HHNC). • Pain from polyneuropathy is treated with standard medications for neuropathic pain. • Cerebrovascular complications from diabetes mellitus (DM) are common, and largely include small-vessel ischemic disease.
Clinical course	Most patients stabilize with improvement in glucose control and resolution of DKA and HHNC. However, long-term complications of the diabetes are inevitable.

Neuropathy

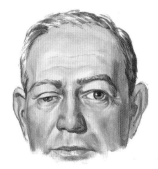

Extra ocular muscle paralysis
(ptosis, strabismus, diplopia)

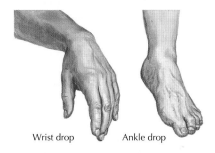

Wrist drop   Ankle drop

Autonomic dysfunction

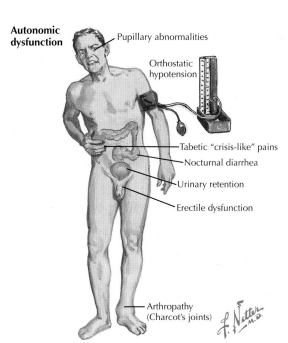

Pupillary abnormalities

Orthostatic hypotension

Tabetic "crisis-like" pains

Nocturnal diarrhea

Urinary retention

Erectile dysfunction

Arthropathy
(Charcot's joints)

THYROID DISORDERS	
Description	Common and can present with cerebral or neuromuscular findings
Pathophysiology	• Thyroid pathology is diverse and both hyperthyroidism and hypothyroidism have neurologic manifestations. • Hyperthyroidism can be caused by autoimmune, medication-related, neoplastic, and idiopathic disorders. • Hypothyroidism can be caused by toxic, metabolic, autoimmune, and idiopathic causes.
Hyperthyroidism	
Clinical findings	• Symptoms include nervousness, irritability, weakness, palpitations, fatigue, and weight loss. • Thyrotoxic myopathy produces weakness that is mainly proximal, with wasting of muscles of the shoulder girdle. Periodic paralysis can develop. Myasthenia gravis also can be associated. • Exam can show the weakness plus tachycardia, exophthalmos, hair loss, and increased sweating.
Laboratory studies	• Routine labs usually are normal. • Thyroid function tests usually show elevated T_3 and T_4 with suppression of thyroid-stimulating hormone (TSH). • Imaging is normal. • Nerve conduction study (NCS) and electromyography (EMG) may show myopathic features.
Diagnosis	• Hyperthyroidism is suspected when a patient presents with weakness, tremor, and/or nervousness. Most patients with these symptoms will not have a thyroid disorder, but this has to be considered. • Thyroid function tests should be considered in patients presenting with the neurologic complaints of tremor, irritability, memory loss, and weakness.
Management	• Some of the symptoms of hyperthyroidism can be treated with medications like β-blockers. • Both radioactive iodine and thyroid surgery can reduce active thyroid hormone production.
Hypothyroidism	
Clinical findings	• Symptoms of hypothyroidism include weakness, fatigue, weight gain, depression, confusion, and irritability. • Exam may show myopathy with weakness—most prominently proximally. Polyneuropathy is common. Ataxia with a cerebellar appearance can be seen. Decreased facial expression with motor findings may suggest parkinsonism.
Laboratory studies	• Routine labs usually are normal. • Thyroid hormone levels typically are low with increased TSH. • Imaging is normal, and often not needed.

Hypothyroidism	
Diagnosis	• Hypothyroidism often is suspected when a patient presents with weakness, fatigue, and weight gain.
	• Diagnosis is confirmed when thyroid function tests show decreased thyroid hormones and increased TSH.
Management	• Replacement with thyroxine results in clinical improvement.
	• Long-term therapy is expected, with rapid worsening if treatment is discontinued.

Hyperthyroidism

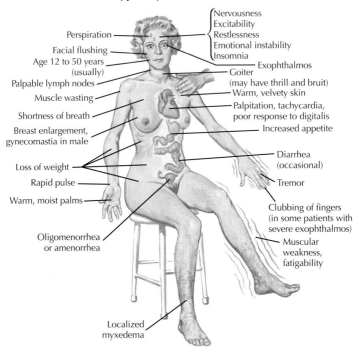

Perspiration

Facial flushing

Age 12 to 50 years (usually)

Palpable lymph nodes

Muscle wasting

Shortness of breath

Breast enlargement, gynecomastia in male

Loss of weight

Rapid pulse

Warm, moist palms

Oligomenorrhea or amenorrhea

Localized myxedema

Nervousness
Excitability
Restlessness
Emotional instability
Insomnia

Exophthalmos

Goiter (may have thrill and bruit)

Warm, velvety skin

Palpitation, tachycardia, poor response to digitalis

Increased appetite

Diarrhea (occasional)

Tremor

Clubbing of fingers (in some patients with severe exophthalmos)

Muscular weakness, fatigability

Hypothyroidism

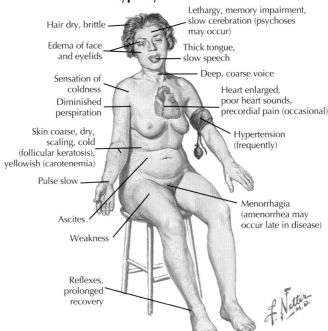

Hair dry, brittle

Edema of face and eyelids

Sensation of coldness

Diminished perspiration

Skin coarse, dry, scaling, cold (follicular keratosis), yellowish (carotenemia)

Pulse slow

Ascites

Weakness

Reflexes, prolonged recovery

Lethargy, memory impairment, slow cerebration (psychoses may occur)

Thick tongue, slow speech

Deep, coarse voice

Heart enlarged, poor heart sounds, precordial pain (occasional)

Hypertension (frequently)

Menorrhagia (amenorrhea may occur late in disease)

ADRENAL DISORDERS	
Description	Can include insufficiency or overactivity
Pathophysiology	• *Hyperadrenalism* often is due to exogenously administered corticosteroids; however, Cushing's syndrome can develop from oversecretion by the adrenal gland. • *Hypoadrenalism (Addison's disease)* often is triggered by a serious illness such as myocardial infarction (MI), major trauma, or sepsis. Withdrawal of exogenously administered corticosteroids is another common cause.
Adrenal Excess	
Clinical features	• Patients with long-standing adrenal insufficiency have weakness, fatigue, hypertension, obesity, and skin striations. This results in a typical cushingoid appearance. • Females have irregular menses and excess hair growth. Males have reduced libido.
Laboratory studies	• Measurement of blood cortisol level initially is performed. The most specific diagnostic test is the 24-hour urinary free-cortisol test. • Dexamethasone suppression test helps to differentiate excessive production of adrenocorticotropin hormone (ACTH) from the pituitary vs. ectopic ACTH production—suppression suggests pituitary production whereas ectopic ACTH-producing tumor is not suppressed. • MRI of the pituitary is performed if a pituitary cause is suspected. • MRI or CT of the abdomen is performed if there is the possibility of adrenal tumor-producing tumor. CT of the chest is performed if ectopic tumor is suspected with a lung origin.
Diagnosis	Adrenal excess is suspected when a patient presents with a cushingoid appearance, especially if they complain of weakness.
Management	Treatment depends on the reason for the adrenal excess. Any one or combination of surgery, chemotherapy, and radiation can be used.
Adrenal Insufficiency	
Clinical features	• Chronic adrenal insufficiency produces weakness, fatigue, anorexia, and weight loss. Hyperpigmentation also is seen, although it can be missed as a complaint—unlike other causes, this hyperpigmentation is prominent in pressured areas and skin folds. • Other less common symptoms include hypotension, nausea, vomiting, diarrhea, and abdominal pain.
Laboratory studies	• Cortisol is measured, but the ACTH stimulation test is standard. Patients with adrenal insufficiency do not respond to ACTH; the corticotropin-releasing hormone (CRH) stimulation test is then performed. Primary adrenal insufficiency patients have high ACTH levels, but do not produce cortisol. Pituitary abnormalities result in absence of an ACTH response. Hypothalamic defects result in delayed ACTH response. • MRI of the brain may be performed to look for destructive lesions of the hypothalamus or pituitary if indicated by the lab results.

Adrenal Insufficiency	
Diagnosis	• Adrenal insufficiency is suspected when a patient presents with weakness and fatigue. Adrenal insufficiency is one of the diagnoses to consider, in addition to hypothyroidism. • Cortisol levels and ACTH stimulation tests make the diagnosis of adrenal insufficiency, with further testing to determine the cause.
Management	• Administration of corticosteroids results in prompt improvement. Oral hydrocortisone can be used, although there are other preparations. • If there also is mineralocorticoid deficiency from adrenal lesion, fludrocortisone also is given.

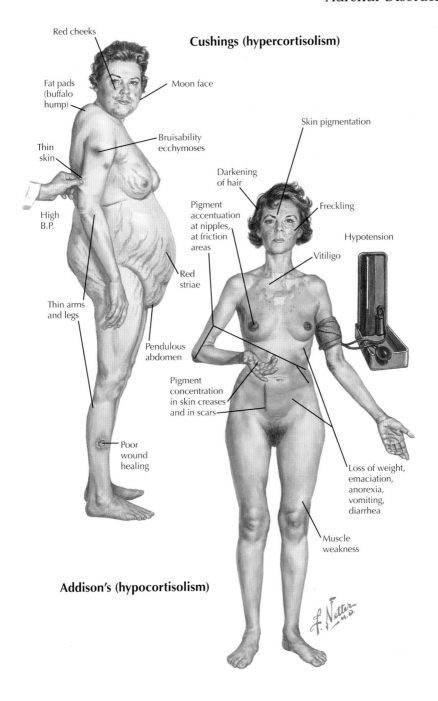

Cushings (hypercortisolism)

Red cheeks

Fat pads (buffalo hump)

Moon face

Thin skin

Bruisability ecchymoses

Skin pigmentation

Darkening of hair

Pigment accentuation at nipples, at friction areas

Freckling

High B.P.

Hypotension

Vitiligo

Red striae

Thin arms and legs

Pendulous abdomen

Pigment concentration in skin creases and in scars

Poor wound healing

Loss of weight, emaciation, anorexia, vomiting, diarrhea

Muscle weakness

Addison's (hypocortisolism)

Pituitary Disorders

PITUITARY DISORDERS	
Description	• Can result from a variety of pathologies, including tumor, infection, infarction, and trauma • Most pituitary tumors are benign and may or may not be functioning. They can produce pituitary hormones or destroy the ability of the pituitary to produce hormones.
Common findings	• All pituitary tumors can produce mass effect in the sella region and impairment in the production of some factors from the pituitary. • Some common features are visual loss from optic nerve and chiasmal compression, headache, and symptoms of hormone deficiency, including fatigue and weakness. • Surgery is performed for all types, although prolactinomas are given a trial of dopamine agonist, which shrinks the lesion in most patients.
Disorder	**Features**
Nonfunctioning pituitary tumor	• Usually presents with visual loss, due to mass effect of the tumor on the optic nerve and chiasm. The tumor can grow to remarkable size before it is diagnosed. • Extensive hormonal analysis is performed to characterize the tumor. • Treatment is with surgery.
Prolactin-producing tumor	• Can induce milk production and amenorrhea in females. The irregularity in menses and galactorrhea usually induces evaluation before the tumor is large. In contrast, men often have no symptoms other than loss of libido, so diagnosis may be delayed until there are symptoms of optic nerve compression or pituitary failure. • MRI of the brain, with special attention to the pituitary, is performed. • Treatment is with dopamine agonists—approximately 89% will respond with medical therapy and may not need surgical therapy.
Growth hormone–producing tumor	• Results in acromegaly. The lower jaw becomes prominent, and if the patient is not fully grown, excessive height is expected. In adults, the hands and feet enlarge along with the jaw. Patients complain of weakness. Distance between teeth can be abnormally wide. • Visual changes can be present with optic nerve compression.
ACTH-producing tumor	• Results in Cushing's syndrome. • Differentiation of pituitary from hypothalamic or adrenal causes is possible with hormonal testing. • Management is surgical. Hormone replacement may be needed following surgery.

Pituitary Tumors

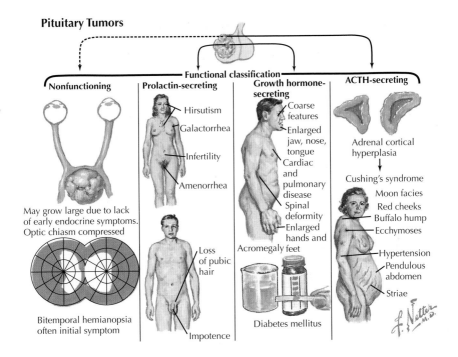

Functional classification

Nonfunctioning

May grow large due to lack of early endocrine symptoms. Optic chiasm compressed

Bitemporal hemianopsia often initial symptom

Prolactin-secreting

Hirsutism

Galactorrhea

Infertility

Amenorrhea

Loss of pubic hair

Impotence

Growth hormone-secreting

Coarse features

Enlarged jaw, nose, tongue

Cardiac and pulmonary disease

Spinal deformity

Enlarged hands and feet

Acromegaly

Diabetes mellitus

ACTH-secreting

Adrenal cortical hyperplasia

Cushing's syndrome

Moon facies

Red cheeks

Buffalo hump

Ecchymoses

Hypertension

Pendulous abdomen

Striae

ANOSMIA	
Description	Lack of smell
	The most common causes of anosmia are:
	• Trauma
	• Olfactory groove meningioma
	• Neurodegenerative disease
Common features	• Patients can be asymptomatic, with identification of anosmia only at exam.
	• Complaint may be of loss of taste, and only on exam is the localization identified as loss of smell rather than loss of elemental taste sensation.
	• There is no treatment for anosmia unless the underlying cause can be cured, and this usually is not the case.

Disorder	Features
Traumatic anosmia	• Can occur in about 10% of patients with significant head injury. Trauma is the most common cause of anosmia in young adults.
	• The cause of the anosmia most commonly is the shearing action of the olfactory fibers at the cribriform plate, but mucosal damage and inferior frontal contusion and hemorrhage also are potential causes.
	• Patients seldom complain of the anosmia at the time of presentation, but subsequently the olfactory defect can be noticed.
Olfactory groove meningioma	• Can occur almost anywhere, but growth in the olfactory groove occurs about 10% of the time
	• Loss of smell is the first symptom. If this is not noticed and evaluated, the tumor may grow to produce visual loss from optic nerve compression or mental status changes from frontal lobe damage.
	• Treatment is surgical.
Neurodegenerative disease	• Alzheimer's disease and Parkinson's disease are associated with loss of smell, which can predate the other neurologic symptoms.
	• Testing of patients with dementia for anosmia is of interest, but there are insufficient data to support the widespread use of this as a screening tool.
	• Testing may be more helpful for patients with parkinsonism, because patients with Parkinson's disease often have impaired smell, whereas patients with vascular parkinsonism do not.

Nerves of Nasal Cavity

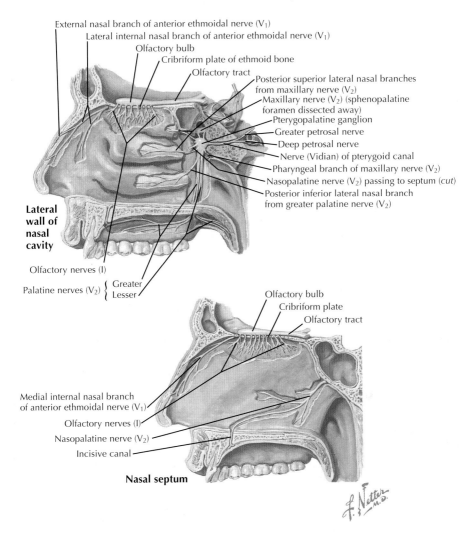

External nasal branch of anterior ethmoidal nerve (V$_1$)
Lateral internal nasal branch of anterior ethmoidal nerve (V$_1$)
Olfactory bulb
Cribriform plate of ethmoid bone
Olfactory tract
Posterior superior lateral nasal branches from maxillary nerve (V$_2$)
Maxillary nerve (V$_2$) (sphenopalatine foramen dissected away)
Pterygopalatine ganglion
Greater petrosal nerve
Deep petrosal nerve
Nerve (Vidian) of pterygoid canal
Pharyngeal branch of maxillary nerve (V$_2$)
Nasopalatine nerve (V$_2$) passing to septum (*cut*)
Posterior inferior lateral nasal branch from greater palatine nerve (V$_2$)

Lateral wall of nasal cavity

Olfactory nerves (I)

Palatine nerves (V$_2$) { Greater / Lesser

Olfactory bulb
Cribriform plate
Olfactory tract

Medial internal nasal branch of anterior ethmoidal nerve (V$_1$)
Olfactory nerves (I)
Nasopalatine nerve (V$_2$)
Incisive canal

Nasal septum

ISCHEMIC OPTIC NEUROPATHY (ION)	
Description	• Results in acute monocular visual loss due to ischemia affecting the optic nerve. There are two subtypes—arteritic and nonarteritic.
	• Arteritic ION is associated with temporal arteritis (TA).
	• Non-arteritic ION is due to cerebrovascular disease.
Pathophysiology	• Patients develop ION because of inflammatory or occlusive disease. Patients with temporal arteritis are predisposed to visual loss, which is a worrisome complication of untreated TA.
	• Patients with vascular risk factors, including hypertension, diabetes, smoking, and hyperlipidemia, are predisposed to develop ION.
Clinical findings	• ION presents with the acute onset of monocular visual loss.
	• Patients with arteritic IONs have findings of TA, including temporal area pain, swelling, and tenderness of the temporal artery, pain in the jaw area, and malaise.
	• Patients with nonarteritic ION have few other symptoms; the arteritic symptoms are distinctly absent.
	• Exam shows papilledema in most patients. Pupil abnormalities are common. Visual fields are severely affected.
	• Bilateral involvement develops in about a third of patients with nonarteritic ION, and in two thirds of patients with arteritic ION, if not treated. Treatment reduces the likelihood of contralateral visual loss.
Laboratory studies	• Erythrocyte sedimentation rate (ESR) is elevated in most patients with arteritic ION.
	• Vascular risk factors, including hyperlipidemia and diabetes, may be identified on labs in patients with nonarteritic ION.
	• Imaging usually is performed to look for infarction. Magnetic resonance imaging (MRI) can show infarctions of the brain, mass lesions in the orbit, and with magnetic resonance angiography (MRA) can show most significant vascular lesions.
	• Lumbar puncture (LP) is performed if the combination of headache, malaise, and visual loss raises suspicions of meningitis or encephalitis, although this usually is not done.
Diagnosis	• ION is suspected when a patient presents with sudden onset of visual loss.
	• Ophthalmologic evaluation can help to differentiate ION from other causes of acute monocular visual loss.
	• MRI often is performed to look for arterial occlusive disease and mass lesions.
	• Elevated ESR and temporal-region pain suggest arteritic ION.

ISCHEMIC OPTIC NEUROPATHY (ION)—cont'd	
Differential diagnosis	• *Optic neuritis.* Can present with monocular or binocular visual loss; however, the onset is not abrupt. Patients tend to be younger than patients with both forms of ION.
	• *Central retinal vein occlusion* (CRVO). Can occur from many causes, including cerebrovascular disease, vasculitis, and hypercoagulable state. The retinal appearance is different. The onset of the visual loss often is slower and is subacute, rather than acute.
Management	• Arteritic ION is treated with corticosteroids. Temporal artery biopsy is recommended for most patients with suspected TA, because secure diagnosis should be established before committing the patient to long-term corticosteroids.
	• Nonarteritic ION is treated only with reduction in risk factors and antiplatelet agents—there is no direct treatment.
Clinical course	• Most patients improve, although this is not universal. If the ION has progressed to blindness, persistent visual loss is expected.
	• Recovery from arteritic ION is much better with early treatment than with late treatment.

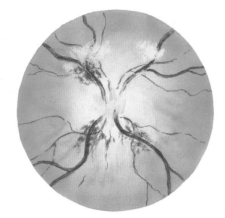

Anterior ischemic optic neuropathy

Anatomy of Optic Nerve

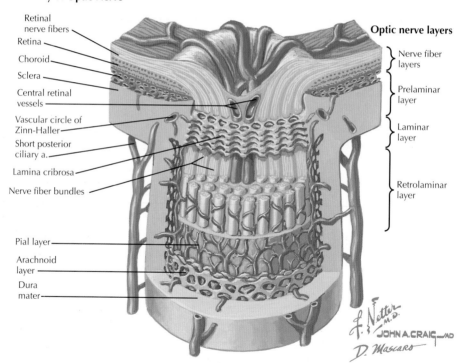

Retinal nerve fibers

Retina

Choroid

Sclera

Central retinal vessels

Vascular circle of Zinn-Haller

Short posterior ciliary a.

Lamina cribrosa

Nerve fiber bundles

Pial layer

Arachnoid layer

Dura mater

Optic nerve layers

Nerve fiber layers

Prelaminar layer

Laminar layer

Retrolaminar layer

HORNER'S SYNDROME	
Description	Loss of sympathetic innervation of the eye
Pathophysiology	• Sympathetic fibers project from the hypothalamus through the brainstem and cervical spine, which then exit to the sympathetic chain. Ascending nerves with the sympathetic chain pass through the cavernous sinus to the orbit and eye. • Lesion of the sympathetic fibers at any point in this long route can produce Horner's syndrome. Associated features help to determine the location of the lesion.
Clinical findings	• Classic presentation is ptosis, miosis, and anhidrosis on the ipsilateral face. • Associated findings can help localization. Hemiataxia suggests brainstem lesion, usually infarction. Hemiparesis suggests carotid lesion. Arm weakness and sensory complaints suggests lesion in the cervical spine or brachial plexus. • Cocaine administration results in prompt dilation in most patients, but not in patients with Horner's syndrome, because there is a paucity of norepinephrine at the terminal. Subsequent administration of hydroxyamphetamine or derivatives can help to distinguish whether the neural lesion is 1st or 2nd vs 3rd order; presynaptic stimulation results in dilation for 1st and 2nd order lesions, but not with 3rd order lesions.
Laboratory studies	• Routine labs are normal. • MRI of the brain can look for brainstem infarction, cervical spine or plexus lesion, cavernous sinus lesion, or orbital lesion. • MRA can look for arterial occlusive disease.
Diagnosis	• Horner's syndrome is a clinical condition with multiple possible causes. When presented with anisocoria, it can be difficult to determine whether the pathologic side is the large or the small side. Associated features such as ptosis and anhidrosis ipsilateral to the miosis make the diagnosis of Horner's syndrome. • Imaging is performed to look for structural causes of Horner's syndrome.
Differential diagnosis	• *Oculomotor (CN-3) palsy.* Can present with anisocoria, but the pathologic side is the dilated side. • *Tonic pupil.* Can present with anisocoria, although this often is a bilateral condition. Pupil responses, associated symptoms, and pharmacologic testing can differentiate these conditions.
Management	• There is no specific management for Horner's syndrome. • Cause of the lesion is treated if possible.
Clinical course	Horner's syndrome is often a persistent finding, largely because the cause is often not reversible; the damage has been done.

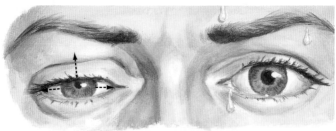

Abnormal eye movements (cranial nerves III, IV and/or VI) Horner's syndrome may be present

BELL'S PALSY AND RAMSAY-HUNT SYNDROME	
Description	• Bell's palsy is an idiopathic facial palsy. • Ramsay-Hunt syndrome is a herpes zoster of the geniculate ganglion with resultant facial palsy.
Pathophysiology	• Inflammation of the facial nerve and geniculate ganglion can produce facial weakness. • In patients with Ramsay-Hunt syndrome, the inflammation is due to varicella zoster virus (VZV) involvement of the geniculate ganglion. In patients with Bell's palsy, about a third also has VZV as the culprit, and, therefore, the term idiopathic facial palsy is not synonymous with Bell's palsy.
Clinical findings	• Patients present with unilateral facial palsy. There is often a history of periauricular pain one or more days prior to the development of the weakness. The pain is more prominent with Ramsay-Hunt than with Bell's palsy. • Vesicles are seen in the external auditory canal (EAC) of patients with RHS. Associated symptoms can be vertigo, and the occasional patient may report hearing loss. • Involvement of the upper and lower face is essential to the diagnosis, because central lesions usually involve only the lower face. Upper face involvement results in inability to close the eye and impaired wrinkling of the forehead—best seen with voluntary upward gaze. • Taste can be impaired from the anterior two thirds of the tongue.
Laboratory studies	• Routine labs are normal. CMP, CBC, ESR, and viral serologies often are done. The viral serologies are of limited value because of the prevalence of these viruses in patients. Hemoglobin (Hg)BA1C may be performed to look for diabetes. • MRI is normal, although enhancement of CN-7 and CN-8 occasionally can be seen.
Diagnosis	• Bell's palsy is suspected when a patient presents with the subacute onset of unilateral facial weakness. • Ramsay-Hunt syndrome is suspected when a patient with Bell's palsy has vesicles in the EAC.
Differential diagnosis	• *Stroke.* Can produce facial weakness, although almost always there are other neurologic deficits. Also, stroke would be expected to produce weakness of the lower face, whereas Bell's palsy and Ramsay-Hunt syndrome produces weakness of the upper and lower face. • *Trigeminal neuralgia.* Can produce pain on the side of the face, although this is not associated with motor loss. • *Hemifacial spasm.* Can produce asymmetric appearance to the face, associated with pain. However, the asymmetry is due to muscle contraction and not weakness. • *Tumors or infections in the ear or cerebellopontine angle.* Can cause pain in the area with facial palsy, but generally has a slower onset than these two entities. However, structural lesions have to be considered.

BELL'S PALSY AND RAMSAY-HUNT SYNDROME—cont'd	
Management	• Corticosteroids are routinely used. • Antivirals such as acyclovir are used, especially for RHS. The use in Bell's palsy is more controversial, but because the adverse effects are few and HSVs are causative, treatment is reasonable. • Physical therapy is helpful for restoration of motor function of the face. • Patients with vertigo can respond to vestibular exercises. • Exposure keratitis is a potential cause of visual loss, so patients with Bell's palsy and Ramsay-Hunt syndrome should be cautioned and instructed on the protection of the eye—patching at night, artificial tears, and taping may be necessary.
Clinical course	• The vast majority of patients with both causes of facial weakness improve. • Residual weakness can occur, and there are some restorative procedures that are tried for this.

Bell's Palsy

Course and distribution of facial (VII) nerve

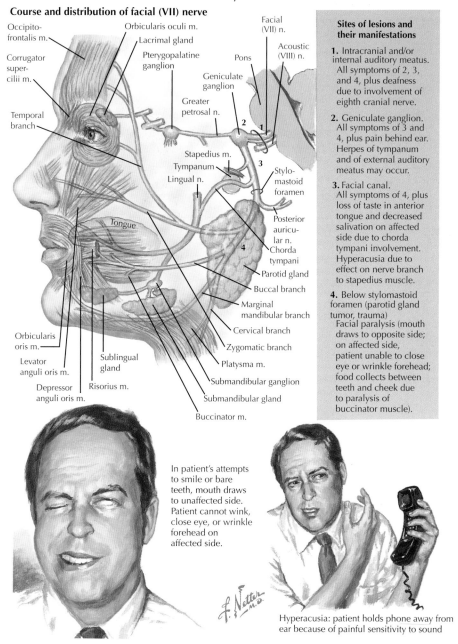

Occipito-frontalis m.
Corrugator supercilii m.
Temporal branch
Orbicularis oculi m.
Lacrimal gland
Pterygopalatine ganglion
Geniculate ganglion
Greater petrosal n.
Facial (VII) n.
Acoustic (VIII) n.
Pons
Stapedius m.
Tympanum
Lingual n.
Tongue
Stylo-mastoid foramen
Posterior auricular n.
Chorda tympani
Parotid gland
Buccal branch
Marginal mandibular branch
Cervical branch
Zygomatic branch
Platysma m.
Submandibular ganglion
Submandibular gland
Buccinator m.
Orbicularis oris m.
Levator anguli oris m.
Depressor anguli oris m.
Risorius m.
Sublingual gland

Sites of lesions and their manifestations

1. Intracranial and/or internal auditory meatus. All symptoms of 2, 3, and 4, plus deafness due to involvement of eighth cranial nerve.

2. Geniculate ganglion. All symptoms of 3 and 4, plus pain behind ear. Herpes of tympanum and of external auditory meatus may occur.

3. Facial canal. All symptoms of 4, plus loss of taste in anterior tongue and decreased salivation on affected side due to chorda tympani involvement. Hyperacusia due to effect on nerve branch to stapedius muscle.

4. Below stylomastoid foramen (parotid gland tumor, trauma) Facial paralysis (mouth draws to opposite side; on affected side, patient unable to close eye or wrinkle forehead; food collects between teeth and cheek due to paralysis of buccinator muscle).

In patient's attempts to smile or bare teeth, mouth draws to unaffected side. Patient cannot wink, close eye, or wrinkle forehead on affected side.

Hyperacusia: patient holds phone away from ear because of painful sensitivity to sound

ACOUSTIC NEUROMA (VESTIBULAR SCHWANNOMA)	
Description	Acoustic neuroma is a really a schwannoma affecting CN-8 between the brainstem and the ear.
Pathophysiology	Acoustic neuroma is a benign tumor with increased incidence in patients with neurofibromatosis.
Clinical findings	• Acoustic neuroma presents with ipsilateral hearing loss, vertigo, and tinnitus. • CN-7 involvement can produce ipsilateral facial weakness. • Patients with neurofibromatois will have other stigmata of the disease. Also, patients with NF also often have bilateral acoustic neuromas.
Laboratory studies	• Routine labs are normal. • Imaging shows the tumor at the cerebellopontine angle (CPA) or IAC, but special attention to the latter must be requested.
Diagnosis	• Acoustic neuroma is suspected when a patient presents with hearing loss and tinnitus. Ear problems always are considered. • Magnetic resonance imaging (MRI) shows the lesion if performed with special attention to the CPA and IAC.
Differential diagnosis	• *Inflammatory and infectious disorders of the inner ear.* Can produce hearing loss and tinnitus. Facial weakness also can develop. These have a slower onset than acoustic neuroma. • *Meningiomas of the cerebellopontine angle.* Can compress and involve CN-8 and CN-7, giving similar symptoms. MRI can help to differentiate, but surgical pathology makes the definitive diagnosis.
Management	Treatment is surgical. Some patients may have lesions that are small enough so they can be followed without resection.
Clinical course	Acoustic neuromas can increase in size, and decisions on resection depend on size, geometry, age, and health of the patient.

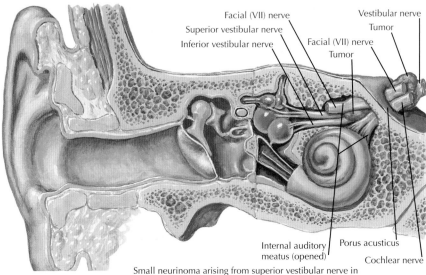

Small neurinoma arising from superior vestibular nerve in
internal auditory meatus and protruding into posterior fossa

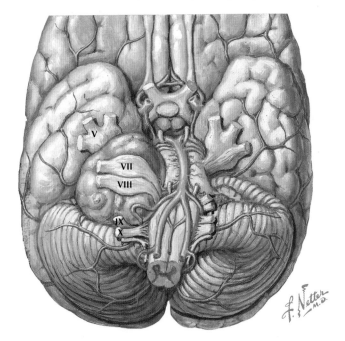

Large acoustic neurinoma filling cerebellopontine angle,
distorting brainstem and cranial nerves V, VII, VIII, IX, X

BENIGN PAROXYSMAL POSITIONAL VERTIGO (BPPV) AND MENIERE'S DISEASE	
Description	Vestibular causes are the most common causes of dizziness. BPPV and Meniere's disease are the most important causes of dizziness.
Common features	• Vertigo is a sensation of motion.
	• Movement commonly exacerbates vertigo.
Benign Paroxysmal Positional Vertigo	
Clinical features	• Patients present with vertigo and imbalance that is precipitated by movement. There may be associated nausea and a sense of lightheadedness, but true syncope is not expected. Head tilt can also trigger vertigo, such as looking upward.
	• Symptoms are temporary, lasting days to a few weeks. Then they abate, although recurrence after a remission is common.
Diagnosis	• BPPV is suspected when a patient complains of positional vertigo with a normal examination.
	• MRI often is not necessary, but is performed if there is suspicion for tumor or stroke.
	• Specialized vestibular tests are performed for documentation of the deficit. Barany maneuvers can be of particular help.
Management	• Meclizine and similar medications are effective for some patients with BPPV.
	• Benzodiazepines can be used if the vertigo is severe, although this should be avoided if possible.
	• Vestibular therapy is the most effective treatment—up to 80% of patients find relief. These can be performed by a physical therapist.
Meniere's Disease	
Clinical features	• Meniere's disease presents with episodic vertigo, hearing loss, and tinnitus.
	• A vague sensation of fullness in the ear is common.
	• Signs of parenchymal brainstem abnormality are absent, including limb ataxia, diplopia, and corticospinal abnormalities.
Diagnosis	• Meniere's disease is suspected with the symptoms of vertigo, hearing loss, and tinnitus. There are few other diagnoses to consider; acoustic neuroma can present with these symptoms; however, there would normally be progressive rather than intermittent symptoms.
	• MRI is performed to look for acoustic neuroma or other tumor at the CPA or IAC.
Management	• Self-help guidelines include dietary changes, including low salt, no caffeine, no alcohol, and no tobacco.
	• Typical treatments for vertigo can help that symptom, but they do not affect the tinnitus or hearing loss.
	• Repositioning maneuvers often are helpful in improving symptoms.
	• Ototoxic drugs can be of help for some individuals.
	• Surgery for Meniere's disease includes removing the labyrinth, although this results in hearing loss, and, therefore, usually it is only considered in patients with existing hearing loss. Vestibular neurectomy can help vertigo without as much risk to hearing.

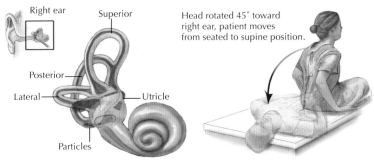

Right ear
Superior
Posterior
Lateral
Utricle
Particles

Head rotated 45° toward right ear, patient moves from seated to supine position.

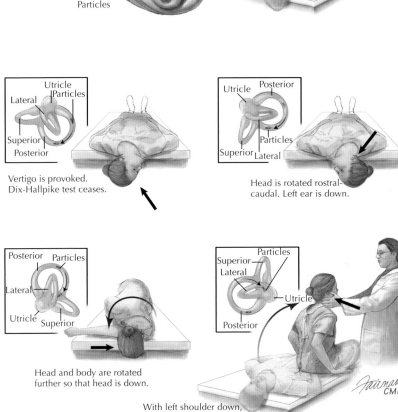

Utricle
Particles
Lateral
Superior
Posterior

Vertigo is provoked.
Dix-Hallpike test ceases.

Utricle
Posterior
Particles
Superior
Lateral

Head is rotated rostral-caudal. Left ear is down.

Posterior
Particles
Lateral
Utricle
Superior

Head and body are rotated further so that head is down.

Particles
Superior
Lateral
Utricle
Posterior

With left shoulder down, patient is brought to a seated position.

CAVERNOUS SINUS THROMBOSIS	
Description	Usually develops from infection in the mouth or face
Pathophysiology	Venous drainage from the face and upper aspect of the mouth is through the cavernous sinus. Infection carried from these locations can result in infectious thrombosis with resultant involvement of vessels and nerves in the sinus.
Clinical findings	• Patients often present with headache and fever, and have signs of a history of facial, oral, ear, or dental infection. A history of trauma may be elicited. • Examination may show orbital edema with signs of venous congestion. With increasing severity, there may be proptosis and eventual ocular motor palsies. • Abducens (CN-6) palsy can be seen before the other ocular motor findings are evident. • Symptoms can be unilateral or bilateral. • Meningeal signs can be seen.
Laboratory studies	• Routine labs often show increased white blood cell count (WBC) and elevated signs of inflammation. • Blood cultures often grow the organism. • Imaging usually shows the cavernous sinus pathology, with computer tomography (CT) and magnetic resonance imaging (MRI) both being effective for diagnosis. • Lumbar puncture (LP) is performed if the patient has any meningeal signs. Cerebrospinal fluid (CSF) may show mild increase in WBC and protein suggestive of parameningeal infection unless the CSF is seeded, in which case typical findings of bacterial meningitis will be seen.
Diagnosis	• Cavernous sinus thrombosis is considered when a patient presents with headache and orbital edema. The diagnosis is most definite when there is proptosis and ophthalmoparesis. • Diagnosis is confirmed by CT or MRI. • LP may be needed if there are symptoms of meningitis.
Differential diagnosis	• *Bacterial meningitis.* Can result in headache and cranial nerve deficits, although proptosis and orbital edema are not expected. It should be noted that bacterial meningitis can develop as a complication of cavernous sinus thrombosis. • *Orbital cellulites.* Can present with proptosis and ocular motor deficit. Trigeminal nerve abnormalities are not expected.
Management	• Antibiotic therapy is needed, and should be initiated with staph coverage. • Heparin often is used to reduce the chance of subsequent thrombosis. • Corticosteroids often are used to reduce tissue edema. • Surgical drainage of a sinus abscess can be helpful.
Clinical course	• Most patients improve with proper medical treatment. • Bilateral involvement can develop.

Intracranial Complications

Cavernous sinus thrombosis

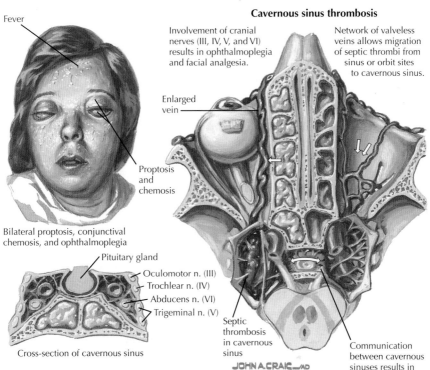

Fever

Involvement of cranial nerves (III, IV, V, and VI) results in ophthalmoplegia and facial analgesia.

Network of valveless veins allows migration of septic thrombi from sinus or orbit sites to cavernous sinus.

Enlarged vein

Proptosis and chemosis

Bilateral proptosis, conjunctival chemosis, and ophthalmoplegia

Pituitary gland

Oculomotor n. (III)
Trochlear n. (IV)
Abducens n. (VI)
Trigeminal n. (V)

Septic thrombosis in cavernous sinus

Communication between cavernous sinuses results in bilateral disease

Cross-section of cavernous sinus

JOHN A. CRAIG—MD

OVERVIEW OF GENETIC DISORDERS	
Description	Inherited disorders affecting the nervous system can be inherited in several ways: • Autosomal dominant • Autosomal recessive • X-linked • Mitochondrial
Mode of Inheritance	**Features**
Autosomal dominant	• A single gene on one of the autosomal chromosomes can cause the disease. • Some autosomal dominant genes have variable penetrance, where there is variable expression of the gene. • Children of one heterozygous parent and one normal parent have a 50% chance of getting the gene and the disease.
Autosomal recessive	• Abnormal genes from both chromosomes, from both parents, are required to produce disease. • Both parents must be at least heterozygous for the gene. • Children of two heterozygous parents have a 25% chance of being homozygous. • All children of an affected homozygous patient and a normal partner will be carriers.
X-linked dominant	• One abnormal X chromosome is needed to produce the disease. • Disease can form in both genders. • All female children of an affected male will have the gene and the disease, but none of the male children of an affected male will be affected. • Half of the female children of an affected female will have the gene and the disease. Half of the male children of an affected female will also be affected.
X-linked recessive	• All X-chromosomes must have the gene to have the disease, so that a female must have two abnormal X-chromosomes, whereas a male has his only X-chromosome abnormal. • Children of a female carrier will have children apportioned as follows: 25% normal male, 25% normal female, 25% affected male, 25% unaffected carrier female. • Children of an affected male will have 50% normal male, 50% unaffected carrier female.
Mitochondrial	• Mitochondria are maternally inherited; therefore, one can consider that mitochondrial DNA is of maternal origin. • Although females pass the affected DNA, both male and female children are affected.

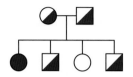

Autosomal recessive
inheritance pattern

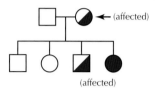

◄— (affected)

(affected)

Autosomal dominant
inheritance pattern

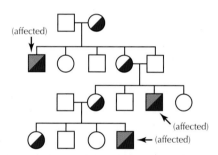

(affected)

(affected)

◄— (affected)

Transmission is **X-linked recessive,**
although some heterozygous females
show decreased IQ

HEREDITARY NEUROPATHIES (HMSN)	
Description	Tendency toward being distal and symmetric, and also can be axonal or demyelinating. There are two major types: • Hereditary sensory-autonomic neuropathy (HSAN) • Charcot-Marie-Tooth (CMT), which includes much of the hereditary motor sensory neuropathy (HMSN) series.
Common features	• There is no treatment that alters the course of any of these conditions. • Neuropathic pain can be treated with many of the available anticonvulsants, tricyclic antidepressants, and a few other medication choices as well.
Neuropathy	Features
CMT-1	• An autosomal dominant disorder with hypertrophic nerves. Neuropathic findings are distal and symmetric with predominant leg involvement. • Patients present with leg weakness and atrophy which is most evident in the tibialis anterior. Foot deformity is typical with pes cavus and hammer toes.
CMT-2	• Resembles CMT-1, but the nerves are not hypertrophic. Inheritance is autosomal dominant. • Patients present with distal weakness, hyporeflexia, and sensory loss.
CMT-3	• Also known as Dejerine-Sottas disease, an autosomal recessive or sporadic disorder. New mutations may be dominant. This is a hypertrophic neuropathy. • Presentation is in childhood with weakness that is disabling. Exam shows areflexia and hypertrophic nerves.
CMT-4	An autosomal recessive disorder that presents with weakness with onset in early childhood
HSAN-1	• Hereditary sensory-autonomic neuropathy type 1 is an autosomal dominant disorder that presents in young adult life. • Loss of sensation with neuropathic pain is typical. There are no motor findings early in the course, although motor deficits are seen in advanced cases.
HSAN-2	• An autosomal recessive disorder that presents in infancy • Severe sensory loss with distal predominance is typical. Spastic paraparesis and peripheral neuropathic weakness can develop in advanced cases. Bladder dysfunction is common.

Neuropathy	Features
HSAN-3	• A familial dysautonomia, an autosomal recessive neuropathy with prominence in patients of Ashkenazi Jewish descent • Autonomic instability presents with esophageal motility disorder with poor feeding, febrile episodes without infection, and fluctuations in blood pressure and heart rate. Later in childhood, there is scoliosis and insensitivity to pain. Fungiform papillae of the tongue are absent.
HSAN-4	• A rare autosomal recessive disorder that presents with congenital insensitivity to pain, episodic fever, anhidrosis, and mild MR. Self-mutilation can be seen. • A subset of these patients have been designated HSAN-5, but this is not clearly a distinct entity.

Hereditary Motor–Sensory Neuropathy Type I

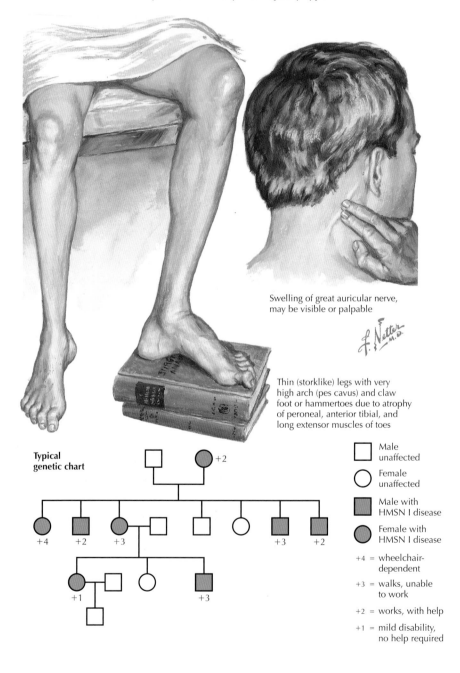

Swelling of great auricular nerve, may be visible or palpable

Thin (storklike) legs with very high arch (pes cavus) and claw foot or hammertoes due to atrophy of peroneal, anterior tibial, and long extensor muscles of toes

Typical genetic chart

□ Male unaffected

○ Female unaffected

■ Male with HMSN I disease

● Female with HMSN I disease

+4 = wheelchair-dependent

+3 = walks, unable to work

+2 = works, with help

+1 = mild disability, no help required

NEUROFIBROMATOSIS	
Description	An inherited disorder that results in neuronal growths that are usually benign
Pathophysiology	• Most patients inherit the NF gene by autosomal dominant transmission. However, at least 30% are new mutations. • NF1 and NF2 are described with separate criteria.
Neurofibromatosis Type 1	
Clinical features	• 6 or more café-au-lait spots larger than 5 mm in diameter • 2 or more neurofibroma or one plexiform neuroma • Multiple axillary or inguinal freckles • Optic glioma • Lisch nodules • Parent or other first-degree relative with NF
Diagnosis	• NF is suspected when a patient presents with café-au-lait spots and neurofibromas. • Clinical diagnosis is sufficient. Genetic testing is available.
Management	• Growths that are rapidly enlarging and may have malignant transformation are removed. • Medications for neuropathic pain are effective.
Neurofibromatosis Type 2	
Clinical features	• Acoustic schwannomas that are often bilateral • Parent or other first-degree relative with schwannoma, meningioma, or glioma • Patients may have spinal tumors, including meningiomas or ependymomas. • Typical skin changes of NF-1 are not expected.
Diagnosis	• NF-2 is suspected when a patient presents with tinnitus and hearing loss and is found on MRI to have bilateral acoustic schwannomas. • Multiple schwannomas or meningiomas suggest this diagnosis. • Genetic testing is available.
Management	• Resection of the schwannoma is sometimes done, especially if there is brainstem compression from extension in the cerebellopontine angle. • Some patients will only require follow-up for progression of their lesions.

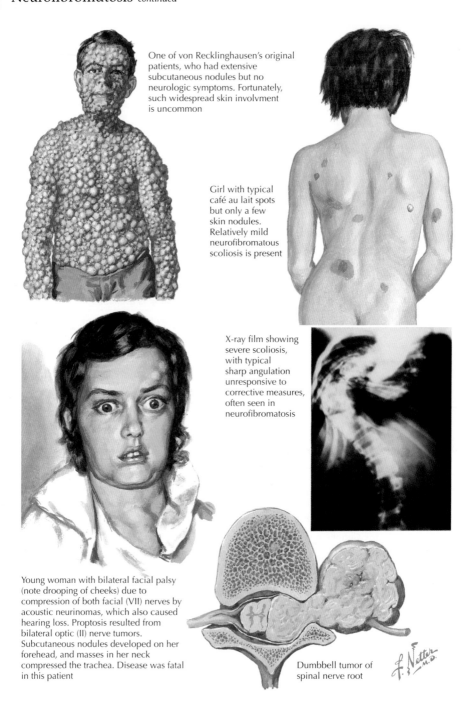

One of von Recklinghausen's original patients, who had extensive subcutaneous nodules but no neurologic symptoms. Fortunately, such widespread skin involvment is uncommon

Girl with typical café au lait spots but only a few skin nodules. Relatively mild neurofibromatous scoliosis is present

X-ray film showing severe scoliosis, with typical sharp angulation unresponsive to corrective measures, often seen in neurofibromatosis

Young woman with bilateral facial palsy (note drooping of cheeks) due to compression of both facial (VII) nerves by acoustic neurinomas, which also caused hearing loss. Proptosis resulted from bilateral optic (II) nerve tumors. Subcutaneous nodules developed on her forehead, and masses in her neck compressed the trachea. Disease was fatal in this patient

Dumbbell tumor of spinal nerve root

STORAGE DISEASES	
Description	• A heterogeneous group of disorders in which metabolic abnormalities are caused by failure in a metabolic pathway • Symptoms can be from accumulation of a product or cessation of neuronal function.
Common features	• The variety of symptoms is vast, but storage diseases can produce several combinations of weakness, discoordination, mental retardation, seizures, short stature, and other abnormalities of body habitus or orthopedic anomalies. • The numbers of disorders are huge, but some of the most important are discussed below.

Disorder	Features
Tay-Sachs disease	• Accumulation of GM2 ganglioside due to deficiency of β-hexosaminidase A • Progressive weakness, slowed growth, macrocephaly, cherry-red spot in the macula, and hyperacusis are seen.
Pompe's disease	• An autosomal recessive disorder, with accumulation of glycogen due to deficiency of acid maltase • Infants present with weakness, hypotonia, poor feeding, and poor suck. There is also cardiomegaly, respiratory failure, and congestive heart failure.
Farber's disease	• Accumulation of gangliosides by deficiency of ceramidase • Painful joint deformities and development of painful subcutaneous modules are seen. Respiratory compromise may require tracheostomy. • Neurologic involvement is variable.
McArdle's disease	• An autosomal recessive disorder, with accumulation of glycogen due to deficiency of muscle glycogen phosphorylase • Presents with myopathy with cramps after exercise, and sometimes with persistent weakness • Myoglobinuria in about half of patients • Patients should avoid strenuous exercise, which aggravates symptoms.
Metachromatic leukodystrophy	• Accumulation of sulfatide due to deficiency of sulfatidase (also known as arylsulfatase A) • There are forms of MLD which present from infancy to adult life. • Patients present with weakness, mental retardation, spasticity, and peripheral neuropathy.

Disorder	Features
Mucopolysaccharidoses (MPS)	• A group of disorders that are mostly autosomal recessive, except for X-linked Hunter's disease. They are all due to deficit in degradation of carbohydrate chains of glycosaminoglycans. • Common symptoms include mental retardation, skeletal abnormalities, and organomegaly to variable degrees. • *Hurler's disease (MPS-1)* is deficiency of α-iduronidase. • *Hunter's disease (MPS-2)* is deficiency of α-iduronate sulfatase. This is X-linked and milder than Hurler's. • *Sanfilippo's disease (MPS-3)* is due to one of four enzymatic defects of heparin sulfate degradation. • *Morquio's disease (MPS-4)* is a skeletal disorder with only secondary neurologic involvement. There are two types—A (N-acetylgalactosamine-6-sulfatase deficiency) and B (β-galactosidase deficiency). • *Maroteaux-Lamy disease (MPS-6)* resembles Hurler's but with relative preservation of intellect. • *B-Glucuronidase deficiency (MPS-7)* has the typical appearance of MPS.
Niemann-Pick disease	• *Type A—Sphingomyelinase deficiency* noted by severe progressive loss of intellectual skills and verbal function. Also present with hepatomegaly and splenomegaly. • *Type B—Sphingomyelinase deficiency* noted with a non-neurologic presentation—hepatosplenomegaly. • *Type C—Sphingomyelinase* reduced in some cells, plus accumulation of low-density lipoprotein (LDL)-cholesterol. Similar to type A, but later in onset and progression, and considered a juvenile form.
Krabbe's disease (globoid cell dystrophy)	• Accumulation of galactosylsphingosine due to deficiency of galactosylceramidase • Loss of myelin centrally and peripherally, with mental retardation, motor deficits with spasticity, and spasms with minor stimuli. Onset in infancy with death in young childhood.

Mucopolysaccharidoses—Signs and Symptoms

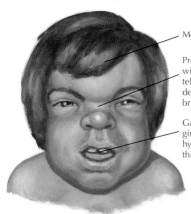

Mental retardation

Prominent eyes, with hyper-telorism and depressed nasal bridge

Gapped teeth, gingival hypertrophy, thickened tongue

Typical features of patient with Hurler syndrome

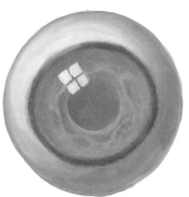

Corneal clouding, which may progress to severe visual loss (prominent feature of the Hurler, Scheie and Morquio syndromes)

Tay-Sachs Disease—Signs and Symptoms

Exaggerated extensor startle response to sound (Moro reflex) early in course

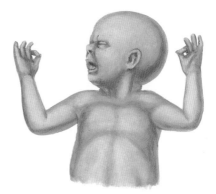

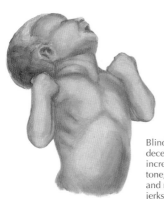

Blindness, decerebration, increased muscle tone, convulsions, and myoclonic jerks as disease progresses

JOHN A.CRAIG—AD

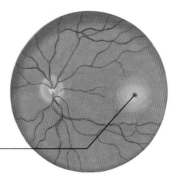

Characteristic cherry-red macular spot surrounded by white opaque area of degenerated retina

OVERVIEW OF SLEEP DISORDERS	
Description	An underdiagnosed group of conditions which have a major impact on quality of life of the patients
Pathophysiology	• Impaired sleep results in daytime fatigue, propensity to sleep, difficulty with concentration and learning, and an increased morbidity for certain other conditions. • Disorders as diverse as hypertension and seizures are made worse by sleep deprivation experienced due to sleep disorders.
Normal sleep	• Normal sleep through the night is punctuated by partial and complete arousals. The patients often are not aware of these, and believe they have slept continuously. • At the extremes of age—youth and elderly—the ability to sleep continuously is impaired, so normal sleep pattern is, to a certain extent, learned.
Sleep interruptions	Interruptions in sleep by periodic movements, sleep apnea, movements of a bed partner, or even external stimuli of light and noise result in impaired sleep with fatigue during the day.

Consequences of poor sleep	Poor sleep can contribute to the following:
	   • Impaired concentration and learning
	   • Exacerbation of pain syndromes such as fibromyalgia
	   • Chronic fatigue syndrome
	• Naps during the day may partially compensate for poor sleep at night.

Testing	• *Nocturnal polysomnography* (PSG) is recording of brain and other physiologic activity overnight. This is used for diagnosis of central and obstructive sleep apnea, periodic limb movements, and insomnia. • *Multiple sleep latency test* (MSLT) involves recording of EEG during the day with multiple naps. The latency to sleep and REM sleep is measured. This is used to evaluate for narcolepsy.
Complaint	**Features**
Excessive daytime sleepiness	• The chief complaint of many patients with sleep disorders • May be due to a primary sleep disorder, such as narcolepsy, or impaired nocturnal sleep from OSA or periodic limb movements
Insomnia	Inability to get to or stay asleep. Wide range of causes include sleep disorder, physical and psychologic factors, and poor sleep hygiene
Hypersomnia	Excessive sleep, common with some degenerative disorders, and seen in patients with certain medical problems such as CHF, COPD, severe metabolic disorders

Disorder	Features
Obstructive sleep apnea	The obstruction to air flow during sleep. The patient awakens because of the interruption, and therefore has poor quality of sleep.
Central sleep apnea	• Cessation of air flow during sleep, which causes arousal • The cause is failure of the drive of the respiratory centers, rather than obstruction.
Narcolepsy	• Sleep attacks that punctuate the daytime. They are more likely to occur during times of excitement than during times of boredom and inattention. • Often associated with cataplexy
Cataplexy	• Episodes of paralysis. Can occur upon awakening, i.e., sleep paralysis, or can develop during the daytime as paralysis without falling asleep, i.e., cataplexy attacks. • Associated with narcolepsy
Periodic limb movements	Episodic involuntary movements, especially of the legs, which interferes with sleep

Periodic Limb Movements

PERIODIC LIMB MOVEMENTS (PLM)	
Description	• Involuntary movements, especially the legs, which result in disturbance of amount and quality of sleep • Associated with restless legs syndrome, although they are distinct clinical entities
Pathophysiology	• *Primary PLM* is of an unknown cause. • *Secondary PLM* can be due to almost any cause of peripheral polyneuropathy, spinal cord lesion, certain medications, or withdrawal of sedative hypnotics.
Clinical findings	• There are episodic movements of the legs, which can range from "writhing and slow" to "fast and jerky." Both legs typically are affected. • The movements may result in partial or complete arousals in both the patient and bed mate. • Exam shows no specific abnormalities unless there is a neurologic cause of secondary PLM.
Laboratory studies	• Routine labs are normal unless the patient has diabetes or some other metabolic disorder. Anemia can be a potential cause of this and restless legs syndrome. • Sleep lab testing shows the periodic movements.
Diagnosis	• PLM is suspected when a patient presents with a history of awakening of the patient or bed mate. • Diagnosis is confirmed by PSG testing.
Differential diagnosis	• *Restless legs syndrome (RLS).* A need to move the legs during the awake state. It can be associated with PLM, but these are distinct entities. • *Nocturnal myoclonus.* Considered by most to be a synonym for PLM. This is jerking of the extremities.
Management	A variety of medications can be helpful to improve the symptoms: • Dopaminergic agents are helpful when given nightly. Levodopa and dopamine agonists are both used. • Benzodiazepines and other sedative hypnotics are used. • Anticonvulsants can be helpful, especially gabapentin.
Clinical course	Most patients improve with treatment, although long-term therapy is needed.

RESTLESS LEGS SYNDROME (RLS)	
Description	Although not strictly a sleep disorder, RLS is considered here because of its relationship to PLM.
Pathophysiology	• There is no specific pathology. Neuropathic abnormalities have been postulated for some patients. • *Primary RLS* is of unknown cause. • *Secondary RLS* is due to polyneuropathy or metabolic disturbance. Medical conditions as diverse as renal failure, Parkinson's disease, and use of various medications can cause secondary RLS.
Clinical findings	• Patients present with a compelling urge to move the legs, with resultant motor restlessness. Symptoms are prominent at rest. • Daytime sleepiness and nocturnal periodic limb movements may be associated with PLM in more than 80% of cases. • Exam is normal unless there is an underlying polyneuropathy or other medical condition.
Laboratory studies	• Routine labs are normal. • Nerve conduction study (NCS) and electromyogram (EMG) may show polyneuropathy in some patients with secondary RLS. • Imaging is normal unless a spinal abnormality is associated, which is quite rare.
Diagnosis	• RLS is a clinical diagnosis. When the typical features of motor restlessness and a compelling urge to move the legs are seen, a search for causes should be initiated. • EMG is performed for patients with symptoms of polyneuropathy. • Lab testing for thyroid, renal, hepatic, or neuropathic disorder is performed when these disorders are suspected. • Testing for iron-deficiency anemia is recommended.
Differential diagnosis	• *Myoclonus.* Can be associated with jerking of the legs and arms, and can be unilateral or bilateral. Motor restlessness is not expected. • *Seizure.* Can be considered if there are repetitive motions of the legs, although the clinical presentation is different. • *Painful legs-moving toes syndrome.* An uncommon condition marked by pain and continuous movement of the toes, with the pain extending to the legs. This often is associated with polyneuropathy. Motor restlessness is not seen.

Management	Medications for symptomatic agents include:
	  • Dopaminergic agents, including levodopa and dopamine agonists are very effective.
	  • Anticonvulsants often are effective, especially gabapentin.
	  • Benzodiazepines commonly are used, especially for nocturnal symptoms, but are of limited use during the day.
	  • Opiate analgesics occasionally are used; however, they are used more for nocturnal symptoms than for daytime symptoms.

Clinical course	Most patients improve with treatment.

SLEEP APNEA	
Description	Cessation of air flow during sleep
Pathophysiology	• *Obstructive sleep apnea (OSA)* is due to mechanical factors in the throat that block air flow, even though there is movement of respiratory muscles. • *Central sleep apnea* is due to failure of respiratory drive from the medullary centers.
Clinical findings	• In both types of sleep apnea, the patient awakens—although there may not be awareness of the awakening, just a general deterioration in the quality of sleep. • Roommates notice the awakenings and often notice the sounds of OSA, if present. • Patients have excessive daytime sleepiness because of their poor quality of sleep. They may fall asleep easily, but true narcoleptic attacks from sleep deprivation are not expected. • Patients with OSA usually are overweight to obese.
Laboratory studies	• Routine labs are normal. Thyroid function tests usually are performed. • Imaging is normal. • Sleep studies show the cessation of air flow. With OSA, there is still movement of chest wall muscles; with central sleep apnea, there is no chest wall movement.
Diagnosis	• Sleep apnea is suggested by the report of excessive daytime sleepiness and the roommate reporting poor sleep or irregular respirations at night. • Diagnosis is confirmed by nocturnal polysomnography (PSG).
Differential diagnosis	• *Periodic limb movements.* Can also produce interruption in sleep, but the clinical and PSG features are different. • *Snoring.* Can produce the respiratory sounds that, with irregular respirations, might suggest OSA to a roommate or physician.
Management	• OSA is treated by nasal continuous positive airway pressure (CPAP). Weight loss is advised, and may be all that is required for many patients. Avoidance of alcohol and sleeping on the side also may be helpful. • Central sleep apnea may require mechanical ventilation to avoid the effects of recurrent hypoxia.
Clinical course	• Both types of sleep apnea are chronic disorders, although they can be treated. • Treatment of the sleep disorder can result in improvement in daytime sleepiness and functioning. However, if patients are not treated, there can be progressive deterioration in functioning.

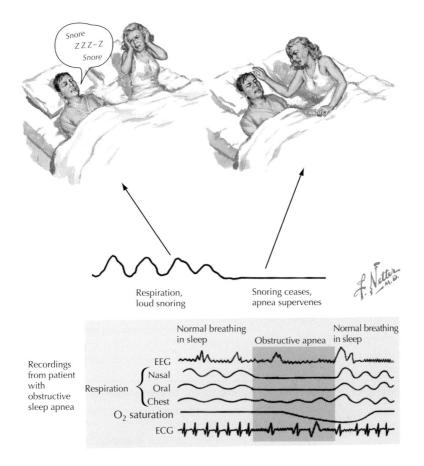

Respiration,
loud snoring

Snoring ceases,
apnea supervenes

Recordings
from patient
with
obstructive
sleep apnea

Respiration
- Nasal
- Oral
- Chest

Normal breathing
in sleep

Obstructive apnea

Normal breathing
in sleep

EEG

O₂ saturation

ECG

NARCOLEPSY	
Description	An uncommon sleep disorder affecting patients in the day with sleep attacks
Pathophysiology	Exact cause is unknown, but genetic predisposition, as well as acquired host factors, cause this disorder of sleep architecture in which patients have abrupt onset of sleep during the day, REM-onset sleep, and sleep paralysis.
Clinical findings	Fundamental features of narcolepsy are: 　· Excessive daytime sleepiness (EDS) 　· Cataplexy 　· Sleep paralysis 　· Hypnagogic hallucinations · The daytime sleepiness may be subtle, with falling asleep during lulls in activity or more prominent with falling asleep during activity. Sleep attacks can occur, without warning. · Cataplexy is a sudden attack of weakness, which may be subtle or cause the patient to fall to the ground, without disturbance of consciousness. This can be triggered by laughter or anger. · Sleep paralysis is the inability to make voluntary movements upon awakening. Respirations, eye movements and other automatic movements are preserved, but there is otherwise paralysis. · Hypnagogic hallucinations can be of any modality and occur as the patient is falling asleep.
Laboratory studies	· Routine labs are normal and imaging is normal. · Nocturnal PSG often is performed to ensure that the EDS is not due to poor nocturnal sleep. · Multiple sleep latency test (MSLT) is diagnostic, with criteria for onset of sleep patterns.
Diagnosis	· Narcolepsy is suspected when a patient presents with excessive daytime sleepiness and a history of cataplexy is obtained. Sleep paralysis can occur in normal patients, and, therefore, is supportive but not confirmatory. · Diagnosis is confirmed by MSLT, often performed by PSG.
Differential diagnosis	· *Poor nocturnal sleep.* Can result in excessive daytime sleepiness and can be associated with an abnormal MSLT. · *Seizures.* Can produce episodes that resemble sleep attacks, although this is uncommon, and is not associated with the other clinical features.
Management	· Narcolepsy is treated with stimulants including methylphenidate, pemoline, modafinil, and sometimes other medications as well. · Cataplexy is treated with sodium oxybate, fluoxetine, clomipramine, imipramine, or venlafaxine.
Clinical course	Most patients improve with treatment. Long-term treatment is needed.

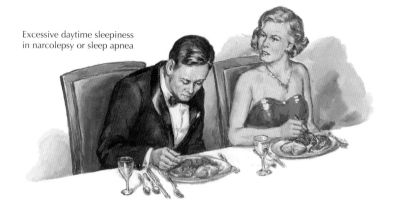

Excessive daytime sleepiness
in narcolepsy or sleep apnea

Cataplexy

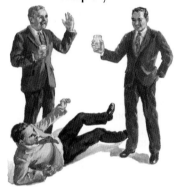

Sudden loss of muscular-postural
tone with laughter or fright

Sleep paralysis

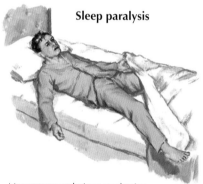

Momentary paralysis on awakening
lasts seconds to minutes

OVERVIEW OF DEVELOPMENTAL DISORDERS	
Description	Developmental disorders are the failure of normal programmed multiplication and migration. Most occur during early gestation.
Pathophysiology	Developmental disorders are of multiple causes. These can be inherited, spontaneous defects; medications; infections; or other illnesses.
Individual entities	Individual diagnostic entities are numerous. Some of the more important are discussed below.
Disorders	**Features**
Anencephaly	• Neural tube abnormality, in which the cerebrum and cerebellum are absent or markedly underdeveloped • Present at birth with absence of higher brain development with preservation of facial features. The lesion may or may not have overlying skin. • No treatment is available, and there is no possibility of neurologic recovery.
Chiari malformation	• Developmental abnormality of the craniocervical junction with extension of the cerebellar tonsils through the foramen magnum • Often an incidental finding, but can present with craniocervical headache, dizziness, cranial nerve abnormalities, diplopia, myelopathic findings • Treated by suboccipital decompression, but often does not need treatment • May be associated with syringomyelia
Craniosynostosis	• Skull deformity due to premature closure of one or more cranial sutures. Cause can be genetic or due to metabolic derangement (e.g., thyroid) or developmental (e.g., microcephaly). • Patients present with an abnormally large head. • Treatment is surgical if the craniosynostosis interferes with normal brain development. The affected suture is opened.
Dandy-Walker anomaly	• Development disorder of the cerebellum in which there is enlargement of the 4th ventricle, partial or complete absence of development of the cerebellar vermis, and cystic fluid collection in the region • The anomaly can be asymptomatic or can result in neuronal compression with signs of increased intracranial pressure (ICP), nausea, vomiting, confusion, and motor abnormalities part of which is cerebellar ataxia. • Treatment is not needed for many patients; however, shunt placement may be needed for patients with fluid collection to the point of neuronal compression.

Disorders	Features
Encephalocele	• Neural tube defect in which there is a skull defect and herniation of the meninges with brain tissue—this from failure of surface ectoderm to separate from neuroectoderm • Treatment is closure of the lesion, but the neural tissue cannot be reconstructed.
Hydrocephalus	• Increased ventricular size usually due to either decreased outflow from the ventricular system (noncommunicating hydrocephalus) or decreased absorption of cerebrospinal fluid (CSF) by the arachnoid granulations (communicating hydrocephalus). Rare cases of hydrocephalus from excess CSF production are seen. • Aqueductal stenosis is one of the abnormalities that can cause hydrocephalus. • Patients present with headache and gait difficulty, but this is difficult to see in infants. Neonates and infants can present with poor feeding, poor head control, and lethargy. Fontanelles may be bulging, and there may be cranial nerve abnormalities, especially ocular motor findings. • Shunting of the hydrocephalus is the definitive treatment; however, shunt failure is common, and, therefore, monitoring is required.
Lissencephaly	• Defective neuronal migration during early brain development results in absence of the normal convolutions of the brain—"smooth brain." • Patients present with severe mental retardation, motor delay, abnormal facial appearance, muscle spasms, seizures. • There is no treatment other than for the seizures and supportive care.
Macrocephaly	• Large head due to abnormal development of the brain. This is different from the head enlargement that occurs with hydrocephalus. • The large brain is not normally developed so that mental function is reduced. Developmental delay, seizures, weakness with corticospinal tract signs is seen. • There is no treatment except supportive care and management of seizures.
Microcephaly	• Small head because of failure of normal development of the brain. The cause can be genetic, and Down syndrome is an important cause. Other causes can be infections, trauma, and maternal drug abuse. • Patients present with mental retardation, motor delay, skeletal abnormalities with short stature, and alteration of facial features. • There is no treatment.
Pachygyria	• Reduction in the number of sulci with resultant enlargement in the size of the gyri • Related to lissencephaly but a more moderate change in the gyration

Disorders	Features
Spina bifida	Neural tube defect where there is failure of the spinal cord to close early in gestation. Severity varies markedly from asymptomatic bony abnormalities to open lesion: • *Spina bifida occulta*—One or more vertebrae are malformed but the underlying neural tissue is normal • *Meningocele*—Meninges protrude through a spinal opening but the spinal cord neural tissue has developed normally. • *Myelomeningocele*—The spinal cord neural tissue and meninges open on the back. Treatment is supportive except for closure of any open lesion after birth.
Syringomyelia	• Fluid-filled cavity within the spinal cord • May be associated with Chiari malformation. Often seen after trauma. • Presents with myelopathy • Can be treated by shunting if syrinx is isolated. If associated with Chiari, decompression of this can result in improvement.

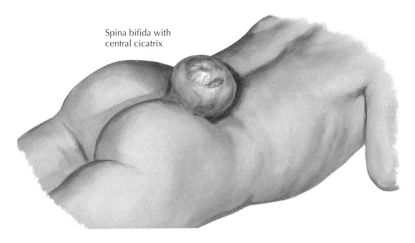

Spina bifida with
central cicatrix

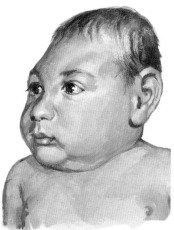

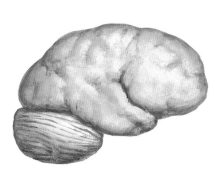

Microcephaly

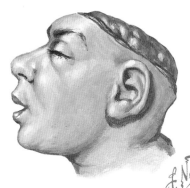

Lissencephalia
(agyria)

Anencephaly

CHIARI MALFORMATION	
Description	Developmental disorder of the craniocervical junction where the cerebellar tonsils extend into the foramen magnum.
Pathophysiology	• Cause is unknown, but there is felt to be a genetic predisposition. • Chiari can also manifest following shunt placement.
Clinical findings	• Patients commonly present with headache at the craniocervical junction. • Most patients have no otherwise neurologic symptoms, but can also develop diplopia, retro-orbital pain, vertigo, nausea, weakness of the limbs, paresthesias in the extremities, or syncope. • Exam may be normal, or ocular motor, other cranial nerve, or myelopathic findings may be identified.
Laboratory studies	• Routine labs are normal. • Magnetic resonance imaging (MRI) makes the diagnosis, by descent of the tonsils into the upper cervical cord. Brainstem compression with or without hydrocephalus can be seen.
Diagnosis	• Chiari malformation is suspected when a patient presents with pain at the craniocervical junction, especially if there are symptoms of dizziness. • MRI confirms the diagnosis. • Chiari is sometimes an incidental finding.
Differential diagnosis	• *Tumor at the foramen magnum.* Can be associated with all of the symptoms of Chiari malformation, although the onset is more rapid than the very slow-progressing Chiari symptoms. • *Multiple sclerosis.* Can produce similar symptoms. MRI diffentiates
Management	• There is no medical therapy for Chiari malformation. Surgery is performed, especially if there is brainstem compression or hydrocephalus. • Surgery for purely subjective symptoms in the absence of objective signs is less urgent, and some patients are followed clinically without surgery.
Clinical course	Surgery results in improvement in most patients.

Arnold-Chiari Malformation

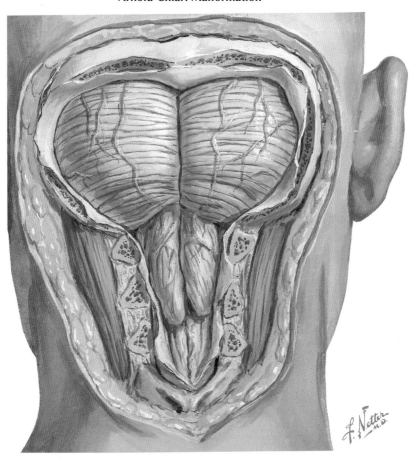

SYRINGOMYELIA	
Description	Fluid within the substance of the spinal cord
Pathophysiology	• Syringomyelia can be from multiple causes including trauma, obstruction of CSF flow, or compression. • There is enlargement of the spinal cord by the fluid with resultant compression of ascending and descending pathways, giving myelopathic signs below the level of the lesion. Damage at the levels of the syrinx can be associated with segmental signs, as well.
Clinical findings	• Myelopathy can produce weakness and loss of sensation below the level of the lesion with corticospinal tract signs. • Segmental deficits can be weakness with decreased reflexes and atrophy at the levels of the syrinx. • Some causes of syringomyelia can be associated with hydrocephalus, which can present with its own symptoms.
Laboratory studies	• Routine labs are normal • MRI shows enlargement of the spinal cord with signal intensities indicating fluid within a confined region of the cord. The anterior-posterior extent of the lesion may extend several segments. • Computed tomography (CT) is less sensitive for syrinx than for MRI. Myelography with postmyelographic CT may be needed for patients who cannot have an MRI because of valve or implanted device.
Diagnosis	• Syringomyelia is suspected when a patient presents with progressive myelopathy. • MRI makes the diagnosis in most patients. • A small syrinx can be seen as an incidental finding.
Differential diagnosis	• *Transverse myelitis and multiple sclerosis.* Considered in patients with myelopathy, although the onset of symptoms is more rapid than with syringomyelia. MRI can differentiate. • *B_{12} deficiency.* Can produce myelopathy, although other findings including peripheral neuropathic, cerebellar, and hematologic are often seen.
Management	• Many patients with small syrinx do not have to be treated. • Syrinx associated with Chiari malformation often improves following decompression for the Chiari. • Syrinx not associated with Chiari often improves with shunting of the fluid. There are a variety of shunt maneuvers that can be effective.
Clinical course	Most patients improve with treatment of the syrinx; however, there are others in whom there are persistent neurologic deficits.

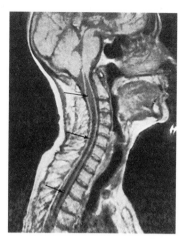

Magnetic resonance image: area of diminished signal within cervical and upper spinal cord (arrows) is fluid-filled syrinx. Cerebellar tonsil extends below foramen magnum

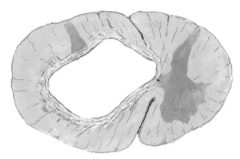

Section of cervical spinal cord showing cavity of syrinx surrounded by gliosis

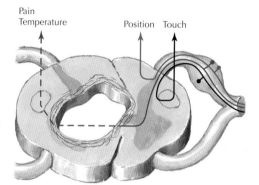

Pain
Temperature   Position   Touch

Diagram demonstrating interruption of crossed pain and temperature fibers by syrinx. Uncrossed light touch and proprioception fibers preserved

LOCALIZATION	
Location	**Clinical Presentation**
Cerebral cortex	• Contralateral hemiparesis, hemisensory loss, hemianopia, depending on the part of the cortex involved • Weakness usually involves the arm more than the leg, although the reverse can be true. • Left hemisphere: aphasia • Right hemisphere: neglect
Internal capsule	• Contralateral hemiparesis and/or hemisensory loss • Weakness involves the face, arm, and leg approximately equally • No aphasia or neglect
Basal ganglia	• Contralateral weakness and coordination difficulty. May have extrapyramidal symptoms with stiffness, dystonia. • No sensory, language, or other cortical abnormalities
Thalamus	• Contralateral sensory disturbance that is usually loss, although can be hyperesthesia or pain • Little or no motor symptoms, although ataxia can develop that resembles cerebellar dysfunction
Midbrain	• Hemiparesis from ventral damage • Diplopia, often with vertical gaze palsy with dorsal damage
Cerebellum	• Gait ataxia from midline cerebellar dysfunction • Ipsilateral limb ataxia from cerebellar hemisphere dysfunction
Pons	• Contralateral hemiparesis or quadriparesis, depending on whether the lesion is unilateral or bilateral • Diplopia often with skew deviation • Often crossed signs—ipsilateral facial palsy and contralateral hemiparesis

Localization

Location	Clinical Presentation
Medulla	• Dysarthria and/or dysphagia • Hemiparesis or hemiataxia • May have crossed sensory findings, ipsilateral facial numbness, and contralateral loss of body pain and temperature sensation
Spinal cord	• Quadriparesis from cervical cord dysfunction • Paraparesis from thoracic or lumbar-cord dysfunction. Hyperreflexia suggests thoracic or higher lesion; flaccid paraparesis suggests lumbar lesion affecting the cauda equina or conus medullaris.
Nerve root	• Pain, sensory loss, and/or weakness in the distribution of one or more nerve roots • Structural lesions are often associated with local and radiating pain.
Plexus	• Weakness and/or sensory loss or pain in one limb, spanning more than one nerve root distribution • Some disorders can affect more than one plexus, so multifocal damage is possible.
Peripheral nerve	• Pain, sensory loss, and/or weakness in the distribution of one peripheral nerve (mononeuropathy) • Distal sensory deficit with or without motor abnormalities occurs with polyneuropathy.

CLINICAL FEATURES OF COMMON NEUROLOGIC DISORDERS	
Disorder	**Features**
VASCULAR DISEASE	
Cerebral infarction	• Acute onset of focal motor or sensory deficit, confusion, visual-field defect, speech defect, or ataxia of gait and/or limb • Diagnosed clinically, confirmed by magnetic resonance imaging (MRI) or computed tomography (CT) • Treated by thrombolytics if early enough. Otherwise, secondary prevention with antithrombotics and risk management.
Venous thrombosis	• Occlusion of intracerebral veins often due to hypercoagulable state • Patients present with focal or multifocal deficits. May have seizures, increased intracranial pressure. • Diagnosed by MRI or CT • Treated by anticoagulation
Subarachnoid hemorrhage (SAH)	• Explosive onset of severe headache. May have confusion, ocular motor palsy, coma. • Diagnosed by CT. Lumbar puncture (LP) may be needed if CT negative. • Treated by prevention of spasm by nimodipine, careful fluid balance, often with anticonvulsants and steroids. Surgery may be needed for aneurysm repair.
Intraparenchymal hemorrhage	• Subacute to acute onset of focal deficit, headache, nausea, and often decreased level of consciousness. May have seizures. • Usually easily seen on CT • Medical management of coagulopathy, blood pressure, or intracranial pressure is often all that is needed. Surgery is rarely needed or helpful.
Subdural hematoma (SDH)	• Acute or subacute onset of headache and hemiparesis. May be traumatic or spontaneous. Chronic SDH can present with confusion with less likelihood of focal signs. • Diagnosed by CT or MRI • Surgical evacuation is needed for substantial SDH, especially if there is midline shift.
Epidural hematoma	• Decreased level of consciousness after a head injury. May be lucid interval before the unconsciousness. • Diagnosed by CT • Surgery is usually needed.
DEMENTIAS	
Alzheimer's disease (AD)	• Progressive degenerative dementia without focal neurologic signs. Most common cause of dementia. • Diagnosed clinically. Imaging and labs are normal. • Treated by cholinesterase inhibitors (donepezil, galantamine, rivastigmine) and/or memantine

Common Disorders

CLINICAL FEATURES OF COMMON NEUROLOGIC DISORDERS	
Disorder	**Features**
DEMENTIAS	
Frontotemporal dementia (FTD)	• Progressive degenerative dementia with prominent frontal lobe dysfunction; otherwise normal exam. • Diagnosed clinically, often with neuropsych testing. Imaging and labs are normal, although frontotemporal atophy may be seen on MRI. • Treated with selective serotonin-uptake inhibitors (SSRIs) for some of the behavioral symptoms, including obsessions. Cholinesterase inhibitors and memantine are tried but unproved.
Dementia with Lewy bodies (DLB)	• Progressive degenerative dementia with parkinsonian features. Looks like the combination of Alzheimer's disease (AD) and Parkinson's disease (PD), although it is pathologically distinct. • Diagnosed clinically. Imaging and labs are normal. • Treated for dementia by cholinesterase inhibitors and/or memantine. Treated for the movement disorder as with PD. Psychosis may be treated by atypical neuroleptics.
MOVEMENT DISORDERS	
Parkinson's disease	• Idiopathic degenerative condition that results in dysfunction of the nigral-striatal pathways • Rigidity and poverty of movement with increased tone, cogwheeling, postural instability, and usually resting tremor • Diagnosed clinically. Imaging and labs are normal. • Treated with anticholinergic agents for tremor, dopaminergic agents for the bradykinesia and rigidity
Dystonia	• Abnormal posture due to focal and asymmetric muscle contraction • Diagnosed clinically. Imaging and labs are usually normal, although structural lesion of the brain or spine can be seen. • Treated mainly by Botox injections, anticholinergics
Dyskinesia	• Abnormal involuntary movements that can be stereotypic and repetitive. No alteration of consciousness. Patient can transiently suppress the movement. • Often related to medications, either long-term neuroleptic use (tardive dyskinesia [TD]) or patients with parkinsonism treated with levodopa or dopamine agonists (peak-dose dyskinesia) • Treated by withdrawal of the offending medication. Older neuroleptic can be replaced by an atypical neuroleptic. For PD, dopamine agonists can be used rather than levodopa. Amantadine can reduce the dyskinesias.
Athetosis and chorea	• Involuntary movements that are slow and writhing (athetosis), rapid and involving the digits (chorea). Can be due to structural lesion or postinfectious (Sydenham's chorea). • Diagnosed clinically, but imaging is done to look for structural lesion • Treated with neuroleptics, benzodiazepines, gabapentin, or tetrabenazine

Hemiballismus	• Flinging movements of usually one side (hemiballismus); rarely bilateral • Due to damage to the subthalamic nucleus, usually infarction • Diagnosed clinically. MRI may show the lesion. • Treated by neuroleptics, gabapentin, and sedatives, including benzodiazepines or barbiturates
Essential tremor (ET)	• Postural and action tremor, disappears at rest. Often familial. Much more common than parkinsonian tremor. • Diagnosed clinically. Imaging and labs are normal. • Treated with primidone, propranolol, gabapentin, topiramate. Botox is occasionally used. Surgery is rarely used for disabling refractory ET.
NEUROMUSCULAR DISORDERS	
Amyotrophic lateral sclerosis (ALS)	• Progressive weakness of the axial, appendicular, and bulbar muscles. Fasciculations and cramps are common. Corticospinal signs are seen. • Diagnosed by the combination of lower-motor neuron and upper-motor neuron deficits. LMN signs include widespread proximal and distal denervation on electromyogram (EMG). • Treatment is supportive. Riluzole is sometimes used, although is of limited benefit. Phenytoin or baclofen may be used for spasms.
Peripheral neuropathy (PN)	• Degeneration of the peripheral nerves that can be sensory and/or motor, due to axonal and/or myelin degeneration, and acute, subacute, or chronic • Causes are multiple. Idiopathic PN may often be familial. DM is the most common cause. • Diagnosed by nerve conduction study (NCS) and EMG that can identify and classify the neuropathy. Blood and urine tests may be needed for diagnosis. Biopsy or nerve and/or muscle is sometimes needed. • Treatment of idiopathic PN is supportive. Neuropathic pain is treated by amitriptyline, gabapentin, duloxetine, pregabalin or similar medications. Symptomatic PN involves this plus treatment of the underlying cause when possible.
Myasthenia gravis (MG)	• Weakness and fatigue often with diplopia, ptosis. No sensory abnormalities. • Diagnosed by NCS with repetitive stimulation, assay for myasthenia antibodies. CT or MRI of the chest is performed to look for thymoma. • Treated by pyridostigmine for acute management of weakness. Steroids or chemotherapy agents are often used for long-term immunosuppression. Intravenous immunoglobulin G (IVIG) or plasma exchange is used for treatment of myasthenic crisis.

Common Disorders

CLINICAL FEATURES OF COMMON NEUROLOGIC DISORDERS	
Disorder	Features
NEUROMUSCULAR DISORDERS contiued	
Lambert-Eaton myasthenic syndrome (LEMS)	• Weakness and fatigue often with autonomic signs, dry mouth. Often associated with cancer, although LEMS may precede identifying the tumor. • Diagnosed by NCS with repetitive stimulation, and assay for paraneoplastic antibodies (voltage-gated calcium channels [VGCC]) • Treatment can be with pyridostigmine or guanidine diaminopyridine. IVIG, steroids, or chemotherapeutic agents have been tried.
AIDP (Guillain-Barre syndrome)	• Acute sensory-motor neuropathy with prominent demyelination. Patients present with weakness and sensory symptoms with areflexia. • Diagnosed by NCS showing slowed conduction especially proximally. CSF protein is usually increased. Assays for other causes of PN and weakness are negative. • Treated with IVIG or plasma exchange initially. No role for steroids. Supportive care is essential, and progression despite early treatment is usual.
CIDP	• Chronic progressive or relapsing PN with weakness and sensory symptoms. Decreased reflexes. • Diagnosed by NCS and EMG. Nerve biopsy may be required. • Treatment is usually with steroids. IVIG is also sometimes used for worsening condition.
Multifocal motor neuropathy (MMN)	• Progressive weakness often with cramps and often asymmetric. No sensory findings. May have fasciculations. Reflexes may be normal or depressed, which helps to distinguish from ALS. • Diagnosed by NCS and EMG, which shows a very different pattern from ALS • Treated usually by IVIG. Cyclophosphamide is also sometimes used for refractory patients.
INFECTIONS	
Herpes simplex encephalitis (HSE)	• Viral infection of the brain usually with HSV1. Patients present with confusion, focal or multifocal signs, often with fever. May have seizures. • Diagnosed clinically, supported by CSF abnormalities, MRI or CT findings. Specific CSF and blood serologies are often positive. • Treatment is with acyclovir. Steroids may be needed for cerebral edema. Anticonvulsants are often needed for seizures, especially phenytoin and valproate, because they can be given parenterally.

Nonherpetic encephalitis	• Viral infection of the brain with a variety of viruses, including West Nile, California, eastern equine, western equine, St. Louis, and others.
	• Patients present with confusion and may have fever. Focal signs and seizures are less common than with HSE.
	• Treatment is supportive. Steroids are sometimes used for cerebral edema. Anticonvulsants are occasionally needed.
Bacterial meningitis	• Bacterial infection of the CSF that often comes from sinuses or overlying one or skin. If the infection involves the brain, it is cerebritis.
	• Patients present with headache, fever, neck pain, meningeal signs with nuchal rigidity. Confusion or coma can develop. Seizures can develop acutely or later.
	• Diagnosis is by CSF that shows pleocytosis and may reveal the organism on smears, cultures, or CIE. Imaging is done especially if there is confusion or focal signs.
	• Treated with antibiotics. The selection depends on host factors. Broad-spectrum CSF-penetrating antibiotics are used first, with narrowing of the selection with identification and characterization of the organism.
Viral meningitis	• Viral infection of the CSF
	• Patients present with headache, often with neck pain. Meningeal signs may be present.
	• Diagnosis is by CSF analysis.
	• Treatment is supportive. Rare patients with viral meningitis due to HSV can be treated with acyclovir.
Cryptococcal meningitis	• Fungal infection due to *Cryptococcus neoformans*. Usually in immunocompromised patients, e.g., AIDS.
	• Patients present with headache and confusion. Ataxia may be present. Papilledema may be present.
	• Diagnosis is by imaging that is normal or shows enhancement of the meninges, especially on MRI. Hydrocephalus can be seen. CSF shows characteristic findings, and the infection is seen on cryptococcal antigen and fungal culture.
	• Treatment depends on the clinical setting. Amphotericin, flucytosine, and fluconazole are among the agents used.
Brain abscess	• Bacterial infection of the brain, which presents as focal or multifocal mass lesions
	• Patients present with headache, confusion, fever. Often with focal deficits. Seizures may be present.
	• Diagnosis is by CT or MRI that shows focal or multifocal enhancing masses. Biopsy is usually needed to differentiate from tumor, and identify the organism.
	• Treatment is with antibiotics. Surgical excision depends on the clinical situation.

Common Disorders

CLINICAL FEATURES OF COMMON NEUROLOGIC DISORDERS	
Disorder	**Features**
INFECTIONS continued	
Creutzfeldt-Jakob disease (CJD)	• Prion disease that presents with progressive dementia, myoclonus, ataxia, and often exaggerated startle • Diagnosed by clinical features, supported by electroencephalogram (EEG) and CSF findings • Treatment is supportive. Seizures and myoclonus can be treated with anticonvulsants and benzodiazepines.
CANCER	
Primary brain tumor	• Neoplasm that starts from supporting or (less likely) neural structures. Gliomas are most common. Can be benign or malignant. • Patients present with focal deficit, seizures, headache, altered mental status, and/or ataxia. Papilledema may be present. • Diagnosis is by MRI or CT, showing a focal lesion. Low-grade neoplasms may not enhance, whereas malignant tumors show enhancement. • Treatment is by surgery when possible. Malignant tumors often require radiation therapy and/or chemotherapy.
Metastatic brain tumor	• Neoplasm that has spread from a distant malignancy. More often multifocal than with primary brain tumors. • Patients present with focal or multifocal deficits, seizures, confusion, ataxia. Papilledema may be seen. Signs of the underlying malignancy are sometimes seen. • Diagnosed by CT or MRI showing focal or multifocal enhancing lesions. Biopsy may be needed if a primary tumor is unknown, or if differentiation from abscess is needed. • Treatment is with resection when a single lesion is accessible. Otherwise, radiation therapy and/or chemotherapy is used.
Limbic encephalitis (a paraneoplastic syndrome)	• Paraneoplastic syndrome that presents with subacute encephalopathy or dementia, often also with weakness and ataxia • Diagnosed by paraneoplastic antibodies. Imaging is done to look for brain metastases. CSF is obtained to look for neoplastic meningitis, and may show a cellular but not neoplastic profile. • Treatment is supportive. Although not proved, steroids, IVIG, and plasma exchange have been tried.
Neoplastic spinal cord compression	• Tumor can spread from outside of the spine into the spinal canal and produce cord compression. • Patients present with pain over the spine, often with percussion tenderness. Weakness is appropriate to the level of the lesion. Sphincter disturbance is common. • Diagnosed by MRI or CT. Confirmed by biopsy if no cancer is known; otherwise, imaging makes the diagnosis in patients with cancer. • Treatment depends on the clinical situation. Surgical stabilization is needed for some patients; otherwise, radiation therapy and high-dose steroids are used.

Neoplastic meningitis	• Some malignancies can spread into the CSF with production of meningitis. • Patients present with multifocal nerve-root pain and deficits, often with headache, confusion, signs of increased intracranial pressure. • Diagnosis is made by CSF cytology after MRI has not shown parenchymal metastases. • Treatment is with systemic and intrathecal chemotherapy. Radiation therapy is used occasionally.
PAIN	
Migraine with aura	• Episodic headache that is unilateral or bilateral associated with nausea, vomiting, photophobia, and/or phonophobia. Most often in young to middle age, more common in females. Inherited predisposition. Sensory aura precedes the headache. • Diagnosed clinically. Imaging and labs are normal. • Acute treatment with analgesics, triptans, antiemetics, ergots • Preventive treatment with β-blockers, some anticonvulsants including valproate and topiramate, some calcium channel blockers, tricyclic antidepressants
Migraine without aura	• Episodic headache but without the sensory aura preceding the headache • Diagnosis and treatment is the same as above.
Muscle contraction/ tension headache	• Intermittent or chronic temporal, occipital, or band-like headache • Diagnosed clinically. Imaging is normal, and is often done to rule out structural lesion, e.g., tumor, Chiari malformation. • Treated by anti-inflammatories, muscle relaxants, tricyclic antidepressants TCAs
Cluster headache	• Multiple brief headache that is centered around the eye. Can wake from sleep. Often associated with nasal congestion. More common in males. • Diagnosed clinically. Imaging and labs are normal. • Acute treatment with analgesics, triptans, steroids, oxygen • Preventive treatment with steroids, calcium-channel blockers
Temporal arteritis	• Arteritis affecting cerebral vessels with temporal predominance. Pain in one or both temporal regions, with thickened and tender temporal artery. Develop in middle-aged to elderly patients. • Diagnosed clinically with support by an elevated erythrocyte sedimentation rate (ESR). Temporal artery biopsy is confirmatory. • Treated by steroids plus analgesics. Can produce blindness and stroke if untreated, so treatment often predates confirmation of the diagnosis.
Neuropathic pain	• Pain due to repetitive electrical discharge of damaged peripheral nerves. Lancinating or burning pain. • Diagnosed clinically. NCS and EMG can identify the neuropathic lesion. • Treated with some anticonvulsants (esp., gabapentin, pregabalin) and TCAs (esp., amitriptyline)

Common Disorders

CLINICAL FEATURES OF COMMON NEUROLOGIC DISORDERS	
Disorder	**Features**
PAIN continued	
Trigeminal neuralgia	• Neuropathic pain affecting one side of the face, often due to microvascular compression of a branch of the trigeminal nerve • Diagnosed clinically. Imaging and labs are normal. • Treated by some anticonvulsants (esp., carbamazepine and gabapentin), baclofen. Surgery can be done for medically refractory patients.
Pseudotumor cerebri	• Increased intracranial pressure not due to mass lesion. Some of these patients have venous occlusive disease. • Patients present with headache, visual blurring, papilledema. Visual loss can be persistent without treatment. • Diagnosed clinically and confirmed by normal imaging and increased CSF pressure on LP. CSF shows no evidence of meningitis. • Treated by CSF drainage, carbonic anhydrase inhibitors (esp., acetazolamide). Lumboperitoneal shunt or optic nerve fenestration can be performed for refractory cases.
Rebound headache	• Chronic headache can develop from the persistent use of certain medications. These are usually analgesics, but can also be triptans or anti-inflammatories. • Patients present with chronic headache that gets worse if medications are not taken. • Diagnosed clinically. Imaging and labs are normal. • Treated by cessation of the offending agents for several weeks. TCAs or other migraine preventative can be used as an adjunct.
IMMUNE-MEDIATED DISORDERS	
Multiple sclerosis (MS)	• Multifocal demyelinating changes in the brain and spine. The lesions develop over time. • Patients present with multifocal neurologic deficits that are either relapsing-remitting or progressive. Common findings are paraparesis, hemiparesis, diplopia with internuclear ophthalmoplegia, and cerebellar ataxia. • Diagnosed clinically with support of MRI and CSF analysis • Acute attacks are treated usually with high-dose steroids. • Long-term treatment is with interferons or glatiramer. Chemotherapy is sometimes used.
Systemic lupus erythematois (SLE)	• Systemic autoimmune disorder with non-neurologic symptoms. PNS can be involved with polyneuropathy. CNS can be affected by vasculopathy or cerebritis. • Common neurologic findings are encephalopathy, neuropathy, stroke, or myopathy

SEIZURES	
Single unprovoked seizure	• Not all patients with an unprovoked seizure have recurrent seizures. Risk is lowest with normal examination, normal imaging, and normal EEG. • Diagnosis is clinical. MRI and EEG are usually normal, unless the seizure was symptomatic of a neurologic disorder. • Treatment with anticonvulsants is usually not needed for a single, unprovoked seizure. If EEG shows interictal activity, anticonvulsants are usually needed.
Absence epilepsy	• Seizures are characterized by episodes of loss of awareness with preservation of postural tone. Automatisms may be present. There is no major motor activity. No post-ictal confusion or somnolence. • Diagnosis is clinical and supported by EEG abnormalities. Imaging is normal. • Treatment is with ethosuximide, valproate, lamotrigine.
Primary generalized tonic/clonic seizures	• Major motor seizures with stiffening and shaking of the extremities with loss of consciousness. Post-ictal confusion and/ or somnolence. • Diagnosed clinically. Confirmed by EEG. Imaging and labs are normal. • Treated by many anticonvulsants, including phenytoin, valproate, carbamazine, and many of the second-generation agents.
Secondarily generalized tonic/clonic seizures	• Major motor seizure that begins with a partial (focal) discharge that then spreads throughout the brain. The focal onset may be simple or complex (see below). Partial symptoms may or may not be seen. • Diagnosis is clinical with support of the EEG. Imaging is usually normal, but may show a structural lesion. Labs are normal. • Treatment can be by phenytoin, carbamazepine, valproate, or many second-generation anticonvulsants.
Juvenile myoclonic epilepsy (JME)	• Patients often have single jerks most prominent upon awakening. Seizures can be generalized tonic/clonic or less likely absence. • Diagnosis is clinical. Imaging is normal. EEG is often abnormal. • Treatment is with valproate, lamotrigine, or some other second-generation anticonvulsants.
Simple partial epilepsy	• Partial (focal) seizure that often begins in the central cortical regions, producing focal motor and/or sensory symptoms. Contralateral jerking is common. There is no disturbance of consciousness. • Diagnosis is clinical, supported by EEG. Imaging is usually normal, but can show a structural lesion. • Treatment is with phenytoin, carbamazepine, but some of the second-generation anticonvulsants can be used.

Common Disorders

CLINICAL FEATURES OF COMMON NEUROLOGIC DISORDERS	
Disorder	**Features**
SEIZURES continued	
Complex partial epilepsy	• Partial (focal) seizure of temporal or frontal origin that presents with disturbance of consciousness, preservation of postural tone, and often complex automatisms. • Diagnosis is clinical, supported by EEG. Imaging is often normal but may show structural lesion such as benign tumor or mesial temporal sclerosis. Labs are normal. • Treatment is with carbamazepine, or many of the second-generation anticonvulsants. Epilepsy surgery is considered for medically refractory patients.

Index

Index

Index

Index

Index

Index

Index

Index

Index

Index

Index

Index

Index

Index

Index

Index